# Cancer Pain

For Alastair
Best Wishes for
Your Future

Michael Bond

March 2011

## Mission Statement

IASP® brings together scientists, clinicians, health care providers, and policy makers to stimulate and support the study of pain and to translate that knowledge into improved pain relief worldwide. IASP Press® publishes timely, high-quality, and reasonably priced books relating to pain research and treatment.

# Cancer Pain:
## *From Molecules to Suffering*

Editors

**Judith A. Paice, RN, PhD, FAAN**
*Division of Hematology and Oncology, Feinberg School of Medicine, Northwestern University, Chicago, Illinois, USA*

**Rae F. Bell, MD, PhD**
*Pain Clinic, Department of Anesthesia and Intensive Care, Haukeland University Hospital, Bergen, Norway*

**Eija A. Kalso, MD, DMedSci**
*Institute of Clinical Medicine, University of Helsinki; Pain Clinic, Department of Anesthesiology, Intensive Care Medicine, Emergency Medicine and Pain Medicine, Helsinki University Central Hospital, Helsinki, Finland*

**Olaitan A. Soyannwo, MBBS, DA, MMed, FWACS, FICS, FAS**
*Department of Anaesthesia, College of Medicine, University of Ibadan, Ibadan, Nigeria*

**IASP PRESS® ◆ SEATTLE**

**Library of Congress Cataloging-in-Publication Data**

Cancer pain : from molecules to suffering / editors, Judith A. Paice ... [et al.].
    p. ; cm.
Includes bibliographical references and index.
Summary: "This book provides an in-depth analysis of basic and clinical research on cancer pain. It describes mechanisms of cancer pain and reviews opioid treatment issues, including tolerance. The book discusses clinical trial designs, covers the psychology of cancer pain, and describes disparities in the availability of cancer care worldwide"--Provided by publisher.
ISBN 978-0-931092-81-7 (pbk. : alk. paper)
1. Cancer pain. I. Paice, Judith A. II. International Association for the Study of Pain.
[DNLM: 1. Neoplasms--complications. 2. Pain. 3. Analgesics, Opioid--therapeutic use. 4. Pain--drug therapy. 5. Palliative Care. QZ 200 C2153636 2010]
RC262.C291185 2010
616.99'4061--dc22
                        2010015700

Published by:
IASP Press®
International Association for the Study of Pain
111 Queen Anne Ave N, Suite 501
Seattle, WA 98109-4955, USA
Fax: 206-283-9403
www.iasp-pain.org

Printed in the United States of America

# Contents

*v*

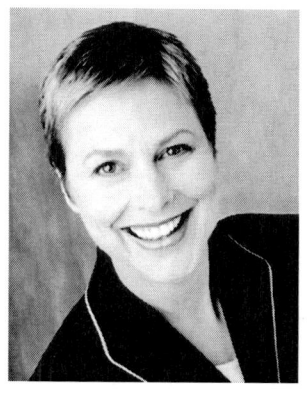

**Judith A. Paice, RN, PhD, FAAN**, is Director of the Cancer Pain Program in the Division of Hematology-Oncology and Research Professor of Medicine at Northwestern University's Feinberg School of Medicine in Chicago, Illinois, USA. She is also a full member of the Robert H. Lurie Comprehensive Cancer Center. Dr. Paice served as President of the American Pain Society from 2006 to 2008 and as a Councilor of the International Association for the Study of Pain until 2008. Much of Dr. Paice's clinical work has been in the relief of pain associated with cancer and HIV disease. In 2002, the American Pain Society honored Dr. Paice with the Narcessian Award for Excellence in Teaching. She has traveled within the People's Republic of China, Indonesia, Japan, Kenya, Korea, Taiwan, Tanzania, and Tajikistan to educate health care professionals regarding cancer pain relief and palliative care. Dr. Paice serves as Associate Editor of the *Journal of Pain* and serves on the editorial board of the *Clinical Journal of Pain* and the *Journal of Pain and Symptom Management*. She is the author of more than 150 scientific manuscripts. She was one of the original consultants in the End of Life Nursing Education Consortium and continues to serve as a faculty member in this program.

**Rae F. Bell, MD, PhD, BA Hons**, is Director of the Pain Clinic at Haukeland University Hospital, Bergen, Norway, and Research Fellow at the Regional Centre of Excellence in Palliative Care, Western Norway. She was leader of the working committee and coauthor of the Norwegian Medical Society Guidelines for Pain Treatment in Norway (2004, 2009) and is an associate editor for the *Scandinavian Journal of Pain*. Dr. Bell is currently chair of the IASP Special Interest group for Systematic Reviews in Pain Relief, a member of the SIG ACTINPAIN writing group, and a Cochrane Pain, Palliative and Supportive Care (PaPaS) review group editor. Her

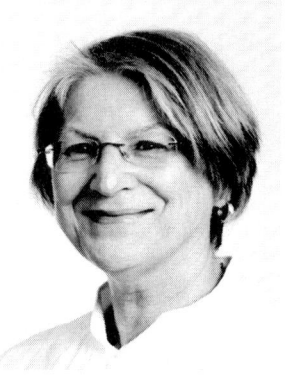

research interests include systematic reviews in pain relief, ketamine, and the relationship between diet and pain.

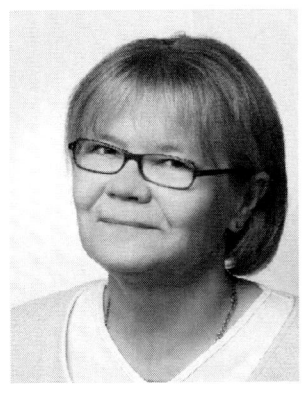

**Eija A. Kalso, MD, DMedSci**, is the Gyllenberg Professor of Pain Medicine at the University of Helsinki and Head of the Multidisciplinary Pain Clinic, Helsinki University Central Hospital, Finland. She is President-Elect of IASP and field editor for clinical science in *PAIN*. She graduated from the Medical School of the University of Helsinki in 1980, defended her thesis in 1983, and became a specialist in anesthesiology in 1986. She was appointed Associate Professor in Anesthesiology in 1992 at the University of Helsinki and received special competence in pain management in 1999. She did postdoctoral work at the Nuffield Dept. of Anaesthetics, Oxford University, with Sir Keith Sykes and Prof. Henry McQuay, and at University College London, with Prof. Anthony Dickenson. She was a clinical teacher of anesthesiology at the Karolinska Institute, Stockholm, Sweden. She was president of the Scandinavian Association for the Study of Pain and founding president of the Finnish Association for the Study of Pain. Her research interests include opioid pharmacology, spinal mechanisms of nociception, cancer pain, clinical trial design, chronic postsurgical pain, and, recently, genetics of pain.

**Olaitan A. Soyannwo, MBBS, DA, MMed, FWACS, FICS, FAS**, is Professor of Anaesthesia, University of Ibadan College of Medicine, and Consultant Anaesthetist, University College Hospital, Ibadan, Nigeria. She is active in advocating effective pain management and opioid availability in developing countries. Since 1996, she has spearheaded the development of pain and palliative care education and services in Nigeria. She cofounded the Society for the Study of Pain, Nigeria, and the Centre for Palliative Care, Nigeria. She has served as consultant to

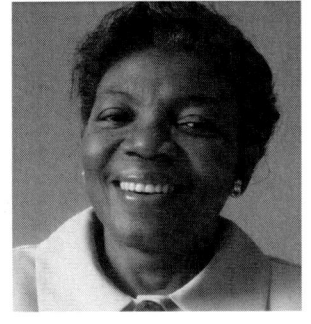

the National Health Development Project in Gambia, President of the Society of Anaesthetists of West Africa, and Head of the Department of Anaesthesia and Dean of Clinical Sciences of the College of Medicine, University of Ibadan. She has served on IASP Council and on several World Health Organization advisory committees. She is a member of the Council of the Nigerian Academy of Science and the West African College of Surgeons and is on the Board of Trustees of the Hospice and Palliative Care Association, Nigeria, and the African Palliative Care Association. Her interests include postoperative pain, cancer pain, and pain education.

# Contributing Authors

**Samantha B. Artherholt, PhD**, *Biobehavioral Sciences, Clinical Research Division, Fred Hutchinson Cancer Research Center, Seattle, Washington, USA*

**Michael I. Bennett, MB ChB, MD, FRCP, FFPMRCA**, *International Observatory on End of Life Care, Lancaster University, Lancaster, United Kingdom*

**Kees Besse, MD**, *Department of Anesthesiology, Pain and Palliative Medicine, University Medical Centre St. Radboud, Nijmegen, The Netherlands*

**Allen W. Burton, MD**, *Department of Anesthesia and Pain Medicine, The University of Texas M.D. Anderson Cancer Center, Houston, Texas, USA*

**Augusto Caraceni, MD**, *Division of Palliative Care, Pain Therapy and Rehabilitation, National Cancer Institute, Milan, Italy*

**Juan P. Cata, MD**, *Department of Anesthesiology, The Cleveland Clinic, Cleveland, Ohio, USA*

**Lesley Colvin, MD**, *Department of Clinical Neurosciences, Western General Hospital, Edinburgh, United Kingdom*

**Patrick M. Dougherty, PhD**, *Department of Anesthesia and Pain Medicine, M.D. Anderson Cancer Center, Houston, Texas, USA*

**Andy Dray, PhD**, *AstraZeneca Research & Development Montreal, Montreal, Quebec, Canada*

**Larry C. Driver, MD**, *Department of Anesthesia and Pain Medicine, The University of Texas M.D. Anderson Cancer Center, Houston, Texas, USA*

**Marie T. Fallon, MB, ChB**, *Institute of Genetics and Molecular Medicine, University of Edinburgh, Edinburgh Cancer Research Centre, Western General Hospital, Edinburgh, United Kingdom*

**Karen Forbes, MBChB, FRCP, EdD**, *Department of Palliative Medicine, Bristol Haematology and Oncology Centre, University of Bristol, Bristol, United Kingdom*

**Sue Gessler, PhD, CPsychol**, *Gynaecological Cancer Centre, University College London, and Elizabeth Garrett Anderson Institute for Women's Health, London, United Kingdom*

**Jane Gibbins, MBChB, MRCP**, *Department of Palliative Medicine, Bristol Haematology and Oncology Centre, University of Bristol, Bristol, United Kingdom*

**Maurice Giezeman, MD, PhD**, *Department of Anesthesiology and Pain Management, Diakonessen Hospital, Utrecht, The Netherlands*

**Sergio Giralt, MD**, *Department of Stem Cell Transplantation, The University of Texas M.D. Anderson Cancer Center, Houston, Texas, USA*

**Ann M. Gregus, PhD**, *Department of Pharmacology, Weill Cornell Medical College, New York, New York, USA; currently Department of Anesthesiology Research, University of California, San Diego, California, USA*

**Basem Hamid, MD**, *Department of Anesthesia and Pain Medicine, The University of Texas M.D. Anderson Cancer Center, Houston, Texas, USA*

**Charles E. Inturrisi, PhD**, *Department of Pharmacology, Weill Cornell Medical College; Pain and Palliative Care Service, Memorial Sloan-Kettering Cancer Center, New York, New York, USA*

**Eija Kalso, MD, DMedSci**, *Institute of Clinical Medicine, University of Helsinki; Pain Clinic, Department of Anesthesiology, Intensive Care Medicine, Emergency Medicine and Pain Medicine, Helsinki University Central Hospital, Helsinki, Finland*

**Francis J. Keefe, PhD**, *Pain Prevention and Treatment Program and Department of Psychiatry and Behavioral Sciences, Duke University Medical Center, Durham, North Carolina, USA*

**Tamara King, PhD**, *Department of Pharmacology, University of Arizona, Tucson, Arizona, USA*

**Ulf E. Kongsgaard, MD, PhD**, *The Norwegian Radium Hospital, Clinic of Emergency Medicine, Oslo University Hospital, Oslo; Medical Faculty, University of Oslo, Oslo, Norway*

**Sejal Kothadia, BS**, *Pain Prevention and Treatment Program and Department of Psychiatry and Behavioral Sciences, Duke University Medical Center, Durham, North Carolina, USA*

**Michaela Kress, Dr med**, *Department of Physiology, Innsbruck Medical University, Innsbruck, Austria*

**Barry J.A. Laird, MBChB, MD, MRCGP**, *Research Fellow in Palliative Medicine, Institute of Genetics and Molecular Medicine, University of Edinburgh, and Edinburgh Cancer Research Centre, Western General Hospital, Edinburgh, United Kingdom*

**Patrick Mantyh, PhD**, *Department of Pharmacology, College of Medicine, University of Arizona, Tucson, Arizona, USA*

**Stephen Morley, PhD**, *Institute of Health Sciences, Leeds, United Kingdom*

**Agustina Pandiani, BA**, *Pain Prevention and Treatment Program and Department of Psychiatry and Behavioral Sciences, Duke University Medical Center, Durham, North Carolina, USA*

**Predrag Petrovic, MD, PhD**, *Department of Clinical Neuroscience, Karolinska Institute, Stockholm, Sweden*

**Frank Porreca, PhD**, *Department of Pharmacology, University of Arizona, Tucson, Arizona, USA*

**Tamara J. Somers, PhD**, *Pain Prevention and Treatment Program and Department of Psychiatry and Behavioral Sciences, Duke University Medical Center, Durham, North Carolina, USA*

**Olaitan A. Soyannwo, MBBS, DA, MMed, FWACS, FICS, FAS**, *Department of Anaesthesia, College of Medicine, University of Ibadan, Medical School, Nigeria*

**Karen L. Syrjala, PhD**, *Biobehavioral Sciences, Clinical Research Division, and Survivorship Program, Fred Hutchinson Cancer Center, πSeattle, Washington, USA; Department of Psychiatry and Behavioral Sciences, University of Washington, Seattle, Washington, USA*

**Marieke H.J. van den Beuken-van Everdingen, MD, PhD**, *Department of Anesthesiology, Pain Management and Research Centre, University Hospital Maastricht, Maastricht, The Netherlands*

**Yvette van der Linden, MD, PhD**, *Radiotherapeutic Institute Friesland, Leeuwarden, The Netherlands*

**Todd W. Vanderah, PhD**, *Department of Pharmacology, University of Arizona, Tucson, Arizona, USA*

**Kris C.P. Vissers, MD, PhD**, *Department of Anesthesiology, Pain and Palliative Medicine, University Medical Centre St. Radboud, Nijmegen, The Netherlands*

**Mads U. Werner, MD, PhD**, *Multidisciplinary Pain Center, Neuroscience Center, Rigshospitalet, Copenhagen, Denmark*

**Amanda C. de C. Williams, PhD**, *Research Department of Clinical, Health and Educational Psychology, University College London, London, United Kingdom*

**Jean C. Yi, PhD**, *Biobehavioral Sciences, Clinical Research Division, Fred Hutchinson Cancer Research Center, Seattle, Washington, USA*

**Haijun Zhang, PhD**, *Department of Anesthesia and Pain Medicine, The University of Texas M.D. Anderson Cancer Center, Houston, Texas, USA*

# Foreword

As readers will appreciate, a quarter, or slightly more, of the world's population will develop some form of cancer, and a high proportion will experience pain, possibly severe pain, as the disease progresses. This problem is particularly relevant in developing countries, where resources for pain relief are often limited or absent.

The battle against cancer involves work including the study of basic mechanisms that cause cells to overgrow or fail to age and to move to different parts of the body to form metastases. Increasingly, the complex genetic processes of cancer cell growth are being unraveled, allowing a move toward more personalized treatment of malignant tumors and away from the derivatives of wartime gases that have been used for many years. Therefore, huge efforts are being made to understand the processes of cell cancer growth and spread and to develop new ways of correcting or eliminating them.

During the past 40 years, much has been learned about the spiritual, psychological, and social consequences of cancer for patients and their families. Advances have been made in these areas in understanding how to help both groups cope with the problems that arise from the diseases and their consequences.

It is against this background that those involved in the management of pain in cancer have developed treatment methods, and the breadth of the field is revealed by the wide-ranging topics covered in the symposium on which the book was based, and reported in this book. The authors are leaders in their respective fields, and as might be expected, the topics, and the volume itself, are at the cutting edge of knowledge in cancer research—be it basic science or clinical research. Relatively recent times have seen increasing awareness of the poor facilities, both in terms of trained personnel and the availability of drugs, especially those of the powerful opioid group, for individuals in severe pain in developing countries. IASP has made this problem one of its major themes with the establishment of education and clinical training for those dealing with people in pain. It is pleasing, therefore, to see that there is a chapter on pain problems in the developing world.

This is not a large book, but it contains a great deal of important and up-to-date information. It is highly recommended to all those from the laboratory to the bedside with an interest in cancer pain.

Sir Michael R. Bond, MD, PhD, DSc, FRSE, FRCS, FRCPsych
University of Glasgow
Glasgow, United Kingdom

# Preface

Cancer pain remains greatly feared. Unfortunately, some of this fear is justified. Studies suggest that cancer pain remains undertreated in both developed and developing countries. However, there is much cause for optimism as scientists and clinicians carefully consider the problem of cancer pain. Extraordinary breakthroughs in our understanding of cancer-related pain have been made in the past few years, and these are leading to new treatment options. This book addresses the most recent findings from the laboratory and the bedside, recognizing that cancer pain encompasses both molecules at the most minuscule level and the larger issue of suffering in the human being with malignancy. Each chapter is based upon presentations delivered at an exceptional research symposium sponsored by the International Association for the Study of Pain. This symposium brought together outstanding basic and clinical scientists from around the world to discuss cutting-edge issues related to cancer pain. The goal of the symposium was to disseminate the most current findings regarding cancer pain and to develop a research agenda to guide future work. This book expands upon these dissemination efforts.

On a molecular level, new findings regarding the underlying neurobiology of malignant bone pain have changed the way we understand and treat pain due to primary or metastatic bone lesions. Several investigators around the world are exploring the neuronal changes underlying chemotherapy-induced painful peripheral neuropathy. This important work has highlighted the role of cancer treatment as a serious cause of persistent pain. Furthermore, it is leading to strategies that might one day be employed in the clinic to prevent such pain, allowing patients to complete potentially curative therapy and improving their quality of life.

As the underlying mechanisms of cancer pain are unraveled, new treatments are being designed that will be targeted to these mechanisms. Examples include anti-nerve growth factor  monoclonal antibodies, such as tanezumab, that bind to tropomyosin-related kinase A receptors on sensory neurons, reducing activation of nociceptors after noxious stimulation. Another example is the reduction of osteoclast activity by osteoprotegerin to reduce malignant bone pain. Many more compounds are currently in development.

Opioids remain crucial to the management of cancer-related pain. One challenge to employing this class of drugs is tolerance. The phenomenon is poorly understood, and findings in the laboratory do not always correlate with what is observed in the clinical setting. Furthermore, in the person with cancer, increasing opioid needs may be the result of changes in absorption or elimination as disease progresses. In addition to opioids, there is greater appreciation for the need to employ multimodal therapies. These include nonopioid and adjunctive agents, along with newer therapies that are currently under investigation. Furthermore, the role of disease-modifying therapies remains essential, including radiotherapy, chemotherapy, biological treatments, interventional approaches, and other techniques.

To fully understand the problem of cancer pain, we must carefully consider research design issues. Starting with the laboratory, the models employed in animals must accurately predict the experience of patients with malignancy. Models such as the tail-flick test rarely emulate the complex experience of patients. Designing clinical trials in the clinical setting can be complicated by disease progression, by the potentially confounding effect of concomitant cancer therapies, and by the heterogeneity of cancer pain syndromes. Conducting these trials can be like shooting at a moving target. Yet there are strategies that can be employed to ensure that cancer pain research is designed to answer the most crucial questions. Collaboration between basic scientists and clinicians is vital. The development of international collaborative groups will help with subject accrual and generalizability of findings.

The psychological context of cancer will greatly affect the entire pain experience and can lead to extraordinary suffering and existential distress. The role of anxiety, helplessness, catastrophizing, and other states may have a neural substrate. Extraordinary work is being conducted to teach patients and families coping skills to improve self-efficacy. More work is clearly needed in this area, and strategies for dissemination into the clinical setting must be encouraged. Education of clinicians is essential, and experts are studying the most effective strategies for teaching new professionals these techniques.

Cancer, with its associated pain, is a universal phenomenon, affecting rich and poor around the world. Obstacles to global relief of cancer pain are primarily issues of access. Lack of access to clinicians who are educated about pain assessment and management is a significant barrier in both developed and developing worlds. In the developing world, limited availability of medications, particularly opioids, precludes good cancer pain control. Educational efforts can begin to address some of the knowledge deficits. Organizations such as IASP can work with governments and other regulatory bodies to develop policies that will improve opioid availability.

*Cancer Pain: From Molecules to Suffering* is unique in that it addresses the most current research related to cancer pain, with chapters written by noted international experts in the field. Each chapter addresses current work along with clinical implications and research that is needed in the future. It is required reading for basic and clinical scientists working in this field, as well as for the health care professionals who care for these patients. A book of this complexity develops only from much dedication and effort. We would like to thank all of the authors who so graciously contributed their time and expertise, as well as the IASP staff, particularly Elizabeth Endres, Associate Editor of IASP Press, whose expert skill and commitment brought this book to realization. And finally, we are grateful to all of those patients who have had cancer pain and have generously shared their experiences with us.

Judith A. Paice, RN, PhD, FAAN
Rae F. Bell, MD, PhD
Eija A. Kalso, MD, DMedSci
Olaitan A. Soyannwo, MBBS, DA, MMed, FWACS, FICS, FAS

# Part I

# Basic Mechanisms of Cancer Pain

# Mechanisms of Chemotherapy-Induced Neuropathic Pain

Juan P. Cata,[a] Haijun Zhang,[b] Larry C. Driver,[b] Basem Hamid,[b] Sergio Giralt,[c] Allen W. Burton,[b] and Patrick M. Dougherty[b]

*[a]Department of Anesthesiology, The Cleveland Clinic, Cleveland, Ohio, USA; Departments of [b]Anesthesia and Pain Medicine and [c]Stem Cell Transplantation, The University of Texas M.D. Anderson Cancer Center, Houston, Texas, USA*

The treatment of a long list of malignancies still depends on the use of various chemotherapy agents. Unfortunately, the development of chemotherapy-related adverse effects limits the total amount of the anticancer agents that can be administered, thus limiting the survival of cancer patients. Nausea, vomiting, anorexia, fatigue, weight loss, and alopecia rank among the most common chemotherapy-related side effects; however, they are usually temporary and subside after treatment cessation. Pain is another common side effect associated with anticancer medications. Chemotherapy-induced pain represents a constellation of symptoms such as myalgias, arthralgias, abdominal pain, pharyngeal spasms, and sensory disturbances such as burning or "electric shock" paresthesias.

In this chapter, we will review current findings from clinical and laboratory studies into the mechanisms of chemotherapy-induced peripheral neuropathy (CIPN). We will also discuss diagnostic methods, preventive interventions, and therapeutic options.

*Cancer Pain: From Molecules to Suffering*
edited by Judith A. Paice, Rae F. Bell, Eija A. Kalso, and Olaitan A. Soyannwo
IASP Press, Seattle, © 2010

3

# Incidence and Risk Factors

Traditionally described as a side effect of older chemotherapeutic medications such as vinca alkaloids, taxanes, platinum-derived compounds, and thalidomide, chemotherapy-induced neuropathy is now also seen after the administration of newer, more effective drugs such as epothilones, bortezomib, and nano-albumin-bounded paclitaxel [8,9,21,63,88]. The incidence of CIPN varies from 10% to 100% among the different anticancer medications, depending on the type of drug, dosage, and pattern of administration [10,26,72,85]. It is clear that similar to cisplatin [16], paclitaxel and oxaliplatin cause a dose-dependent peripheral neuropathy [8,15,26,72]. Low doses of paclitaxel are not associated with significant neuropathy (grade III or IV as defined by the National Cancer Institute's common toxicity criteria) in patients with non-small-cell lung carcinoma [51].

Pharmacokinetic factors associated with the pattern of chemotherapy administration also influence the incidence of CIPN. For instance, prolonged infusions of paclitaxel that were given over 6–24 hours were associated with worse neuropathy than were shorter regimens (lasting only 3 hours) [87]. The incidence of neuropathic symptoms varies among antitumor agents with similar mechanisms of cytotoxicity. Paclitaxel is more neurotoxic than docetaxel, and cisplatin causes more sensorimotor disturbances than carboplatin and oxaliplatin [14,74]. Epothilones, a new class of microtubule inhibitor, may be associated with severe CIPN [110]; however, the neuropathy associated with ixabepilone, a novel epothilone B analogue, is reversible and mild [63].

Clinical studies remain controversial regarding the impact of older age and preexisting comorbidities such as inherited neuropathies, carpal tunnel syndrome, diabetes mellitus, and alcoholism on the incidence of CIPN [15,27,62,66,79,84]. It is plausible to infer from these studies that the use of antitumor agents with a safer neurotoxic profile is recommended in patients with preexisting non-chemotherapy-induced neuropathy. Less disputed are data suggesting that paraneoplastic sensory neuropathy and previous exposure to or co-administration of chemotherapeutic agents are risk factors in the development of CIPN. Coadministration of cisplatin and paclitaxel to women with breast cancer caused neuropathy in 35% of patients [37]. Peripheral neuropathy occurred in approximately 45–50% of ovarian cancer patients receiving cisplatin alone [103]; however, peripheral sensorimotor disturbances occurred in almost all patients who were previously exposed to taxanes and platinum-based agents [78]. Contrary to the previously mentioned studies, prior exposure to cisplatin, vincristine, and thalidomide was not associated with a higher incidence of bortezomib-induced neuropathy compared to patients who had not previously received other chemotherapeutic drugs [78]. Age may be a related risk factor for this type of neuropathy because the risk increases by 6% per year of age [28].

# Pathogenesis

There is no consensus about the exact pathogenesis of CIPN. Several investigators have proposed different theories based on experimental and clinical studies. It was initially suggested that CIPN was the result of the direct action of chemotherapy agents on neuronal microtubules because of the known effects of vincristine and paclitaxel on cancer cell microtubules [46,93]. Histological studies showed structural defects at the microtubular level, as well as axonal degeneration and demyelination in peripheral sensory neurons of animals treated with vincristine and humans treated with paclitaxel [25,75,99]. These structural abnormalities would lead to axonal transport disturbances causing metabolic and excitatory disturbances in the affected neurons. Unfortunately, this theory cannot explain CIPN associated with the administration of cisplatin, thalidomide, and bortezomib, which do not act on microtubules. Furthermore, this theory does not explain the early histological signs of neuropathy, such as the swollen and vacuolated mitochondria seen in both C fibers and myelinated axons after the administration of low doses of paclitaxel or vincristine [34,97].

The toxic effects of cisplatin on sensory neurons might be related to its actions on mitogen-activated protein kinases (MAPKs), which are known to control a wide variety of cellular functions such as proliferation, differentiation, and regulation of apoptosis. Specifically, cisplatin activated p38 and extracellular signal-related kinase (ERK) types 1 and 2 and reduced the activated form of c-Jun N-terminal kinase (JNK)/stress-activated protein kinase (Sapk) in sensory neurons [92]. Activation of gene expression ERK in peripheral and central neurons plays an important role in the pathogenesis of pain behaviors in different animal models. The induction of ERK modulates the expression of neurokinin-1 (NK1) and tyrosine kinase B (TrkB) receptors and cyclooxygenase [52]. Thus, it is plausible that MAPK activation by antitumor medications may be responsible for the development of acute hyperalgesia followed by prolonged sensitization.

Mitochondrial dysfunction has also been proposed as a potential cause of CIPN. Bortezomib and oxaliplatin cause mitochondrial injury due to an increase in the production of reactive oxygen species and greater inner mitochondrial membrane potential [53,65]. Moreover, the administration of bortezomib causes mitochondrial vacuolization in rats with CIPN [25]. The administration of drugs such as acetyl-L-carnitine and olesoxime (cholest-4-en-3-one, oxime), which are known to have mitochondrial protective effects, has proven effective in the treatment of vincristine- and paclitaxel-induced painful neuropathy in animals [35]. Thus, neuroprotective agents might have short-term effects in improving metabolic imbalance in sensory neurons and could ameliorate acute allodynia and hyperalgesia. The long-term treatment effects of mitochondrial protective agents may prevent axonal degeneration [35]. In contrast to these studies, the administration of inhibitors of the mitochondrial electron transport chain and antioxidants did not ameliorate cisplatin-induced painful neuropathy [34,53].

Inflammation around sensory fibers has also been indicated in the etiology of CIPN. Early evidence indicates that the administration of chemotherapeutic agents in combination with granulocyte-macrophage colony-stimulating factor (GM-CSF), a cytokine secreted by immune system cells, produces worse symptoms of CIPN [86]. The exposure of mice to vincristine not only increased levels of GM-CSF but caused macrophage invasion and interleukin-6 (IL-6) expression around the sciatic nerve and dorsal root ganglia (DRG) [73]. Furthermore, the coadministration of anti-IL-6 and cyclooxygenase inhibitors prevented vincristine-induced mechanical allodynia [22,59]. Paradoxically, the exogenous administration of IL-6 provided neuroprotection in rodents with cisplatin-, paclitaxel-, and vincristine-induced neuropathy [18]. These results are not surprising because IL-6 has shown to be protective in other models of neuronal damage [49]. It is possible that after toxic nerve damage, increased levels of IL-6 are responsible for both hyperalgesia and an attempted mode of neuroprotection [57]. Cisplatin may also induce inflammation around peripheral neurons. Gene mapping of DRG from rats treated with cisplatin showed increased expression of genes such as *MMP9*, the gene expressing matrix metallopeptidase 9, which is known to be involved in inflammation [2]. Moreover, the coadministration of minocycline, an antimicrobial agent with anti-inflammatory effects, prevented paclitaxel-induced CIPN [20]. Based on the fact that bradykinins cause hyperalgesia, Bujalska et al. investigated the effect of a bradykinin receptor antagonist in animals with vincristine neuropathy. Interestingly, the systemic administration of a B1- and B2-receptor antagonist showed antihyperalgesic effects [17].

A deficiency in neurotrophic factors can contribute to CIPN. Treatment with chemotherapeutic agents decreases circulating levels of nerve growth factor (NGF), and administration of NGF was effective in the prevention of toxic sympathetic nerve injury induced by vincristine and paclitaxel but was not protective against cisplatin-induced nerve cell injury [24,25,45]. In rodents with paclitaxel-induced neuropathy, the administration of NGF restored levels of neuropeptides in sensory neurons [91]. The administration of NGF ameliorated CIPN, and cotreatment with acetyl-L-carnitine also improved neuropathic symptoms by restoring NGF levels [77].

Brain-derived neurotrophic factor (BDNF) might also be implicated in chemotherapy-induced neurotoxicity [105]. Cisplatin-treated animals showed decreased levels of BDNF in peripheral tissues, and these levels were restored by the exogenous administration of NGF [4]. Interestingly, cisplatin-treated rodents had increased NGF and BDNF levels in the spinal cord as a result of abnormal utilization of these growth factors by affected sensory neurons [4].

In summary, it is possible that the coexistence of several mechanisms involving inflammation, direct cytotoxicity, and a deficiency in growth factor may be responsible for this syndrome.

# Peripheral and Central Sensitization

Tissue injury causes the release of pronociceptive mediators that sensitize peripheral nerve terminals (peripheral sensitization) and thus leads to neurochemical, electrical, and phenotypic alterations of sensory neurons and increased excitability of spinal cord dorsal horn neurons (central sensitization). All these abnormalities have been found in experimental models of CIPN.

A high incidence of abnormal spontaneous discharge in A-fiber and C-fiber cells has been described in animals with paclitaxel- and vincristine-induced neuropathic pain [108]. In vincristine-treated rodents, Tanner et al. found a subset of high-firing nociceptors (C fibers) that were hyperresponsive to both mechanical and heat stimulation [96]. The origin of the ectopic spontaneous discharge from peripheral sensory neurons may be located in injured or normal sensory terminal arbors or at the level of the axon or DRG. Potential pain generators responsible for peripheral sensitization include ion channels, cytokines, and intracellular enzymes, all of which have been implicated in CIPN. For instance, the transient receptor potential vanilloid (TRPV) ion channels are a family of cation channels that participate in the sensory process and are activated by a diverse range of stimuli, including heat, protons, lipids, phorbols, phosphorylation, changes in extracellular osmolarity or pressure, and depletion of intracellular $Ca^{2+}$ stores. TRPV4 located in peripheral sensory neurons is a transducer of osmotic and mechanical stimuli that contributes to enhanced paclitaxel- and vincristine-induced hyperalgesia by an unclear mechanism. Recently, a group of researchers demonstrated that TRPV4$^{-/-}$ mice did not develop hyperalgesia after treatment with paclitaxel and vincristine [3].

Expression of the voltage-dependent calcium channel $\alpha_2\delta_1$ subunit is increased in the DRG of oxaliplatin- and paclitaxel-treated rats [40], specifically in medium- and large-diameter neurons, which may underlie the allodynia present in the animals with CIPN [68]. Also, expression of the 5-HT$_{2A}$ receptor in nociceptive DRG neurons is increased in vincristine-treated rats, and mechanical hypersensitivity in these animals can be reduced with a 5-HT$_{2A}$-receptor antagonist [98]. Proinflammatory mediators may also contribute to peripheral sensitization. Interleukin-6 is present in the DRG of chemotherapy-treated animals, and the administration of cyclooxygenase inhibitors ameliorates vincristine-induced hyperalgesia [22].

The continuous and abnormal barrage of electrical signals in peripheral sensory neurons alters the sensory coding of spinal dorsal horn neurons, leading to central sensitization. Briefly, wide-dynamic-range neurons of animals with CIPN show high spontaneous activity, increased evoked responses to acute natural stimuli (except in cisplatin-treated rats), continued discharge following removal of cutaneous stimuli (afterdischarges), and wind-up (Fig. 1). In rats with CIPN, central sensitization has several causes. First, glutamate reuptake is abnormal [19]. Second, expression of cation channels, such as the voltage-dependent calcium channel $\alpha_2\delta_1$ subunit, increases [40]. Third, expression of the 5-HT$_{2A}$ receptor is increased throughout the dorsal horn [98]. Fourth, modulation of cannabinoid receptors is altered [81]. Fifth, dysfunction of the nitrous oxide–cyclic

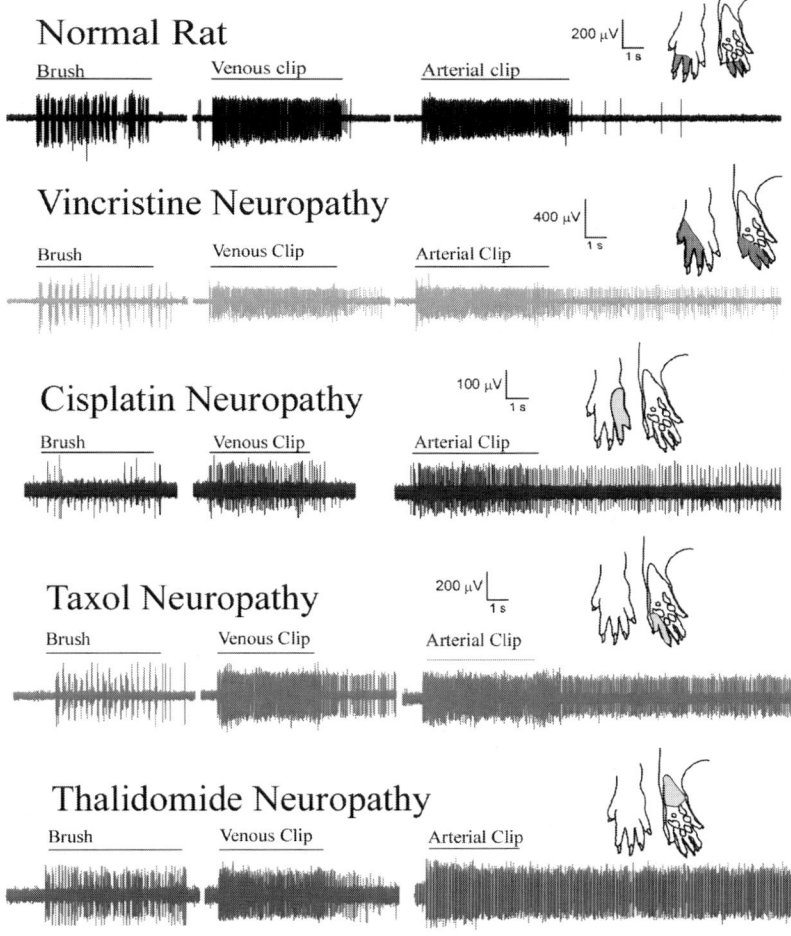

**Fig. 1.** Electrophysiological data from spinal cord recordings in animals with chemotherapy-induced peripheral neuropathy (CIPN). Note that the response of wide-dynamic-range neurons is abnormal in rats with CIPN. The most remarkable finding is the presence of prolonged and intense afterdischarges after the application of a noxious stimulus (venous and arterial clip) to the hindpaw of the animals.

guanosine monophosphate (NO/cGMP) pathway can be responsible for neuronal hyperexcitability and central sensitization [16]. This statement is corroborated by an experimental study that showed that the protein level of neuronal nitric oxide synthase (nNOS), but not inducible nitric oxide synthase (iNOS), in the spinal cord of vincristine-treated mice was significantly decreased compared to the level in vehicle-treated naive mice. Moreover, the administration of a nitric oxide precursor reversed vincristine CIPN [54]. And last, central sensitization may involve glial activation and further release of inflammatory cytokines such as TNF-α [59]. It is likely that all these disturbances contribute simultaneously to the development of central sensitization, making it complicated to understand the mechanisms of CIPN.

# Clinical Findings in Patients with CIPN

Patients with CIPN usually report sensory, motor, and autonomic disturbances. Unfortunately, these signs and symptoms are worsened by side effects caused by opiates and adjuvant analgesics given to relieve neuropathic pain. Therefore, the quality of life of patients with CIPN is generally rated as poor, not only with regard to basic functioning, but also because patients may be prevented from working or enjoying other aspects of life.

## Sensory Disturbances

The onset of sensory symptoms generally occurs early in treatment, between the first and third cycle of chemotherapy administration, with the peak in severity occurring approximately 3 months into therapy [31,48,103]. A recent study demonstrated that after three, six, and nine cycles, sensory neuropathy was seen in 61%, 57%, and 76% of the patients, respectively; however, some patients may have a delayed onset (also known as the "coasting effect") occurring 2–4 months after chemotherapy [55,71]. Importantly, the presence of CIPN during treatment with paclitaxel was found to be a predictor of the development of neuropathic pain after treatment cessation in a study showing that those who had experienced CIPN were three times more likely to develop neuropathic pain [83].

Symptoms characteristically appear in a distal stocking-and-glove pattern [21,30,31] and are described as numbness and tingling by more than 90% of patients and as overtly painful in 26% of cases [66]. It has been suggested that the numbness and tingling reflect the involvement of large myelinated fibers and that the progression to burning sensations represents damage to small unmyelinated fibers [21]. Symptoms are usually worse at night and interfere with sleep. Some patients with cutaneous allodynia complain of pain when bed sheets touch their feet. Patients with severe neuropathy also complain of cold allodynia, which is reported as extremely painful sensations during cold weather or avoidance of cold liquids or reaching into the refrigerator or freezer.

Other sensory symptoms such as pharyngolaryngeal and cold dysesthesias and Lhermitte's sign (tingling sensations traveling down the limbs or torso on neck flexion) are reported to occur in 67%, 47%, and 3%, respectively, of patients receiving oxaliplatin.

## Motor Neuropathy

Motor neuropathy is usually less frequent and milder than sensory neuropathy, but muscle strength can be abnormal after the administration of large doses of chemotherapy [42,95]. Common complaints are muscle weakness [60,87]. Argyriou et al. reported mild to moderate weakness, mainly involving the distal muscles, in patients with oxaliplatin-induced neuropathy [8].

## Autonomic Neuropathy

The presence of autonomic neuropathy is not uniform in all patients with CIPN. Patients with autonomic neuropathy may experience dryness of the mouth, nose, and eyes; orthostatic dizziness; ileus; diarrhea; sweating; and red or white skin discoloration [26,33].

# Evaluation of Patients

## Clinical Examination

The first sign of sensory neuropathy is an elevated vibratory detection threshold in distal extremities, followed by loss of deep tendon reflexes in the ankles and impaired temperature sensation [102]. The vibratory perception threshold increases more in the feet than in the hands in patients with symptomatic or asymptomatic chemotherapy-induced neuropathy [36,80,87]. Another common finding is the loss of sense of position (proprioception) in the fingers and toes; however, this finding is a sign of severe neuropathy and underlies symptoms such as gait disturbances. Motor neuropathy presents as muscle wasting, weakness, and fasciculation [10].

## Quantitative Sensory Testing

Quantitative sensory testing measures the detection threshold of accurately calibrated sensory stimuli in patients with (or at risk of) peripheral sensory neuropathy. It is worth noting that as many as 50% of subjects in some studies show signs of a mild sensory peripheral neuropathy prior to chemotherapy [36,66]. The three main components of the test are detection of vibratory, thermal, and painful stimuli, which relate to distinct neuroanatomic pathways with discrete fiber populations [94]. Quantitative sensory testing in patients with CIPN shows similar features; however, subtle differences exist among the chemotherapy agents. It is clear that vibratory touch detection thresholds are increased in most patients with CIPN, regardless of the chemotherapy agent, representing deficits in the function of larger myelinated fibers (Fig. 2) [10,31]. This abnormality is further expressed as reduced dexterity and deteriorated performance in tests such as the slotted-peg-board test, along with elevated touch detection (Fig. 2). Sharpness detection is also impaired in patients with CIPN, representing dysfunction in small myelinated fibers (Fig. 3) [31]. However, the impairment is limited to the area of paresthesias or dysesthesias (pain area in Fig. 3). Contrary to touch and pinprick detection, the thresholds for heat pain are preserved and minimally affected in patients with paclitaxel- and cisplatin-induced neuropathy [31]. A particular distinction applies to patients with vincristine- and bortezomib-induced painful neuropathy who have major impairment of both myelinated and unmyelinated sensory fibers [21] (Fig. 4). Cold allodynia is also present in some patients with painful neuropathies. In those with paclitaxel-induced neuropathy, skin cooling triggers paradoxical burning pain [31], whereas patients with vincristine- and cisplatin-induced neuropathy do not have significant alterations in cold detection [21].

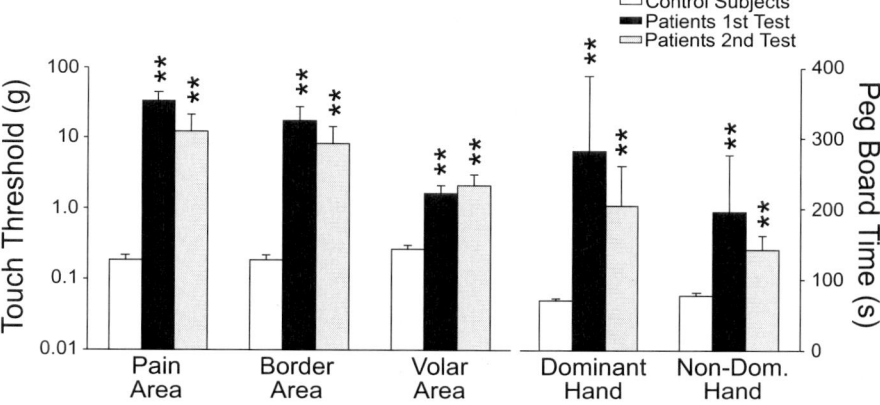

**Fig. 2.** The left panel shows statistically significant differences in touch detection perception thresholds between control subjects (open bars) and patients with bortezomib-related neuropathic pain (filled black and gray bars). The abnormal thresholds extend not only to the painful (pain area) or paresthetic area (border area) of the extremities but also to more proximal nonpainful areas of skin (volar area). The right panel depicts the performance of control subjects and patients in the pegboard test. It can be seen that subjects with chemotherapy-induced peripheral neuropathy have significantly reduced dexterity compared to controls. Similar findings have been reported for patients with paclitaxel-, vincristine-, and cisplatin-induced neuropathy. Comparison of the data shown in the black bars (Patients 1st Test) with the gray bars (Patients 2nd Test) indicates that at the 1-year follow-up examination there was no improvement in sensory function. * P < 0.05, *** P < 0.01, *** P < 0.001.

## Nerve Conduction Studies

### Sensory Nerve Conduction Studies

Sensory nerve conduction studies are performed by electrical stimulation of a peripheral nerve and recording from a purely sensory portion of the nerve. Common findings consistent with the presence of sensory neuropathy include prolonged latency and slowed conduction velocity [62,90]. Given the predominantly distal onset of the sensory symptoms, the loss of distal (ankle) reflexes, and the findings in nerve conduction studies, several authors have agreed that most of the neurotoxic chemotherapy drugs induce a "dying-back" type of neural degeneration, suggesting axonopathy [23,87]. However, this hypothesis has been challenged by a recent study that could not find a pattern dependent on axon length in patients with cisplatin-induced neuropathy [60,61].

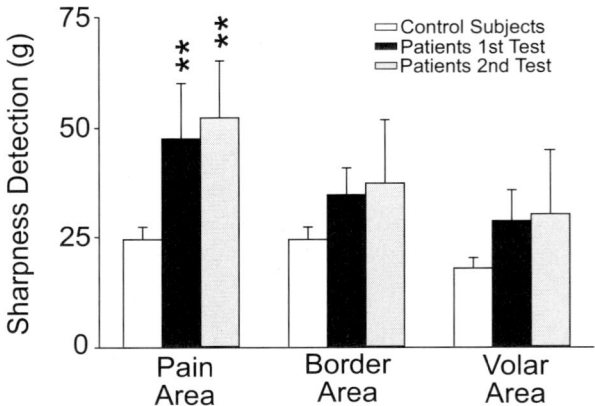

**Fig. 3.** Patients with chemotherapy-induced peripheral neuropathy (filled black and gray bars) have significantly higher detection thresholds to sharp stimuli than control subjects (open bars). This finding represents abnormal function of Aδ fibers. Similar findings have been reported for patients with paclitaxel-, vincristine-, and cisplatin-induced neuropathy. Comparison of the data shown in the black bars (Patients 1st Test) with the gray bars (Patients 2nd Test) indicates that at the 1-year follow-up examination there was no improvement in sensory function. * $P < 0.05$, *** $P < 0.01$, *** $P < 0.001$.

## *Motor Nerve Conduction Studies*

Motor nerve conduction studies are performed by electrically stimulating a peripheral nerve and recording from a muscle supplied by this nerve. Usually, the peroneal and ulnar nerves are used to assess amplitudes and conduction velocities. In a recent study in oxaliplatin- and cisplatin-treated patients, motor nerve conduction tests failed to show motor neuropathy [61,76]. Electrophysiological findings similar to those in platinum-treated patients have been reported recently in patients with bortezomib-induced neuropathy who presented sensory nerve fiber abnormalities with a normal motor fiber pattern [85]. Interestingly, acute oxaliplatin-induced peripheral neuropathy is characterized by repetitive motor discharges along with spontaneous high-frequency firing, with spared involvement of sensory nerves [106].

# Prognosis

The time course for resolution of chemotherapy-induced peripheral neuropathy is highly variable and may be related to the type and amount of chemotherapy received during treatment. A recent study showed that

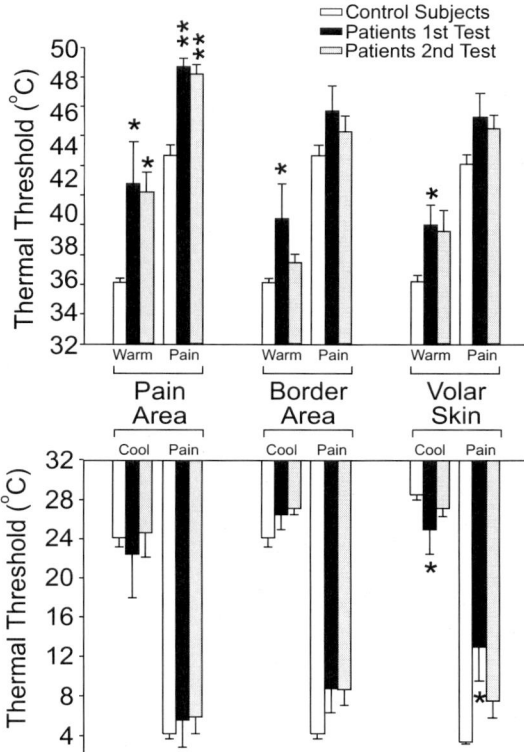

**Fig. 4.** The upper graphic shows that patients with chemotherapy-induced peripheral neuropathy (CIPN) have significantly impaired detection of warm and heat pain stimuli compared to control subjects. This sensory abnormality extends not only to the painful or paresthetic area of the extremities but also to more proximal nonpainful areas of skin (border and volar areas). The lower graphic shows that detection of cold stimuli is also abnormal in subjects with CIPN. In fact, cold allodynia is present in the volar area. Similar findings have been reported for patients with paclitaxel-, vincristine-, and cisplatin-induced neuropathy. Comparison of the data shown in the black bars (Patients 1st Test) with the gray bars (Patients 2nd Test) indicates that at the 1-year follow-up examination there was no improvement in sensory function. * $P < 0.05$, *** $P < 0.01$, *** $P < 0.001$.

one-third of the patients with bortezomib-induced neuropathy had resolution or improvement during treatment, while one-third improved after treatment and the rest did not experience any improvement. The median duration from the last dose to resolution or improvement of peripheral neuropathy was 47 days [85]. In a different study, resolution or improvement of bortezomib-induced peripheral neuropathy occurred in half of the patients within a median period of 3 months. However, Chaudry et al. found an 80% rate of improvement of symptoms after bortezomib treatment [26]. The data shown in Figs. 1–4 indicate that a cohort of patients studied at the M.D. Anderson Cancer Center with chronic bortezomib neuropathy (presenting with pain lasting for 3 months or more) showed no improvement in any measure at a 1-year follow-up examination.

Symptoms of CIPN can be permanent after chemotherapy. For instance, persistent peripheral neuropathy was found in 20–60% of patients treated with cisplatin. In patients with vincristine-induced peripheral neuropathy, the mean duration of pain and sensory complaints was 40.6 months, with some patients experiencing pain for 10 years or longer [30]. In another subset of patients with paclitaxel- and bortezomib-induced neuropathy, the mean duration of pain was 14.9 and 22 months, respectively [21,31]. In general, paresthesias and abnormal physical signs in patients with chemotherapy-induced peripheral neuropathy do not resolve simultaneously, and abnormal detection thresholds may persist even when paresthesias or pain have improved or disappeared [50].

# Prevention and Treatment

Pharmacological interventions have targeted potential receptors or nociceptive pathways involved in CIPN. Unfortunately, the results are worrisome because of the lack of efficacy of most of the therapies attempted.

## Anti-Inflammatory and Immune-Modulatory Drugs

Anti-inflammatory and immune-modulatory drugs have been tried with the goal of reducing inflammatory changes associated with CIPN. In rodents, the administration of cyclooxygenase (COX) inhibitors was shown to ameliorate vincristine-induced neuropathy [22]. Thalidomide has pleiotropic actions in the immune system. Cata et al. demonstrated that the coadministration of low doses of thalidomide to rats with paclitaxel- and vincristine-induced neuropathy diminished allodynia and hyperalgesia [20,22].

The role of COX inhibitors and thalidomide in the prevention and treatment of CIPN has not been studied in humans. Moreover, thalidomide has itself been associated with the development of CIPN. COX inhibitors are generally used as adjuvant analgesics for chemotherapy-induced myalgias; however, no randomized, controlled trials have evaluated the use of these mild analgesics on CIPN.

As described above, IL-6 is involved in the pathogenesis of CIPN. Researchers thus theorized that the administration of recombinant human leukemic inhibitor factor (rhuLIF)—a cytokine involved in nerve injury and repair—might help prevent CIPN. In a randomized, double-blind, placebo-controlled trial, patients with CIPN were randomized to receive rhuLIF or placebo. Unfortunately, rhuLIF was not effective in the prevention of CIPN, based on neurophysiological findings and quantitative sensory tests [29].

## Anticonvulsants

Anticonvulsants have been studied in the context of prevention and treatment of CIPN, based on evidence of their efficacy in other pain syndromes [11]. Gabapentin is the most commonly used anticonvulsant drug in cancer patients with neuropathic pain [13]. It causes analgesia by binding the $\alpha_2\delta_1$ subunit of voltage-dependent calcium channels, and in studies in rodents, it ameliorates paclitaxel- and oxaliplatin-induced hyperalgesia [40,64,68]. In a small study of patients with bortezomib-induced neuropathy, more than 80% of patients were receiving gabapentin plus opioids. In this group of patients, pain was rated as moderate [21]. In contrast, only half of another group of patients with vincristine-induced pain were being treated with gabapentin [30]. CIPN symptoms were not alleviated in a randomized, double-blind, placebo-controlled trial by Rao et al. in which patients received a maximum dose of 2700 mg/day of gabapentin or placebo [82]. In a recent unblinded and uncontrolled study of patients undergoing chemotherapy, gabapentin was administered at the onset of neuropathic pain symptoms. Interestingly, gabapentin caused at least partial improvement of symptoms in approximately 70% of patients [100]. Pregabalin is commonly administered in patients who cannot tolerate gabapentin. A recent open-label study suggested that pregabalin may be effective in the treatment of CIPN [104].

Carbamazepine and oxcarbazepine are anticonvulsant drugs commonly administered to patients with neuropathic pain. One small trial that evaluated the neuroprotective efficacy of each drug in subjects receiving oxaliplatin found little, if any, protection [77]. Topiramate has shown analgesic effects in experimental CIPN. However, there are no clinical studies evaluating the effects of this anticonvulsant in patients with CIPN [107]. Lamotrigine, a newer anticonvulsant, demonstrated analgesic effects in animals with vincristine-induced peripheral neuropathy [67]. Lamotrigine has also been clinically tested in patients with CIPN by Rao et al., who showed that lamotrigine was not effective for relieving neuropathic symptoms [82]. The effect of other anticonvulsant agents such as levetiracetam, tiagabine, and valproic acid in the prevention and treatment of CIPN is unknown.

## Antidepressants

Many types of antidepressants, including amitriptyline, nortriptyline, imipramine, duloxetine, mirtazapine, citalopram, and venlafaxine have also been used to treat neuropathic pain. Amitryptiline is the most commonly used antidepressant in cancer patients with neuropathic pain [13]. In a rodent study, amitryptiline was effective in treating paclitaxel- and vincristine-induced hyperalgesia [107]. In patients with CIPN, amitryptiline did not show greater analgesic effects compared to placebo; however, subjects experienced improved quality of life [56]. A recent clinical trial investigated the preventive properties of amitryptiline versus placebo in patients without previous neuropathy, who were receiving vinca alkaloids, platinum derivatives, or taxanes. The authors concluded that amitryptiline did not prevent chemotherapy-induced neuropathy [55]. Nortriptyline, also a commonly used antidepressant, blocks the synaptic reuptake of serotonin and norepinephrine and has a better side-effect profile than amitriptyline. Based on a randomized controlled trial by Mayo Clinic investigators, the analgesic effect of nortriptyline in patients with cisplatin-induced neuropathy is moderate compared to placebo [44]. In rodents, venlafaxine has shown antiallodynic effects in oxaliplatin-induced neuropathy [64]. A report of a small clinical study by Durant et al. suggested that venlafaxine was effective in preventing oxaliplatin-induced paresthesias [32]. However, randomized trials demonstrating a prophylactic or therapeutic effect of venlafaxine on CIPN neurotoxicity are still lacking.

## Opioids

Opioids are the most commonly used analgesics in cancer patients with neuropathic pain [13]. Three studies showed that more than 80% of CIPN patients were receiving opioids [21,30,31]. Experimental studies demonstrate that opioids and opioid degradation inhibitors are at least partially effective in relieving allodynia and hyperalgesia in rodents with CIPN, although large doses are usually needed to produce analgesia [41,89,107]. A more recent study demonstrated that cisplatin may increase opioid efflux from neurons due to its interaction with glycoprotein-P, thus creating a potential multidrug-resistant stage [12]. This evidence may explain the so-called refractoriness of CIPN to opioids and the large amounts of these analgesics need to partially relive pain [21,30,31]. So far there have been no randomized controlled trials to assess the efficacy of opioids in CIPN.

## Acetyl-L-Carnitine

Acetyl-L-carnitine is an acetylated derivative of L-carnitine that has shown preventive effects in animal models of neuronal injury, possibly by restoring levels of NGF [1,77]. This agent both helped prevent and ameliorated hyperalgesia in rodents with CIPN [77,108], and thus attracted the attention of clinicians. In fact, based on a small clinical study, it was recommended for prevention or treatment of CIPN. Unfortunately, there is no randomized controlled trial that strongly suggests the use of acetyl-L-carnitine as a preventive or therapeutic agent in patients who have CIPN or are at risk for developing it.

## Amifostine

Amifostine was one the earliest drugs tested in the prevention of CIPN [69]. In animals with cisplatin-induced peripheral neuropathy, amifostine had preventive effects comparable to those of recombinant human erythropoietin [109]. Clinical studies provide little evidence to recommend the use of amifostine for the prevention of CIPN, although one study reported promising results [58,69,70].

## Magnesium and Calcium

An infusion of magnesium and calcium can reduce acute pain-related behaviors associated with the administration of oxaliplatin [64]. It was hypothesized that the active agent of this combination is the magnesium, which stabilizes neuron membranes, while the calcium would act as an oxalate-chelating agent [43]. It is unclear whether the combination of magnesium and calcium is effective in preventing CIPN in the clinic [38], because the only randomized studied conducted by Hochster et al. was stopped earlier than planned because of untoward oncological outcomes [47].

## Vitamin E

One of the most promising agents in the prevention of CIPN is vitamin E, which may exert this action due to its antioxidant properties. Small studies in patients have demonstrated that vitamin E was preventive against cisplatin- and paclitaxel-induced neuropathy [5-7]. Specifically, a small randomized trial showed that 600 mg/day of vitamin E prevented CIPN.

## Glutamine and Glutamate

In rodents, glutamine and glutamate prevented vincristine-induced neuropathy. This effect was speculated to be related to their to their anti-inflammatory properties and their ability to assemble microtubules and induce the release of NGF [39,95]. Thus, investigators suggested that glutamine and glutamate could prevent paclitaxel- and vincristine-induced neuropathy [95,101]. However, a multicenter, randomized, placebo-controlled, double-blinded pilot study failed to show evidence of protection [66].

# Conclusions

Neuropathic pain is a common and dose-limiting side effect of several chemotherapy agents. CIPN not only limits the amount of chemotherapy that patients receive, and thus the chances of cure, but can also result in permanent pain and associated symptoms that negatively affect quality of life. The pathophysiological mechanisms underlying CIPN remain unclear, and thus effective preventive and therapeutic interventions are still lacking. Unfortunately, the few pharmacological treatments that have suggested efficacy in small trials have failed to demonstrate benefit in large randomized controlled trials. Therefore, more basic, translational, and clinical research is essential.

# References

[1] Al Majed AA, Sayed-Ahmed MM, Al Omar FA, Al Yahya AA, Aleisa AM, Al Shabanah OA. Carnitine esters prevent oxidative stress damage and energy depletion following transient forebrain ischaemia in the rat hippocampus. Clin Exp Pharmacol Physiol 2006;33:725–33.

[2] Alaedini A, Xiang Z, Kim H, Sung YJ, Latov N. Up-regulation of apoptosis and regeneration genes in the dorsal root ganglia during cisplatin treatment. Exp Neurol 2008;210:368–74.

[3] Alessandri-Haber N, Dina OA, Joseph EK, Reichling DB, Levine JD. Interaction of transient receptor potential vanilloid 4, integrin, and SRC tyrosine kinase in mechanical hyperalgesia. J Neurosci 2008;28:1046–57.

[4] Aloe L, Manni L, Properzi F, DeSantis S, Fiore M. Evidence that nerve growth factor promotes the recovery of peripheral neuropathy induced in mice by cisplatin: behavioral, structural and biochemical analysis. Auton Neurosci 2000;86:84–93.

[5] Argyriou AA, Chroni E, Koutras A, Ellul J, Papapetropoulos S, Katsoulas G, Iconomou G, Kalofonos HP. Vitamin E for prophylaxis against chemotherapy-induced neuropathy: a randomized controlled trial. Neurology 2005;64:26–31.

[6] Argyriou AA, Chroni E, Koutras A, Iconomou G, Papapetropoulos S, Polychronopoulos P, Kalofonos HP. A randomized controlled trial evaluating the efficacy and safety of vitamin E supplementation for protection against cisplatin-induced peripheral neuropathy: final results. Support Care Cancer 2006;14:1134–40.

[7] Argyriou AA, Chroni E, Koutras A, Iconomou G, Papapetropoulos S, Polychronopoulos P, Kalofonos HP. Preventing paclitaxel-induced peripheral neuropathy: a phase II trial of vitamin E supplementation. J Pain Symptom Manage 2006;32:237–44.

[8] Argyriou AA, Polychronopoulos P, Iconomou G, Koutras A, Makatsoris T, Gerolymos MK, Gourzis P, Assimakopoulos K, Kalofonos HP, Chroni E. Incidence and characteristics of peripheral neuropathy during oxaliplatin-based chemotherapy for metastatic colon cancer. Acta Oncol 2007;46:1131–7.

[9] Argyriou AA, Polychronopoulos P, Koutras A, Xiros N, Petsas T, Argyriou K, Kalofonos HP, Chroni E. Clinical and electrophysiological features of peripheral neuropathy induced by administration of cisplatin plus paclitaxel-based chemotherapy. Eur J Cancer Care (Engl) 2007;16:231–7.

[10] Augusto C, Pietro M, Cinzia M, Sergio C, Sara C, Luca G, Scaioli V. Peripheral neuropathy due to paclitaxel: study of the temporal relationships between the therapeutic schedule and the clinical quantitative score (QST) and comparison with neurophysiological findings. J Neurooncol 2008;86:89–99.

[11] Backonja M, Beydoun A, Edwards KR, Schwartz SL, Fonseca V, Hes M, LaMoreaux L, Garofalo E. Gabapentin for the symptomatic treatment of painful neuropathy in patients with diabetes mellitus: a randomized controlled trial. JAMA 1998;280:1831–6.

[12] Balayssac D, Cayre A, Ling B, Maublant J, Penault-Llorca F, Eschalier A, Coudore F, Authier N. Increase in morphine antinociceptive activity by a P-glycoprotein inhibitor in cisplatin-induced neuropathy. Neurosci Lett 2009;465:108–12.

[13] Berger A, Dukes E, Mercadante S, Oster G. Use of antiepileptics and tricyclic antidepressants in cancer patients with neuropathic pain. Eur J Cancer Care (Engl) 2006;15:138–45.

[14] Beuselinck B, Wildiers H, Wynendaele W, Dirix L, Kains JP, Paridaens R. Weekly paclitaxel versus weekly docetaxel in elderly or frail patients with metastatic breast carcinoma: a randomized phase-II study of the Belgian Society of Medical Oncology. Crit Rev Oncol Hematol 2009; Epub Aug 1.

[15] Brouwers EE, Huitema AD, Boogerd W, Beijnen JH, Schellens JH. Persistent neuropathy after treatment with cisplatin and oxaliplatin. Acta Oncol 2009;48:832–41.

[16] Bujalska M, Gumulka SW. Effect of cyclooxygenase and nitric oxide synthase inhibitors on vincristine induced hyperalgesia in rats. Pharmacol Rep 2008;60:735–41.

[17] Bujalska M, Tatarkiewicz J, Gumulka SW. Effect of bradykinin receptor antagonists on vincristine- and streptozotocin-induced hyperalgesia in a rat model of chemotherapy-induced and diabetic neuropathy. Pharmacology 2008;81:158–63.

[18] Callizot N, Andriambeloson E, Glass J, Revel M, Ferro P, Cirillo R, Vitte PA, Dreano M. Interleukin-6 protects against paclitaxel, cisplatin and vincristine-induced neuropathies without impairing chemotherapeutic activity. Cancer Chemother Pharmacol 2008;62:995–1007.

[19] Cata JP, Weng HR, Chen JH, Dougherty PM. Altered discharges of spinal wide dynamic range neurons and down-regulation of glutamate transporter expression in rats with paclitaxel-induced hyperalgesia. Neuroscience 2006;138:329–38.

[20] Cata JP, Weng HR, Dougherty PM. The effects of thalidomide and minocycline on taxol-induced hyperalgesia in rats. Brain Res 2008;1229:100–10.

[21] Cata JP, Weng H-R, Burton AW, Villareal H, Giralt S, Dougherty PM. Quantitative sensory findings in patients with bortezomib-induced pain. J Pain 2007;8:296–306.

[22] Cata JP, Weng H-R, Dougherty PM. Cyclooxygenase inhibitors and thalidomide ameliorate vincristine-induced hyperalgesia in rats. Cancer Chemother Pharmacol 2004;54:391–7.

[23] Cata JP, Weng H-R, Dougherty PM. Clinical and experimental findings in humans and animals with chemotherapy-induced peripheral neuropathy. Minerva Anestesiol 2006;72:151–69.

[24] Cavaletti G, Bogliun G, Marzorati L, Zincone A, Piatti M, Colombo N, Franchi D, La Presa MT, Lissoni A, Buda A, et al. Early predictors of peripheral neurotoxicity in cisplatin and paclitaxel combination chemotherapy. Ann Oncol 2004;15:1439–42.

[25] Cavaletti G, Gilardini A, Canta A, Rigamonti L, Rodriguez-Menendez V, Ceresa C, Marmiroli P, Bossi M, Oggioni N, D'Incalci M, De Coster R. Bortezomib-induced peripheral neurotoxicity: a neurophysiological and pathological study in the rat. Exp Neurol 2007;204:317–25.

[26] Chaudhry V, Cornblath DR, Polydefkis M, Ferguson A, Borrello I. Characteristics of bortezomib- and thalidomide-induced peripheral neuropathy. J Peripher Nerv Syst 2008;13:275–82.

[27] Chauvenet AR, Shashi V, Selsky C, Morgan E, Kurtzberg J, Bell B. Vincristine-induced neuropathy as the initial presentation of a Charcot-Marie-Tooth disease in acute lymphoblastic leukemia: a pediatric oncology group study. J Pediatr Hematol Oncol 2003;25:316–20.

[28] Corso A, Mangiacavalli S, Varettoni M, Pascutto C, Zappasodi P, Lazzarino M. Bortezomib-induced peripheral neuropathy in multiple myeloma: a comparison between previously treated and untreated patients. Leuk Res 2009; Epub Aug 10.

[29] Davis ID, Kiers L, MacGregor L, Quinn M, Arezzo J, Green M, Rosenthal M, Chia M, Michael M, Bartley P, et al. A randomized, double-blinded, placebo-controlled phase ii trial of recombinant human leukemia inhibitory factor (rhuLIF, Emfilermin, AM424) to prevent chemotherapy-induced peripheral neuropathy. Clin Cancer Res 2005;11:1890–8.

[30] Dougherty PM, Cata JP, Burton AW, Vu K, Weng HR. Dysfunction in multiple primary afferent fiber subtypes revealed by quantitative sensory testing in patients with chronic vincristine-induced pain. J Pain Symptom Manage 2007;33:166–79.

[31] Dougherty PM, Cata JP, Cordella JV, Burton A, Weng HR. Taxol-induced sensory disturbance is characterized by preferential impairment of myelinated fiber function in cancer patients. Pain 2004;109:132–42.

[32] Durand JP, Brezault C, Goldwasser F. Protection against oxaliplatin acute neurosensory toxicity by venlafaxine. Anticancer Drugs 2003;14:423–5.

[33] Ferrara F, Annunziata M, Pollio F, Palmieri S, Copia C, Mele G, Pocali B, Schiavone EM. Vincristine as treatment for recurrent episodes of thrombotic thrombocytopenic purpura. Ann Hematol 2002;81:7–10.

[34] Flatters SJ, Bennett GJ. Studies of peripheral sensory nerves in paclitaxel-induced painful peripheral neuropathy: evidence for mitochondrial dysfunction. Pain 2006;122:245–57.

[35] Flatters SJ, Xiao WH, Bennett GJ. Acetyl-L-carnitine prevents and reduces paclitaxel-induced painful peripheral neuropathy. Neurosci Lett 2006;397:219–23.

[36] Forsyth PA, Balmaceda C, Peterson K, Seidman AD, Brasher P, DeAngelis LM. Prospective study of paclitaxel-induced peripheral neuropathy with quantitative sensory testing. J Neurooncol 1997;35:47–53.

[37] Frasci G, Comella P, Rinaldo M, Iodice G, Di Bonito M, D'Aiuto M, Petrillo A, Lastoria S, Siani C, Comella G, D'Aiuto G, Preoperative weekly cisplatin-epirubicin-paclitaxel with G-CSF support in triple-negative large operable breast cancer. Ann Oncol 2009;20:1185–92.

[38] Gamelin L, Boisdron-Celle M, Delva R, Guerin-Meyer V, Ifrah N, Morel A, Gamelin E. Prevention of oxaliplatin-related neurotoxicity by calcium and magnesium infusions: a retrospective study of 161 patients receiving oxaliplatin combined with 5-fluorouracil and leucovorin for advanced colorectal cancer. Clin Cancer Res 2004;10:4055–61.

[39] Garrett-Cox RG, Stefanutti G, Booth C, Klein NJ, Pierro A, Eaton S. Glutamine decreases inflammation in infant rat endotoxemia. J Pediatr Surg 2009;44:523–9.

[40] Gauchan P, Andoh T, Ikeda K, Fujita M, Sasaki A, Kato A, Kuraishi Y. Mechanical allodynia induced by paclitaxel, oxaliplatin and vincristine: different effectiveness of gabapentin and different expression of voltage-dependent calcium channel alpha-2-delta-1 subunit. Biol Pharm Bull 2009;32:732–4.

[41] Genedani S, Bernardi M, Bertolini A. Influence of antineoplastic drugs on morphine analgesia and on morphine tolerance. Eur J Pharmacol 1999;367:13–7.

[42] Graziano SL, Herndon JE, Socinski MA, Wang X, Watson D, Vokes E, Green MR. Phase II trial of weekly dose-dense paclitaxel in extensive-stage small cell lung cancer: cancer and leukemia group B study 39901. J Thorac Oncol 2008;3:158–62.

[43] Grolleau F, Gamelin L, Boisdron-Celle M, Lapied B, Pelhate M, Gamelin E. A possible explanation for a neurotoxic effect of the anticancer agent oxaliplatin on neuronal voltage-gated sodium channels. J Neurophysiol 2001;85:2293–7.

[44] Hammack JE, Michalak JC, Loprinzi CL, Sloan JA, Novotny PJ, Soori GS, Tirona MT, Rowland KM Jr, Stella PJ, Johnson JA. Phase III evaluation of nortriptyline for alleviation of symptoms of cis-platinum-induced peripheral neuropathy. Pain 2002;98:195–203.

[45] Hayakawa K, Itoh T, Niwa H, Mutoh T, Sobue G. NGF prevention of neurotoxicity induced by cisplatin, vincristine and taxol depends on toxicity of each drug and NGF treatment schedule: in vitro study of adult rat sympathetic ganglion explants. Brain Res 1998;794:313–9.

[46] Hiser L, Herrington B, Lobert S. Effect of noscapine and vincristine combination on demyelination and cell proliferation in vitro. Leuk Lymphoma 2008;49:1603–9.

[47] Hochster HS, Grothey A, Childs BH. Use of calcium and magnesium salts to reduce oxaliplatin-related neurotoxicity. J Clin Oncol 2007;25:4028–9.

[48] Holland JF, Scharlau C, Gailani S, Krant MJ, Olson KB, Horton J, Shnider BI, Lynch JJ, Owens A, Carbone PP, et al. Vincristine treatment of advanced cancer: a cooperative study of 392 cases. Cancer Res 1973;33:1258–64.

[49] Holliday J, Parsons K, Curry J, Lee SY, Gruol DL. Cerebellar granule neurons develop elevated calcium responses when treated with interleukin-6 in culture. Brain Res 1995;673:141–8.

[50] Iniguez C, Larrode P, Mayordomo JI, Gonzalez P, Adelantado S, Yubero A, Tres A, Morales F. Reversible peripheral neuropathy induced by a single administration of high-dose paclitaxel. Neurology 1998;51:868–70.

[51] Jeremic B, Milicic B, Acimovic L, Milisavljevic S. Concurrent hyperfractionated radiotherapy and low-dose daily carboplatin/paclitaxel in patients with early-stage (I/II) non-small-cell lung cancer: long-term results of a phase II study. J Clin Oncol 2005;23:6873–80.

[52] Ji RR, Gereau RW, Malcangio M, Strichartz GR. MAP kinase and pain. Brain Res Rev 2009;60:135–48.

[53] Joseph EK, Levine JD. Comparison of oxaliplatin- and cisplatin-induced painful peripheral neuropathy in the rat. J Pain 2009;10:534–41.

[54] Kamei J, Tamura N, Saitoh A. Possible involvement of the spinal nitric oxide/cGMP pathway in vincristine-induced painful neuropathy in mice. Pain 2005;117:112–20.

[55] Kautio AL, Haanpaa M, Leminen A, Kalso E, Kautiainen H, Saarto T. Amitriptyline in the prevention of chemotherapy-induced neuropathic symptoms. Anticancer Res 2009;29:2601–6.

[56] Kautio AL, Haanpaa M, Saarto T, Kalso E. Amitriptyline in the treatment of chemotherapy-induced neuropathic symptoms. J Pain Symptom Manage 2008;35:31–9.

[57] Kawasaki Y, Zhang L, Cheng JK, Ji RR. Cytokine mechanisms of central sensitization: distinct and overlapping role of interleukin-1beta, interleukin-6, and tumor necrosis factor-alpha in regulating synaptic and neuronal activity in the superficial spinal cord. J Neurosci 2008;28:5189–94.

[58] Kemp G, Rose P, Lurain J, Berman M, Manetta A, Roullet B, Homesley H, Belpomme D, Glick J. Amifostine pretreatment for protection against cyclophosphamide-induced and cisplatin-induced toxicities: results of a randomized control trial in patients with advanced ovarian cancer. J Clin Oncol 1996;14:2101–12.

[59] Kiguchi N, Maeda T, Kobayashi Y, Kondo T, Ozaki M, Kishioka S. The critical role of invading peripheral macrophage-derived interleukin-6 in vincristine-induced mechanical allodynia in mice. Eur J Pharmacol 2008;592:87–92.

[60] Krarup-Hansen A, Fugleholm K, Helweg-Larsen S, Hauge EN, Schmalbruch H, Trojaborg W, Krarup C. Examination of distal involvement in cisplatin-induced neuropathy in man. An electrophysiological and histological study with particular reference to touch receptor function. Brain 1993;116:1017–41.

[61]  Krarup-Hansen A, Helweg-Larsen S, Schmalbruch H, Rorth M, Krarup C. Neuronal involvement in cisplatin neuropathy: prospective clinical and neurophysiological studies. Brain 2007;130:1076–88.

[62]  Lanzani F, Mattavelli L, Frigeni B, Rossini F, Cammarota S, Petro D, Jann S, Cavaletti G. Role of a pre-existing neuropathy on the course of bortezomib-induced peripheral neurotoxicity. J Peripher Nerv Syst 2008;13:267–74.

[63]  Lee JJ, Low JA, Croarkin E, Parks R, Berman AW, Mannan N, Steinberg SM, Swain SM. Changes in neurologic function tests may predict neurotoxicity caused by ixabepilone. J Clin Oncol 2006;24:2084–91.

[64]  Ling B, Authier N, Balayssac D, Eschalier A, Coudore F. Behavioral and pharmacological description of oxaliplatin-induced painful neuropathy in rat. Pain 2007;128:225–34.

[65]  Ling YH, Liebes L, Zou Y, Perez-Soler R. Reactive oxygen species generation and mitochondrial dysfunction in the apoptotic response to bortezomib, a novel proteasome inhibitor, in human H460 non-small cell lung cancer cells. J Biol Chem 2003;278:33714–23.

[66]  Loven D, Levavi H, Sabach G, Zart R, Andras M, Fishman A, Karmon Y, Levi T, Dabby R, Gadoth N. Long-term glutamate supplementation failed to protect against peripheral neurotoxicity of paclitaxel. Eur J Cancer Care (Engl) 2009;18:78–83.

[67]  Lynch JJ, III, Wade CL, Zhong CM, Mikusa JP, Honore P. Attenuation of mechanical allodynia by clinically utilized drugs in a rat chemotherapy-induced neuropathic pain model. Pain 2004;110:56–63.

[68]  Matsumoto M, Inoue M, Hald A, Xie W, Ueda H, Inhibition of paclitaxel-induced A-fiber hypersensitization by gabapentin. J Pharmacol Exp Ther 2006;318:735–40.

[69]  Mollman JE, Glover DJ, Hogan WM, Furman RE. Cisplatin neuropathy. Cancer 1988;61:2192–5.

[70]  Moore DH, Donnelly J, McGuire WP, Almadrones L, Cella DF, Herzog TJ, Waggoner ST. Limited access trial using amifostine for protection against cisplatin- and three-hour paclitaxel-induced neurotoxicity: a phase II study of the gynecologic oncology group. J Clin Oncol 2003;21:4207–13.

[71]  Nardone R, Buratti T, Golaszewski S, Bratti A, Caleri F, Tezzon F, Ladurner G, Mitterer M. Delayed oxaliplatin-induced sensorimotor polyneuropathy. Onkologie 2009;32:283–5.

[72]  Nurgalieva Z, Xia R, Liu CC, Burau K, Hardy D, Du XL, Risk of chemotherapy-induced peripheral neuropathy in large population-based cohorts of elderly patients with breast, ovarian, and lung cancer. Am J Ther 2009; Epub May 15.

[73]  Ogura K, Ohta S, Ohmori T, Takeuchi H, Hirose T, Horichi N, Okuda K, Ike M, Ozawa T, Siba K, et al. Vinca alkaloids induce granulocyte-macrophage colony stimulating factor in human peripheral blood mononuclear cells. Anticancer Res 2000;20:2383–8.

[74]  Paccagnella A, Favaretto A, Oniga F, Barbieri F, Ceresoli G, Torri W, Villa E, Verusio C, Cetto GL, Santo A, et al. Cisplatin versus carboplatin in combination with mitomycin and vinblastine in advanced non small cell lung cancer. A multicenter, randomized phase III trial. Lung Cancer 2004;43:83–91.

[75]  Persohn E, Canta A, Schoepfer S, Traebert M, Mueller L, Gilardini A, Galbiati S, Nicolini G, Scuteri A, Lanzani F, et al. Morphological and morphometric analysis of paclitaxel and docetaxel-induced peripheral neuropathy in rats. Eur J Cancer 2005;41:1460–6.

[76]  Pietrangeli A, Leandri M, Terzoli E, Jandolo B, Garufi C. Persistence of high-dose oxaliplatin-induced neuropathy at long-term follow-up. Eur Neurol 2006;56:13–6.

[77]  Pisano C, Pratesi G, Laccabue D, Zunino F, Lo Giudice P, Bellucci A, Pacifici L, Camerini B, Vesci L, Castorina M, et al. Paclitaxel and cisplatin-induced neurotoxicity: a protective role of acetyl-L-carnitine. Clin Cancer Res 2003;9:5756–67.

[78]  Polyzos A, Tsavaris N, Gogas H, Lagadas A, Polyzos K, Giannakopoulos K, Felekouras E, Tsigris C, Karatzas T, Papadopoulos O, Giannopoulos A. Cisplatin-ifosfamide-gemcitabine as salvage chemotherapy in ovarian cancer patients pretreated with platinum compounds and paclitaxel. Anticancer Res 2009;29:2681–6.

[79]  Porter CC, Carver AE, Albano EA. Vincristine induced peripheral neuropathy potentiated by voriconazole in a patient with previously undiagnosed CMT1X. Pediatr Blood Cancer 2009;52:298–300.

[80]  Postma TJ, Vermorken JB, Liefting AJM, Pinedo HM, Heimans JJ. Paclitaxel-induced neuropathy. Ann Oncol 1995;6:489–94.

[81]  Rahn EJ, Makriyannis A, Hohmann AG. Activation of cannabinoid CB1 and CB2 receptors suppresses neuropathic nociception evoked by the chemotherapeutic agent vincristine in rats. Br J Pharmacol 2007;152:765–77.

[82]  Rao RD, Michalak JC, Sloan JA, Loprinzi CL, Soori GS, Nikcevich DA, Warner DO, Novotny P, Kutteh LA, Wong GY. Efficacy of gabapentin in the management of chemotherapy-induced peripheral neuropathy: a phase 3 randomized, double-blind, placebo-controlled, crossover trial (N00C3). Cancer 2007;110:2110–8.

[83]  Reyes-Gibby CC, Morrow PK, Buzdar A, Shete S. Chemotherapy-induced peripheral neuropathy as a predictor of neuropathic pain in breast cancer patients previously treated with paclitaxel. J Pain 2009;10:1146–50.

[84]  Richardson P, Clinical update: proteosome inhibitors in hematologic malignancies. Cancer Treat Rev 2003;29:33–9.

[85]  Richardson PG, Briemberg H, Jagannath S, Wen PY, Barlogie B, Berenson J, Singhal S, Siegel DS, Irwin D, Schuster M, et al. Frequency, characteristics, and reversibility of peripheral neuropathy during treatment of advanced multiple myeloma with bortezomib. J Clin Oncol 2006;24:3113–20.

[86]  Rowinsky EK, Chaudhry V, Forastiere AA, Sartorius SE, Ettinger DS, Grochow LB, Lubejko BG, Cornblath DR, Donehower RC. Phase I and pharmacologic study of paclitaxel and cisplatin with granulocyte colony-stimulating factor: neuromuscular toxicity is dose-limiting. J Clin Oncol 1993;11:2010–20.

[87]  Rowinsky EK, Chaudry V, Cornblath DR, Donehower RC. Neurotoxicity of taxol. J Nat Cancer Inst Monogr 1993;15:107–15.

[88]  Roy V, LaPlant BR, Gross GG, Bane CL, Palmieri FM. Phase II trial of weekly nab (nanoparticle albumin-bound)-paclitaxel (nab-paclitaxel) (Abraxane) in combination with gemcitabine in patients with metastatic breast cancer (N0531). Ann Oncol 2009;20:449–53.

[89]  Saika F, Kiguchi N, Kobayashi Y, Fukazawa Y, Maeda T, Ozaki M, Kishioka S. Suppressive effect of imipramine on vincristine-induced mechanical allodynia in mice. Biol Pharm Bull 2009;32:1231–4.

[90]  Sarosy G, Stone DA, Rothenberg M, Jacob J, Adamo DO, Ognibene FP, Cunnion RE, Reed E. Phase I of taxol and granulocyte colony-stimulating factor in patients with refractory ovarian cancer. J Clin Oncol 1992;10:1165–70.

[91]  Schmidt J, Unger JW, Bartke I, Reiter R. Effect of nerve growth factor on peptide neurons in dorsal root ganglia after taxol or cisplatin treatment and in diabetic (db/db) mice. Exp Neurol 1995;132:16–23.

[92]  Scuteri A, Galimberti A, Maggioni D, Ravasi M, Pasini S, Nicolini G, Bossi M, Miloso M, Cavaletti G, Tredici G. Role of MAPKs in platinum-induced neuronal apoptosis. Neurotoxicology 2009;30:312–9.

[93]  Scuteri A, Nicolini G, Miloso M, Bossi M, Cavaletti G, Windebank AJ, Tredici G. Paclitaxel toxicity in post-mitotic dorsal root ganglion (DRG) cells. Anticancer Res 2006;26:1065–70.

[94]  Shy ME, Frohman EM, So YT, Arezzo JC, Cornblath DR, Giuliani JL, Kincaid JC, Ochoa JL, Parry GJ, Weimer LH. Quantitative sensory testing. Neurology 2003;60:898–904.

[95]  Stubblefield MD, Vahdat LT, Balmaceda CM, Troxel AB, Hesdorffer CS, Gooch CL. Glutamine as a neuroprotective agent in high-dose paclitaxel-induced peripheral neuropathy: a clinical and electrophysiologic study. Clin Oncol (R Coll Radiol) 2005;17:271–6.

[96]  Tanner KD, Reichling DB, Levine JD. Nociceptor hyper-responsiveness during vincristine-induced painful peripheral neuropathy in the rat. J Neurosci 1998;18:6480–91.

[97]  Thant M, Hawley RJ, Smith MT, Cohen MH, Minna JD, Bunn PA, Ihde DC, West W, Matthews MJ. Possible enhancement of vincristine neuropathy by VP-16. Cancer 1982;49:859–64.

[98]  Thibault K, Van Steenwinckel J, Brisorgueil MJ, Fischer J, Hamon M, Calvino B, Conrath M. Serotonin 5-HT2A receptor involvement and Fos expression at the spinal level in vincristine-induced neuropathy in the rat. Pain 2008;140:305–22.

[99]  Topp KS, Tanner KD, Levine JD. Damage to the cytoskeleton of large diameter sensory neurons and myelinated axons in vincristine-induced painful peripheral neuropathy in the rat. J Comp Neurol 2000;424:563–76.

[100] Tsavaris N, Kopterides P, Kosmas C, Efthymiou A, Skopelitis H, Dimitrakopoulos A, Pagouni E, Pikazis D, Zis PV, Koufos C. Gabapentin monotherapy for the treatment of chemotherapy-induced neuropathic pain: a pilot study. Pain Med 2008;9:1209–16.

[101] Vahdat L, Papadopoulos K, Lange D, Leuin S, Kaufman E, Donovan D, Frederick D, Bagiella E, Tiersten A, Nichols G, et al. Reduction of paclitaxel-induced peripheral neuropathy with glutamine. Clin Cancer Res 2001;7:1192–7.

[102] Valero V, Holmes FA, Walters RS, Theriault RL, Esparza L, Fraschini G, Fonseca GA, Bellet RE, Buzdar AU, Hortobagyi GN. Phase II trial of docetaxel: a new, highly effective antineoplastic agent in the management of patients with anthracycline-resistant metastatic breast cancer. J Clin Oncol 1995;13:2886–94.

[103] Verstappen CCP, Postma TJ, Hoekman K, Heimans JJ. Peripheral neuropathy due to therapy with paclitaxel, gemcitabine and cisplatin in patients with advanced ovarian cancer. J Neurooncol 2003;63:201–5.

[104] Vondracek P, Oslejskova H, Kepak T, Mazanek P, Sterba J, Rysava M, Gal P. Efficacy of pregabalin in neuropathic pain in paediatric oncological patients. Eur J Paediatr Neurol 2009;13:332–6.

[105] Wick A, Wick W, Hirrlinger J, Gerhardt E, Dringen R, Dichgans J, Weller M, Schulz B. Chemotherapy-induced cell death in primary cerebellar granule neurons but not in astrocytes: in vitro paradigm of differential neurotoxicity. J Neurochem 2004;91:1067–74.

[106] Wilson RH, Lehky T, Thomas RR, Quinn MG, Floeter MK, Grem JL. Acute oxaliplatin-induced peripheral nerve hyperexcitability. J Clin Oncol 2002;20:1767–74.

[107] Xiao W, Naso L, Bennett GJ, Experimental studies of potential analgesics for the treatment of chemotherapy-evoked painful peripheral neuropathies. Pain Med 2008;9:505–17.

[108] Xiao WH, Bennett GJ, Chemotherapy-evoked neuropathic pain: abnormal spontaneous discharge in A-fiber and C-fiber primary afferent neurons and its suppression by acetyl-L-carnitine. Pain 2008;135:262–70.

[109] Yalcin S, Kilickap S, Temucin CM, Erman M. Recombinant human erythropoietin in comparison to amifostine against cisplatin-induced peripheral sensorial neurotoxicity in rats. J Exp Clin Cancer Res 2006;25:523–7.

[110] Yardley DA. Proactive management of adverse events maintains the clinical benefit of ixabepilone. Oncologist 2009;14:448–55.

*Correspondence to:* Patrick M. Dougherty, PhD, Department of Anesthesia and Pain Medicine, The University of Texas M.D. Anderson Cancer Center, 1400 Holcombe Boulevard, Houston, TX 77030, USA. Tel: 1-713-745-0438; fax: 1-713-792-7591; email: pdougherty@mdanderson.org.

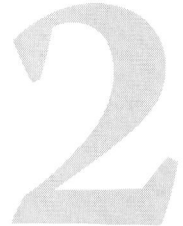

# Mechanisms of Radiotherapy-Induced Pain Relief

Yvette M. van der Linden

*Radiotherapeutic Institute Friesland, Leeuwarden, The Netherlands*

Radiotherapy is an important treatment modality that is often used in the treatment of patients with various types of primary cancers. About half of all cancer patients receive some form of radiotherapy during their illness. Radiotherapy can be applied either curatively (with the intention of curing the patient by destroying the cancer) or palliatively (to treat complaints such as pain due to the primary tumor, local/regional recurrence, or metastatic disease) in patients in whom a cure is no longer possible. Radiotherapy can be applied as the sole treatment, but it is also often included as part of an extended treatment protocol using different treatment modalities either sequentially or concomitantly. The choice of treatment and the intention with which it is started in each patient will depend on interacting factors such as the type, location, and stage of the tumor, as well as the condition, comorbidities, and life expectancy of the patient. Optimally, a multidisciplinary team of health care professionals will decide on the course of treatment for each patient individually. Evidence-based treatment protocols are essential tools to help in the decision-making process.

*Cancer Pain: From Molecules to Suffering*
edited by Judith A. Paice, Rae F. Bell, Eija A. Kalso, and Olaitan A. Soyannwo
IASP Press, Seattle, © 2010

27

Over time, the treatment of a given patient may change from curative to palliative. For both curative and palliative purposes, patients may be
treated with a mixture of options, which may include surgery, radiotherapy, and chemotherapy. The rationale behind the use of combined protocols is to achieve equal treatment outcome with fewer side effects, to spare
vital organs, to gain higher rates of clinically relevant responses, and/or
to improve survival. For example, neoadjuvant chemoradiotherapy for
locally advanced rectal tumors may reduce the size of the tumors and facilitate radical surgery. Postoperative radiotherapy after breast-conserv-
ing surgery diminishes the occurrence of a local/regional recurrence. In
locally advanced laryngeal tumors, chemoradiotherapy may provide a
cure and spare the patient a debilitating laryngectomy with permanent
loss of normal speech.

When primarily focusing on the complaint pain in patients that
is caused by a primary tumor, by a local/regional recurrence, or by metastatic cancer, radiotherapy is an effective noninvasive treatment modality
for pain. This chapter first describes the technical, biological, and practical
aspects of radiotherapy and then discusses the mechanisms of radiotherapy-induced pain relief and its effectiveness in patients with various types
of cancer.

# Mechanisms of Radiotherapy

## Technical Aspects

Two types of radiotherapy are distinguished: external beam radiotherapy (EBRT) and brachytherapy. For EBRT, radiotherapy departments
worldwide mostly use modern linear accelerators (LINAC units) that
instantly generate ionizing radiation to treat their patients (Fig. 1).
LINAC units have replaced the old-fashioned Cobalt machines because
they are more reliable, more accurate, and, importantly, they produce
no nuclear waste. In addition, when shut down at the end of the day,
LINAC units no longer emit radiation, and thus they require fewer special security procedures and less heavy shielding of rooms and buildings
to prevent leakage.

The gantry of a LINAC is capable of rotating 360° around the patient, and the collimator (the head of the gantry) can rotate 360° as well.

Thus, virtually all field sizes and contours are possible using multi-leaf collimators that shape the beams (Fig. 1). LINAC units produce beams of highly energetic photons or electrons that can be focused toward the patient. These beams can penetrate deeply into the patient's body to allow the cancerous tissue to absorb their energy.

In brachytherapy, for a calculated time period a radioactive source is placed within the body very close to the tumor. In cervical or esophageal cancer, this endoluminal treatment irradiates the tumor with a very localized high dose without exposing the surrounding normal tissues to excessive radiation. In localized prostate cancer, permanent radioactive seeds are implanted to destroy the tumor.

## Biological Aspects

Photon or electron beams cause damage in both healthy and malignant cells at a cellular level by creating single- or double-strand breakages in the DNA. Because malignant cells have a diminished ability to repair these breakages, tumors are much more vulnerable to ionizing radiation than most healthy tissues. Non-repair in tumor cells leads to cumulative cell death and eventually reduction and possibly total eradication of the tumor.

The tolerance of the surrounding healthy tissue to ionizing radiation is often the dose-limiting factor in radiotherapy. Consequently, the total dose in Gray (Gy) is divided into smaller daily portions (fractions) to allow for repair of the normal cells. The use of fractionation diminishes long-term side effects (e.g., fibrosis, edema, and vascular sclerosis) as much as possible. In curative radiotherapy, doses range from 20 Gy in 10 fractions in radiosensitive tumors (lymphoma, testicular seminoma) to 60–78 Gy in 30–39 fractions in lung cancer or prostate cancer. In palliative radiotherapy, patients often have a limited life expectancy or a deteriorating condition. Therefore, the goal of treatment is to achieve a substantial palliative effect in as short a time as possible. Usually, single doses or short courses of treatment are given (8 Gy in a single fraction, or 20 Gy in 5 fractions). Acute side effects of radiotherapy depend on the localization of the treatment and may include a skin rash, mucosal damage, nausea, diarrhea, and loss of hair. Most acute side effects are mild and are self-limiting within a few weeks.

a

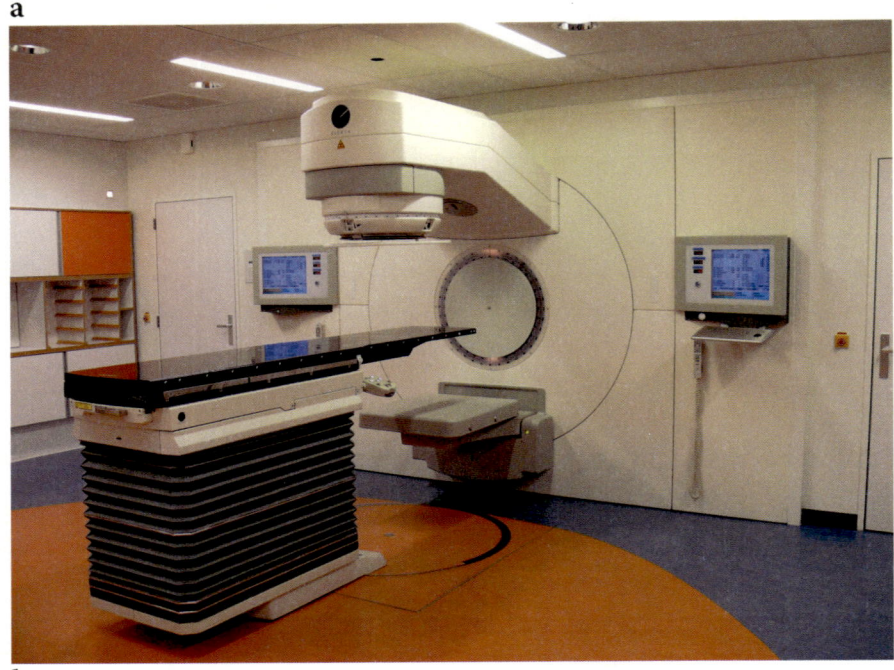

b

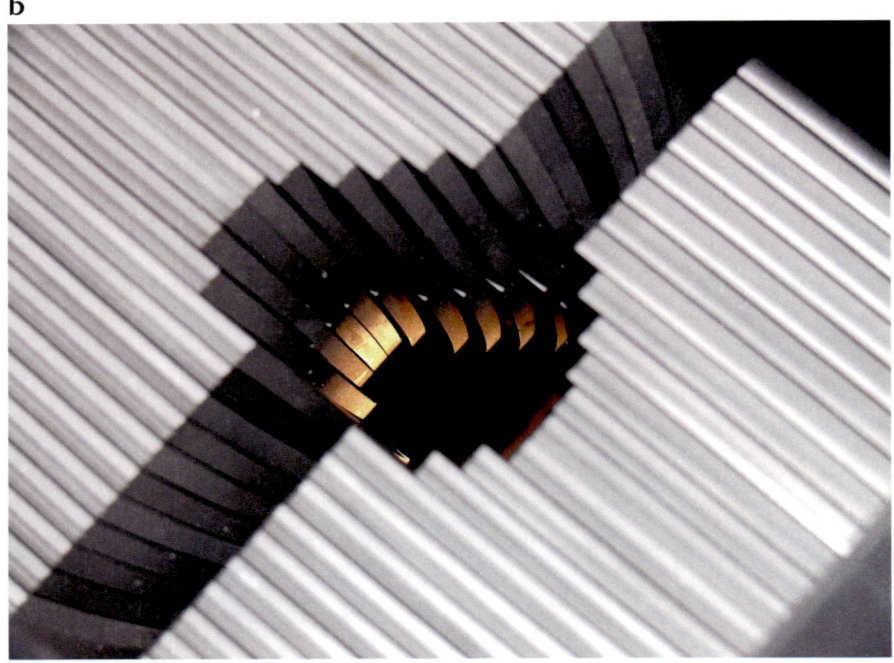

c

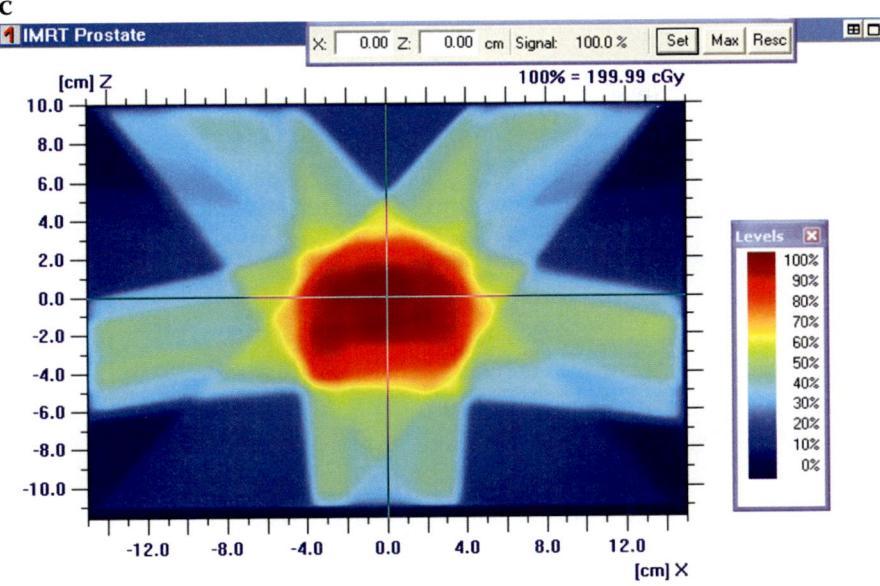

**Fig. 1.** Radiotherapy treatment at the Radiotherapeutic Institute Friesland, Leeuwarden, The Netherlands. (a) Linear accelerator with a gantry arm that can rotate 360°. (b) The multileaf collimator is shaped to form a radiation beam for an intensity-modulated radiotherapy (IMRT) five-field treatment of prostate cancer. (c) Dose distribution for an IMRT five-field treatment of prostate cancer.

## Simulation and Dose-Planning Aspects

Before a radiotherapy treatment can start, the patient must see the radiation oncologist to discuss the treatment plan, the possible acute and long-term side effects of treatment, and the expected treatment outcome. A simulation procedure is then performed using a special X-ray machine or a computed tomography (CT) scan in the treatment position in order to simulate the actual treatment. The individual treatment planning volume is created on the computer using additional information from diagnostic imaging studies such as bone scintigraphy, magnetic resonance imaging (MRI), and/or positron emission tomography (PET) and CT scans. Around the treatment target, a certain margin is usually included to allow for uncertainties in daily set-up and tumor or organ motion. Planning may take about 10–15 minutes for relatively simple single-field or two opposing field techniques for mostly palliative indications in which sparing of healthy organs is of less importance, such as palliative treatment of bone metastases or bulky mediastinal lymph nodes in advanced non-small-cell lung cancer (Fig. 2a,b). More sophisticated planning of treatment such as intensity-modulated radiotherapy (IMRT) or high-dose stereotactic radiotherapy may take several hours or days. Examples are curative treatment of a prostate cancer or palliative treatment of a single brain metastasis (Fig. 2c,d).

When several beams are delivered from various angles, the highest dose is delivered to the target tissues, and normal surrounding tissues are spared as much as possible to diminish acute and chronic side effects. After a number of quality assurance checks of the treatment plans, the patient may then start LINAC treatment. Depending on the number of fractions that are to be applied, patients visit the radiotherapy department daily on an outpatient basis, with the actual treatment time ranging from a few minutes for simple techniques, to 10 minutes for IMRT, and up to 45 minutes for stereotactic radiotherapy. With online portal imaging techniques and patient set-up correction protocols, the stability of both the patient and the volume of target tissues are closely monitored, and, if necessary, daily adjustments are made in order to irradiate as precisely as possible (Fig. 3). Examples of target tissues that can change in volume or position are lung cancers, which can move during inhalation and exhalation, or the prostate in prostate cancer, which can move depending on the filling of the bladder or rectum.

# Mechanisms of Radiotherapy-Induced Pain Relief

Primary tumors, local/regional recurrences, and distant metastases may cause pain, either directly when the expanding tumor infiltrates into the surrounding tissues, or indirectly when it compresses the surrounding tissues or nerves (Table I). If a growing tumor blocks adjacent blood vessels or lymph nodes, accumulation of blood flow or lymphatic flow may occur, causing thrombosis or edema. If bowel movements are distorted, pain and progressive constipation may occur. The pain-relieving effect of an anticancer treatment, whether it consists of radiotherapy alone or combined with other treatment modalities, is due to the reduction of infiltration or pressure caused by shrinkage of the tumor (Table II). In addition, surrounding edema may resolve, and inflammatory cells, such as chemical

Table I
Possible causes of pain in patients with primary or metastatic cancer

| Site | Pathophysiology | Type of Pain |
|------|-----------------|--------------|
| *Primary Tumors* | | |
| Brain | Compression of intracranial cavities, causing increased intracranial pressure | Headache |
| | Adjacent reactive edema | Headache |
| Breast | Skin infiltration, lymph node involvement | Swelling, pain |
| Lung | Pleural infiltration, growth into adjacent ribs | Local pain, visceral pain, bone pain |
| Cervix | Compression of urinary tract, rectum | No spontaneous emptying of bladder; constipation |
| Head and neck | Infiltration of mucosa, cartilage, muscle | Pain with speech or swallowing |
| Esophagus | Narrowing of lumen | Pain with swallowing or vomiting |
| Colorectal | Narrowing of lumen, bowel adhesions | Bowel pain, cramping, constipation |
| Kidney | Capsular involvement | Abdominal pain or back pain |
| *Metastases* | | |
| Brain | Compression of intracranial cavities, causing increased intracranial pressure | Headache |
| | Adjacent reactive edema | Headache |
| Skin | Infiltration | Pain |
| Liver | Enlargement | Pain |
| Bone | Stretching of periosteum, microfractures, surrounding edema | Local pain, pathological fracturing |
| | Infiltration or compression of spinal cord or cauda equina | Pain, motor and/or sensory weakness, paraplegia |
| | Infiltration or compression of peripheral nerves | Neuropathic pain |
| Lymph nodes | Obstruction or infiltration | Peripheral edema |
| Blood vessels | Obstruction or infiltration, causing thrombosis | Peripheral edema |

pain mediators and prostaglandins, will diminish. This process may take several weeks to months to occur, mostly with some degree of permanent fibrosis (scarring).

In patients with bone metastases, the initial pain response may take place several hours after the treatment, sooner than would be expected due to tumor shrinkage alone (Table II). It is thought that a fast response to pain in bone metastases is caused by a rapid drop in chemical pain mediators [40].

**a**

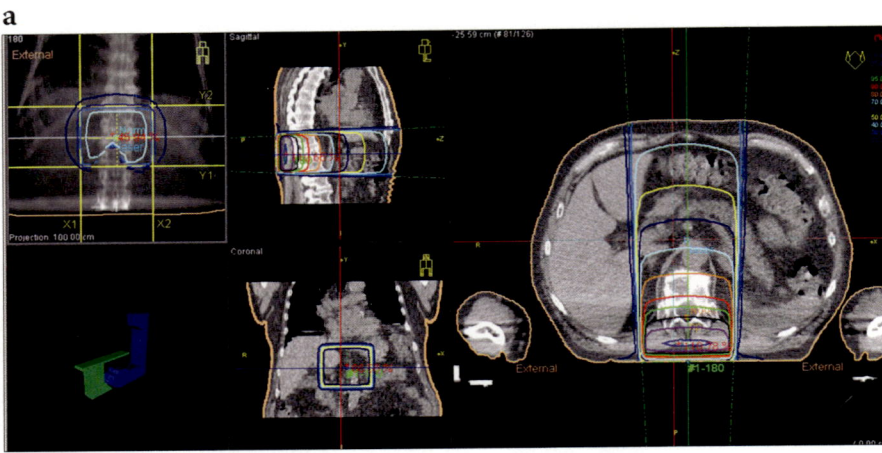

**b**

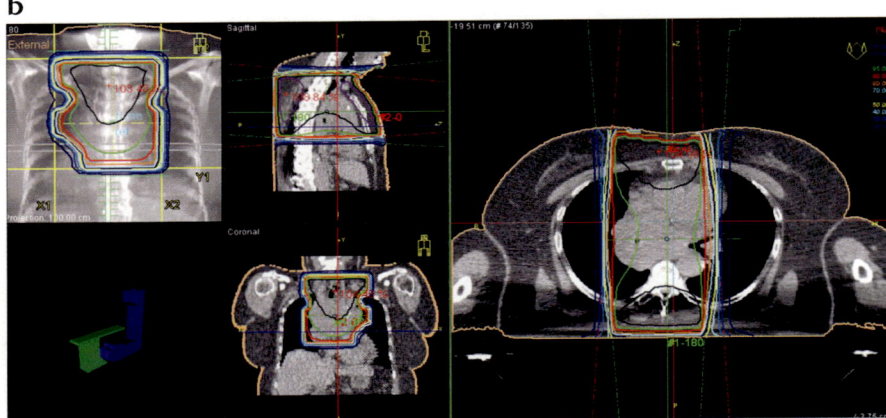

***Fig. 2.*** Examples of radiotherapy treatment planning at the Radiotherapeutic Institute Friesland. (a) Bone metastasis in the spinal column, treated with a single posterior photon beam, with a dose schedule of 8 Gy in a single fraction. Orange line isodose = 80% of the prescribed dose. (b) Mediastinal lymph node metastases of a non-small-cell lung cancer, treated with two opposed fields, with a dose schedule of 30 Gy in 10 fractions. Green line isodose indicates 95% of the prescribed dose. (c) Prostate cancer, treated with an intensity-modulated radiotherapy (IMRT) technique using five non-collinear beams, with a dose schedule of 78 Gy in 39 fractions. (d) Single brain metastasis, treated with highly conformal (or best fit) stereotactic radiotherapy consisting of 14 beams, with a dose schedule of 20 Gy in one fraction.

c

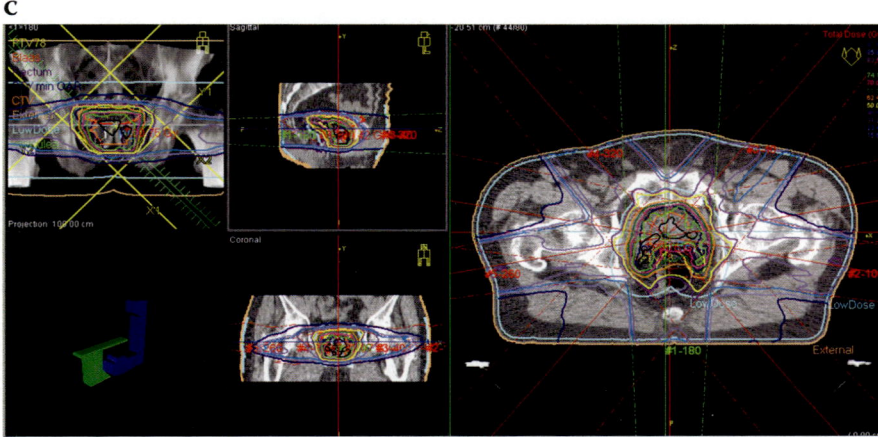

d

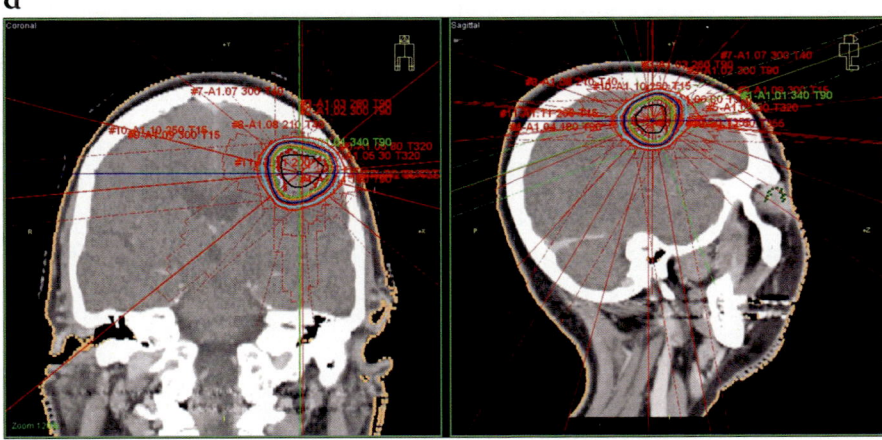

# Evidence-Based Effectiveness of Radiotherapy for Pain

## Primary Tumor or Local/Regional Recurrence

In the treatment of painful primary cancers or local/regional recurrences, radiotherapy can be effective in reducing pain. The literature includes a large number of studies on the effectiveness of radiotherapy in esophageal cancer [16,17,51], non-small-cell lung cancer [10,22,24,38], rectal cancer [9,50], pancreatic cancer [9], and cancers of the head and neck [1,8,27].

a

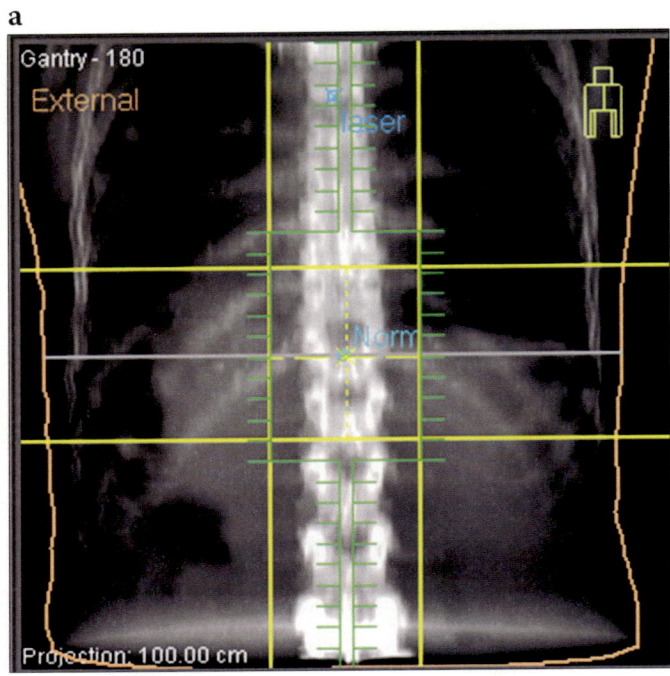

b

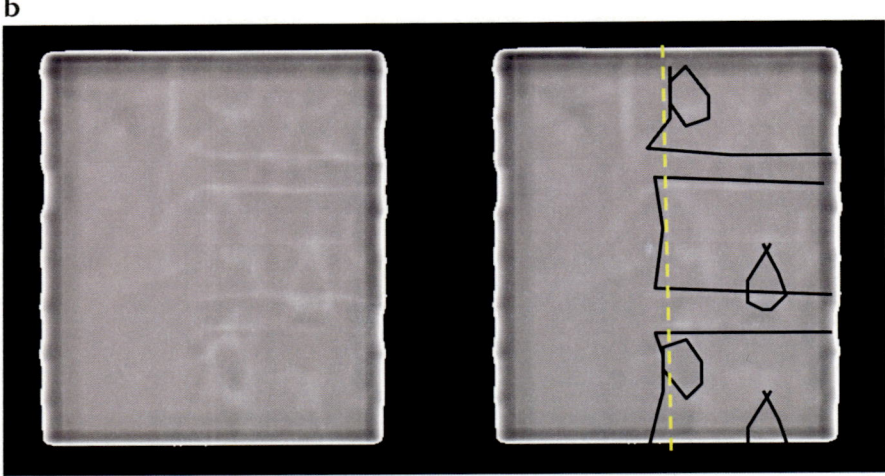

**Fig. 3.** Online portal imaging of radiation delivery in a patient with painful spinal me-tastases who was treated with 20 Gy in five fractions. (a) Planned treatment field using a computed tomography simulator. (b) Delivery of the first fraction of treatment; due to severe pain, the patient could not remain immobile. A lateral shift of 2 cm is visible. The isocenter was shifted and checked again, and the patient was irradiated.

Table II
Possible mechanisms of radiotherapy-induced pain relief
for pain caused by bone metastases

| Pain Caused by Bone Metastases: Relatively Rapid Response* | | | Pain Caused by Other Metastases: Relatively Delayed Response** | | |
|---|---|---|---|---|---|
| 1 | Inflammatory cells | ↓↓↓ | 1 | Tumor cell destruction | ↓↓↓↓ |
| | Chemical pain mediators (prostaglandins) | ↓↓↓ | 2 | Inflammatory cells | ↓↓↓ |
| | Edema | ↓↓ | | Chemical pain mediators (prostaglandins) | ↓↓ |
| 2 | Tumor cell destruction | ↓ | | Edema | ↓↓ |

* Rapid onset of pain relief, within hours to days after radiotherapy is applied;
median time to response is about 3–4 weeks [52].
** Delayed onset of pain relief, within days to weeks after radiotherapy is applied.

In these studies, pain was reported as a primary or secondary outcome measure. Randomized or large retrospective trials on other primary tumors are lacking, but clinical experience shows good results from radiotherapy for treatment of pain in patients with other types of cancer, including painful, ulcerating, infectious, or bleeding tumors with skin infiltration, such as malignant lymphomas or locally advanced breast cancer. After radiotherapy, shrinkage of such tumors also causes re-epithelization and hence cleaner wounds. Other examples are painful, bleeding cancers of the stomach, gynecological cancers, bladder cancer, and anal cancer, which may well respond to radiotherapy.

## Metastases

### Bone Metastases

About 20–50% of patients with cancer will experience bone metastases at some time during their illness. A single fraction of 8 Gy is considered to be the standard radiotherapy schedule for patients with uncomplicated bone pain, that is for bone lesions without neurological complaints and without a high risk of pathological fracture [3,13,49,52]. Three to four weeks after treatment, 65–72% of patients will respond. In patients with longer survival (>1 year), 80% will benefit from single-dose radiotherapy [47]. Optimally, the intake, simulation procedure, and treatment will take place on the same day. This "one-stop treatment" is optimal for patients with a deteriorating condition and a limited life expectancy (a median of 7 months)

[46]. Most side effects that are reported by patients are self-limiting, such as pain flare or nausea. If pain recurs after an initial response or if it does not respond at all, a second treatment can be applied, with a response rate of 46–83% [20,26,46,48]. An ongoing randomized, controlled international trial is studying the effectiveness of retreatment [5]. There is no evidence that more prolonged radiotherapy schedules with higher total doses (20 Gy in 5 fractions, or 30 Gy in 10 fractions) lead to higher response rates or a longer duration of response [49]. Even in patients with neuropathic pain, a single dose was as effective as 20 Gy in 5 fractions, with a response in 53–61% of 272 randomized patients [34]. Some patients (24–44%) may experience a pain flare shortly after single-dose or short-schedule radiotherapy [14,23]. Retrospective studies have shown that oral dexamethasone may prevent such a flare [6,15]. Two dose-finding randomized trials are currently investigating the role of dexamethasone.

Despite numerous publications on the effectiveness of the single-fraction regimen, its convenience for patients, its cost-effectiveness and advantages regarding sparing of resources [42,52], higher doses are still being favored by many radiation oncologists worldwide [11,35]. Some reasons for not adapting are previous education, the influence of reimbursement, and unfamiliarity with large fraction sizes. Continuous efforts should be focused on the education of health care professionals and the implementation of the single-dose schedule for pain.

Higher total doses are probably more effective than single-fraction radiotherapy in extensive osteolytic metastases, in lesions with concomitant swelling of adjacent soft tissues, or in large lesions with an increased risk of pathological fracturing. A higher total dose reduces the tumor load and also induces remineralization and thus may strengthen the bone [21,45]. In high-risk patients with femoral metastases, prophylactic surgery should always be considered to prevent the occurrence of a pathological fracture, which can be very distressing and can cause considerable morbidity. Prediction of pathological fracturing is difficult, however, and overestimation of risk may lead to unnecessary prophylactic surgical stabilizations [43]. An ongoing study on fracture risk prediction is investigating the use of finite-element computer modeling in patients with femoral lesions [36].

In patients with pain and neurological complaints due to compression of the spinal cord or adjacent nerves, prompt intervention with surgery and/or radiotherapy is necessary to prevent worsening of symptoms. The majority of patients presenting with neurological complaints are not surgical candidates due to their deteriorating condition, comorbidity, and short life expectancy, and they are well palliated with noninvasive radiotherapy [30]. The duration of the neurological complaints predicts the chance of full or partial recovery after radiotherapy, with a slow onset of symptoms being favorable [33]. Overall, patients with a relatively poor prognosis are treated with single or short schedules [25,32]. Patients with relatively radiosensitive tumors, such as breast cancer or myeloma, probably will not benefit more from higher total doses [31]. In patients with an expected survival of more than 1 year, however, higher total doses will prevent a recurrence of spinal cord compression [30]. A recent randomized trial in 101 patients with spinal cord compression studied surgery plus radiotherapy versus radiotherapy alone and showed a significant improvement in mobility for the combined treatment [28]. There is still debate about these results, however, because these patients were a highly selected group [41]. Ideally, more studies should be performed with the same research questions. There is general consensus on operating on unstable spinal vertebrae prior to radiotherapy in operable patients who are in relatively good condition.

### Brain Metastases

Metastases to the brain occur more frequently, probably due to increased life expectancy, in patients with improved systemic therapies such as chemotherapy, hormonal therapy, and immunotherapy. Depending on the number and localization of the metastases, the patient may suffer from headaches, epilepsy, loss of vision, neurological deficits including peripheral paresis, and changes in personality. The psychological impact of having metastases to the brain is high and should not be underestimated. Depending on the severity of symptoms, patients may start with steroids such as dexamethasone to treat the edema, and/or anticonvulsants. Without treatment, median survival is short, only 1–2 months. Short-schedule whole-brain radiotherapy, usually 20 Gy in 5 fractions, reduces symptoms and improves survival to a median of 6–7 months; an important side effect is reversible hair loss [39]. In patients with up to three small brain metastases, highly conformal single-dose stereotactic radiotherapy diminishes hair loss and may lead to long-term remission (see Fig. 2d) [2]. The exact role or sequence of whole-brain radiotherapy, stereotactic treatment, or surgery in the treatment of one or more brain metastases is still being explored in ongoing studies.

### Lymph Node Metastases

If lymph node enlargement in the upper abdomen or pelvis leads to blocked lymphatic flow, patients may experience peripheral edema in both legs, along with a higher chance of vascular thrombosis. Pain can also be a major complaint, and sometimes back pain can be the only indication of growing lymph node metastases. Palliative radiotherapy (20–30 Gy in 5–10 fractions) early on may be effective, however, if radiotherapy is still possible, depending on whether radiation treatment was used earlier in the curative phase. If large parts of the bowel are within the radiation treatment fields, patients should be warned about possible nausea, diarrhea, and bowel pain, and prophylactic medication should be provided. In addition, manual pressure therapy and elastic stockings may help these patients to walk around without too much difficulty.

## Life Expectancy

Patients, their relatives, and their radiation oncologists should always balance the expected benefit of a treatment versus the time spent in the hospital and the expected duration and severity of the side effects. In palliative patients, radiotherapy schedules should preferably be as short as possible, with maximum effectiveness and minimum side effects. Prediction of life expectancy remains a difficult but necessary task to enable the optimal choice of treatment for individual patients [4,29,44].

# International Consensus Meetings

In 2009 and 2010, at the annual meetings of the American Society for Radiation Therapy and Oncology (ASTRO), an international consensus group of experts gave an update on palliative radiotherapy and formulated goals for research for the near future. At earlier meetings in 1990 and 2000, consensus statements were published to inform all health care professionals in palliative medicine on ongoing issues in palliative radiotherapy [7,12,18,19,37]. Such international consensus meetings are extremely valuable in helping to focus attention toward optimizing palliative radiotherapy.

# Conclusions

Radiotherapy is an effective and noninvasive treatment modality for patients with pain caused by the primary tumor or by metastatic disease. Optimally, all patients with cancer should be advised and treated by a multidisciplinary team of health care professionals, including radiation oncologists. Awareness should be focused on the education of all health care professionals on the numerous possibilities of pain treatment in patients with cancer, using evidence-based treatment guidelines.

More research is needed in order to treat the complaints of cancer patients as a whole, focusing not only on alleviating pain, but also on improving quality of life. Topics for future research are: (1) Optimization of pain management through a combination of therapies: systemic anti-cancer therapies, surgery, analgesic medication, and steroid medication. (2) Education of patients and their relatives to increase their knowledge about pain and teach self-management skills. (3) Adequate prediction of life expectancy to choose the best palliative treatments. (4) Psychological distress studies, focusing on identifying patients at risk of psychological distress early on in their disease process and on ways to treat psychological distress. (5) Cost-effectiveness analyses of the use of conformal techniques (IMRT and stereotactic radiotherapy) for metastatic disease.

# References

[1]    Allal A, Nicoucar K, Mach N. Quality of life in patients with oropharynx carcinomas: assessment after accelerated radiotherapy with or without chemotherapy versus radical surgery and postoperative radiotherapy. Head Neck 2003;25:833–9.
[2]    Aoyama H, Shirato H, Tago M, Nakagawa K, Toyoda T, Hatano K, Kenjyo M, Oya N, Hirota S, Shioura H, et al. Stereotactic radiosurgery plus whole-brain radiation therapy vs. stereotactic radiosurgery alone for treatment of brain metastases: a randomized controlled trial. JAMA 2006;295:2483–91.
[3]    Chow E, Harris K, Fan G, Tsao M, Sze WM. Palliative radiotherapy trials for bone metastases: a systematic review. J Clin Oncol 2007;25:1423–36.
[4]    Chow E, Harth T, Hruby G, Finkelstein J, Wu J, Danjoux C. How accurate are physicians' clinical predictions of survival and the available prognostic tools in estimating survival times in terminally ill cancer patients? A systematic review. J Clin Oncol (R Coll Radiol) 2001;13:209–18.

[5]  Chow E, Hoskin PJ, Wu J, Roos DE, van der Linden YM. A phase III international randomised trial comparing single with multiple fractions for re-irradiation of painful bone metastases: National Cancer Institute of Canada Clinical Trials Group (NCIC CTG) SC 20. J Clin Oncol 2006;18:125–8.

[6]  Chow E, Loblaw A, Harris K, Doyle M, Goh P, Chiu H, Panzarella T, Tsao M, Barnes EA, Sinclair E, et al. Dexamethasone for the prophylaxis of radiation-induced pain flare after palliative radiotherapy for bone metastases: a pilot study. Support Care Cancer 2007;15:643–7.

[7]  Chow E, Wu J, Hoskin P, Coia L, Bentzen S, Blitzer P. International consensus on palliative radiotherapy endpoints for future clinical trials in bone metastases. Radiother Oncol 2002;64:275–80.

[8]  Corry J, Peters LJ, Costa ID. The 'QUAD SHOT': a phase II study of palliative radiotherapy for incurable head and neck cancer. Radiother Oncol 2005;77:137–42.

[9]  Crane CH, Willett CG. Stereotactic radiotherapy for pancreatic cancer? Cancer 2009;115:468–72.

[10] Erridge S, Gaze M, Price A. Symptom control and quality of life in people with lung cancer: a randomised trial of two palliative radiotherapy fractionation schedules. J Clin Oncol (R Coll Radiol) 2005;17:61–7.

[11] Fairchild A, Barnes E, Ghosh S, Ben-Josef E, Roos D, Hartsell W, Holt T, Wu J, Janjan N, Chow E. International patterns of practice in palliative radiotherapy for painful bone metastases: evidence-based practice? Int J Radiat Oncol Biol Phys 2009;75:1501–10.

[12] Hanks GE, Maher EJ, Coia L. An overview of the First International Consensus Workshop on Radiation Therapy in the Treatment of Metastatic and Locally Advanced Cancer. Int J Radiat Oncol Biol Phys 1992;23:201.

[13] Hartsell WF, Scott CB, Bruner DW. Randomized trial of short- versus long-course radiotherapy for palliation of painful bone metastases. J Natl Cancer Inst 2005;97:798–804.

[14] Hird A, Chow E, Zhang L, Wong R, Wu J, Sinclair E, Danjoux C, Tsao M, Barnes E, Loblaw A. Determining the incidence of pain flare following palliative radiotherapy for symptomatic bone metastases: results from three Canadian cancer centers. Int J Radiat Oncol Biol Phys 2009;75:193–7.

[15] Hird A, Zhang L, Holt T, Fairchild A, DeAngelis C, Loblaw A, Wong R, Barnes E, Tsao M, Danjoux C, Chow E. Dexamethasone for the prophylaxis of radiation-induced pain flare after palliative radiotherapy for symptomatic bone metastases: a phase II study. J Clin Oncol (R Coll Radiol) 2009;21:329–35.

[16] Homs M, Essink-Bot M, Borsboom GJ. Quality of life after palliative treatment for oesophageal cancer: a prospective comparison between stent placement and single dose brachytherapy. Eur J Cancer 2004;40:1862–71.

[17] Homs M, Steyerberg EW, Eijkenboom WM. Single-dose brachytherapy versus metal stent placement for the palliation of dysphagia from oesophageal cancer. Lancet 2004;364:1497–504.

[18] Hoskin PJ, Brada M. Radiotherapy for brain metastases. J Clin Oncol (R Coll Radiol) 2001;13:91–4.

[19] Hoskin PJ, Yarnold JR, Roos DR, Bentzen S. Radiotherapy for bone metastases. J Clin Oncol (R Coll Radiol) 2001;13:88–90.

[20] Jeremic B, Shibamoto Y, Igrutinovic I. Single 4 Gy re-irradiation for painful bone metastasis following single fraction radiotherapy. Radiother Oncol 1999;52:123–7.

[21] Koswig S, Buchali A, Bohmer D, Schlenger L, Budach V. [Palliative radiotherapy of bone metastases. A retrospective analysis of 176 patients]. Strahlenther Onkol 1999;175:509–14.

[22] Kramer GW, Wanders SL, Noordijk EM. Results of the Dutch national study of the palliative effect of irradiation using two different treatment schemes for non–small-cell lung cancer. J Clin Oncol 2005;22:2962–70.

[23] Loblaw DA, Wu JS, Kirkbride P, Panzarella T, Smith K, Aslanidis J, Warde P. Pain flare in patients with bone metastases after palliative radiotherapy—a nested randomized control trial. Support Care Cancer 2007;15:451–5.

[24] Macbeth F, Toy E, Coles B. Palliative radiotherapy regimens for non-small cell lung cancer. Cochrane Database Syst Rev 2001;CD002143.

[25] Maranzano E, Trippa F, Casale M, Costantini S, Lupattelli M, Bellavita R, Marafioti L, Pergolizzi S, Santacaterina A, Mignogna M, et al. 8-Gy single-dose radiotherapy is effective in metastatic spinal cord compression: results of a phase III randomized multicentre Italian trial. Radiother Oncol 2009;93:174–9.

[26] Mithal NP, Needham PR, Hoskin PJ. Retreatment with radiotherapy for painful bone metastases. Int J Radiat Oncol Biol Phys 1994;29:1011–4.

[27] Mohanti BK, Umapathy H, Bahadur S. Short course palliative radiotherapy of 20 Gy in 5 fractions for advanced and incurable head and neck cancer: AIIMS study. Radiother Oncol 2004;71:275–80.

[28] Patchell R, Tibbs PA, Regine WF, Payne R. Direct decompressive surgical resection in the treatment of spinal cord compression caused by metastatic cancer: a randomised trial. Lancet 2005;366:643–8.

[29] Rades D, Dunst J, Schild S. The first score predicting overall survival in patients with metastatic spinal cord compression. Cancer 2008;112:157–61.

[30] Rades D, Lange M, Veninga T, Rudat V, Bajrovic A, Stalpers LJ, Dunst J, Schild SE. Preliminary results of spinal cord compression recurrence evaluation (score-1) study comparing short-course versus long-course radiotherapy for local control of malignant epidural spinal cord compression. Int J Radiat Oncol Biol Phys 2009;73:228–34.

[31] Rades D, Rudat V, Veninga T, Stalpers LJ, Basic H, Karstens JH, Hoskin PJ, Schild SE. A score predicting posttreatment ambulatory status in patients irradiated for metastatic spinal cord compression. Int J Radiat Oncol Biol Phys 2008;72:905–8.

[32] Rades D, Stalpers L, Veninga T. Evaluation of five radiation schedules and prognostic factors for metastatic spinal cord compression in a series of 1304 patients. J Clin Oncol 2005;23:3366–75.

[33] Rades D, Heidenreich F, Karstens JH. Final results of a prospective study of the prognostic value of the time to develop motor deficits before irradiation in metastatic spinal cord compression. Int J Radiat Oncol Biol Phys 2002;53:975–9.

[34] Roos DE, Turner SL, O'Brien PC, Smith JG, Spry NA, Burmeister BH, Hoskin PJ, Ball DL. Randomized trial of 8 Gy in 1 versus 20 Gy in 5 fractions of radiotherapy for neuropathic pain due to bone metastases (Trans-Tasman Radiation Oncology Group, TROG 96.05). Radiother Oncol 2005;75:54–63.

[35] Szumacher E, Llewellyn-Thomas H, Franssen E, Chow E, DeBoer G, Danjoux C, Hayter C, Barnes E, Andersson L. Treatment of bone metastases with palliative radiotherapy: patients' treatment preferences. Int J Radiat Oncol Biol Phys 2004;61:1473–81.

[36] Tanck E, van Aken JB, van der Linden YM, Schreuder HW, Binkowski M, Huizenga H, Verdonschot N. Pathological fracture prediction in patients with metastatic lesions can be improved with quantitative computed tomography based computer models. Bone 2009;45:777–83.

[37] Timothy AR, Girling DJ, Saunders MI, Macbeth F, Hoskin PJ. Radiotherapy for inoperable lung cancer. Clin Oncol (R Coll Radiol) 2001;13:86–7.

[38] Toy E, Macbeth F, Coles B. Palliative thoracic radiotherapy for non-small cell lung cancer: a systematic review. Am J Clin Oncol 2003;26:112–20.

[39] Tsao MN, Lloyd N, Wong R, Chow E, Rakovitch E, Laperriere N. Whole brain radiotherapy for the treatment of multiple brain metastases. Cochrane Database Syst Rev 2006;3:CD003869.

[40] Vakaet LA, Boterberg T. Pain control by ionizing radiation of bone metastasis. Int J Dev Biol 2004;48:599–606.

[41] van den Bent MJ. Comment on: Surgical resection improves outcome in metastatic epidural spinal cord compression. Patchell et al., Lancet 2005;366:643–648. Lancet 2005;366:609–10.

[42] van den Hout WB, van der Linden YM, Steenland E, Wiggenraad RG, Kievit J, de Haes H, Leer JW. Single- versus multiple-fraction radiotherapy in patients with painful bone metastases: cost-utility analysis based on a randomized trial. J Natl Cancer Inst 2003;95:222–9.

[43] van der Linden YM, Dijkstra PD, Kroon HM, Lok JJ, Noordijk EM, Leer J, Marijnen CA. Comparative analysis of risk factors for pathological fracture with femoral metastases. J Bone Joint Surg Br 2004;86:566–73.

[44] van der Linden YM, Dijkstra PDS, Vonk EJA, Marijnen CAM, Leer JWH. Prediction of survival in patients with metastases in the spinal column. Cancer 2005;103:320–8.

[45] van der Linden YM, Kroon HM, Dijkstra SP, Lok JJ, Noordijk EM, Leer JW, Marijnen CA; Dutch Bone Metastasis Study Group. Simple radiographic parameter predicts fracturing in metastatic femoral bone lesions: results from a randomized trial. Radiother Oncol 2003;69:21–31.

[46] van der Linden YM, Lok JJ, Steenland E, Martijn H, van Houwelingen H, Marijnen CA, Leer JW; Dutch Bone Metastasis Study Group. Single fraction radiotherapy is efficacious: a further analysis of the Dutch Bone Metastasis Study controlling for the influence of retreatment. Int J Radiat Oncol Biol Phys 2004;59:528–37.

[47] van der Linden YM, Steenland E, van Houwelingen HC, Post WJ, Oei B, Marijnen CA, Leer JW; Dutch Bone Metastasis Study Group. Patients with a favourable prognosis are equally palliated with single and multiple fraction radiotherapy: results on survival in the Dutch Bone Metastasis Study. Radiother Oncol 2006;48:245–53.

[48] van Helvoirt R, Bratelli K. Both immediate and late retreatment with single fraction radiotherapy are effective in palliating patients with painful skeletal metastases: a prospective cohort analysis. Radiother Oncol 2008;88(Suppl):S51.
[49] Wai Man Sze, Mike S, Ines H, Malcolm M. Palliation of metastatic bone pain: single fraction versus multifraction radiotherapy: a systematic review of the randomised trials. Cochrane Database Syst Rev 2004;CD004721.
[50] Wong R, Thomas G, Cummings B. The role of radiotherapy in the management of pelvic recurrence of rectal cancer. Can J Oncol 1996;6(Suppl 1):39–47.
[51] Wong R, Malthaner R. Esophageal cancer: a systematic review. Curr Probl Cancer 2000;24:297–373.
[52] Wu JS, Wong R, Johnston M, Bezjak A, Whelan T. Meta-analysis of dose-fractionation radiotherapy trials for the palliation of painful bone metastases. Int J Radiat Oncol Biol Phys 2003;55:594–605.

**Correspondence to:** Yvette M. van der Linden, MD, PhD, Radiotherapeutic Institute Friesland, Borniastraat 36, 8934 AD Leeuwarden, The Netherlands. Email: y.m.linden@skf-rif.nl.

# 3

# Mechanisms of Malignant Bone Pain

## Patrick Mantyh

*Department of Pharmacology, College of Medicine,
University of Arizona, Tucson, Arizona, USA*

Cancer-associated pain can be present at any time during the course of the disease, but the frequency and intensity of cancer pain tends to increase with advancing stages of cancer. In patients with advanced cancer, 62–86% experience significant pain that is described as moderate to severe in approximately 40–50% and as very severe in 25–30% [72]. Bone cancer pain is the most common pain in patients with advanced cancer, and two-thirds of patients with metastatic bone disease experience severe pain [13,43]. Although bone is not a vital organ, many of the most common tumors (breast, prostate, thyroid, kidney, and lung) have a strong predilection for bone metastasis (Fig. 1). Tumor metastases to the skeleton are major contributors to morbidity and mortality in metastatic cancer. Tumor growth in bone results in pain, hypercalcemia, anemia, increased susceptibility to infection, skeletal fractures, compression of the spinal cord, spinal instability, and decreased mobility, all of which compromise the patient's survival and quality of life [13,14]. Once tumor cells have metastasized to the skeleton, tumor-induced bone pain is usually described as dull in character, constant in presentation, and gradually increasing in intensity with time [20]. As tumor-induced bone remodeling progresses, severe incident pain frequently occurs [42], and because the onset of this pain is both acute and unpredictable, this component of bone cancer

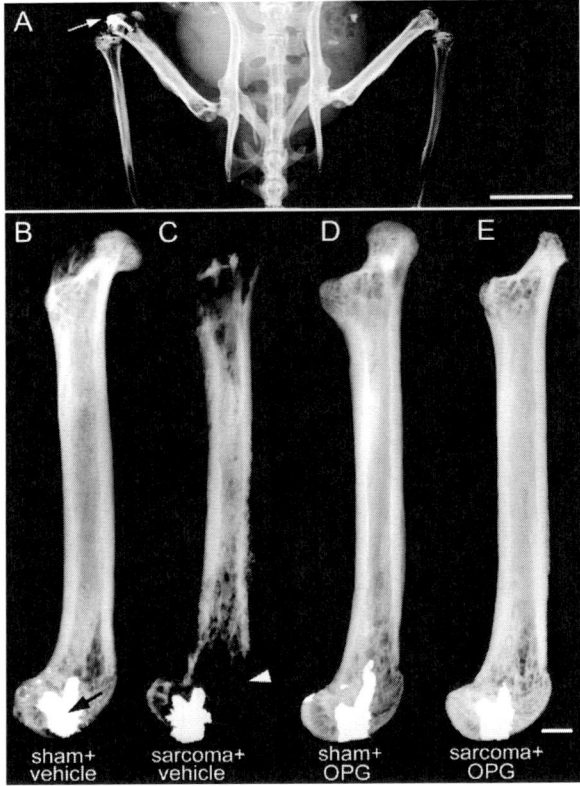

**Fig. 1.** Blockade of interactions between receptor activator for nuclear factor κB (RANK) and its ligand (RANKL) attenuates sarcoma-induced bone destruction in a mouse model of bone cancer pain. (A) Lower power frontal radiograph of mouse pelvis and hindlimbs following unilateral injection of 2472 murine osteosarcoma cells into the distal end of the femur and closure of the injection with a dental amalgam plug (arrow). The amalgam plug was used to prevent tumor cells from growing outside the bone. High-resolution radiographs of sham-injected (B and D) and sarcoma-injected (C and E) femurs from mice that received vehicle (B and C) or osteoprotegerin (OPG) (D and E). Note that at day 17 after the injection of the osteosarcoma cells, there is significant bone destruction in the distal femur without OPG (C; white arrowhead), whereas tumor-induced bone destruction is not evident in a sarcoma-injected mouse that received OPG (E). OPG is a decoy receptor that prevents the activation and proliferation of osteoclasts by binding to and sequestering OPG ligand (OPGL; also known as receptor for activator of the nuclear factor κB [NFκB] ligand, RANKL). Scale bars represent 10 mm (a) and 0.5 mm (b–e; bottom panel). Reprinted with permission of *Nature Medicine* from Honore et al. [28].

pain can be highly debilitating to the patient's functional status and quality of life [15,42]. Incident or breakthrough pain, which is defined as an intermittent episode of extreme pain, can occur spontaneously, or more commonly is induced by movement of, or weight-bearing by, the tumor-bearing bone(s) [44].

Currently, the treatment of pain from bone metastases involves the use of multiple complementary approaches, including radiotherapy applied to the painful area, surgery, chemotherapy, bisphosphonates, calcitonin, and analgesics [42,43]. However, bone cancer pain is one of the most difficult of all persistent pains to fully control [42], as the metastases are generally not limited to a single site, and the analgesics that are most commonly used to treat bone cancer pain—nonsteroidal anti-inflammatory drugs (NSAIDs) [42] and opioids [11,38,42,59]—are limited by significant adverse side effects [27,76].

Over the last decade, a major focus of our laboratory has been to investigate the mechanisms underlying cancer pain (mostly due to bone cancer) and to develop mechanism-based therapies to attenuate the pain and reduce disease progression [25,29,66]. These efforts have provided a new understanding of the factors that drive bone cancer pain and disease progression and have provided preclinical data that have resulted in several clinical trials of these mechanism-based therapies.

# Development of a Murine Model of Bone Cancer

Given the enormous consequences in terms of human suffering that cancer pain can cause, it was surprising to us when we first began exploring the mechanisms that drive cancer pain that there simply was not a well-established animal model for studying any form of cancer pain. However, two in vivo models were commonly used to study tumor-induced bone destruction. In the first model, tumor cells are injected into the left ventricle of the heart and then spread to multiple sites including the bone marrow where they multiply, grow, and destroy the surrounding bone [2,77]. This model replicates the observation that most tumor cells metastasize to multiple sites including bone, but a major problem with this model is the animal-to-animal variability in the sites, size, and extent of the metastases.

Since the tumors frequently metastasize to vital organs such as the lungs or liver, the general health of the animal is also variable, making behavioral assessment difficult. Additionally, the tumors frequently metastasize to bone in the vertebral column, and tumor growth in the vertebrae can result in collapse of the vertebral column and compression of the spinal cord with resultant spinal dysfunction and paralysis. Given these problems, the development of a model of bone cancer pain using intracardiac injection proved difficult at best.

The second major model used to study tumor-induced bone destruction involves the direct injection of lytic sarcoma cells into the intramedullary space of the mouse tibia or femur. The major problem with this model was that the injection site could not be plugged using conventional sealing agents (as it is a wet, bony surface), and the tumor cells rapidly escaped and grew avidly in nearby skin and joints, resulting in large extraskeletal tumor masses that not only interfered with behavioral analysis, but also destroyed nerves passing though these sites and generated a neuropathic pain state. We chose to adapt and modify this model by plugging the injection hole with a dental amalgam that tightly binds and seals the injection hole in the proximal head of the femur. This plugging of the injection site allowed us to contain the tumor cells within the intramedullary space and prevent tumor invasion into surrounding soft tissue (Fig. 1) [29]. This advance, along with the immunohistochemical techniques that allowed us to simultaneously measure bone-cancer-induced pain behaviors, tumor growth, and tumor-induced bone remodeling, provided us with the first preclinical cancer pain model. We then used this model to define the mechanisms that generate and maintain bone cancer pain.

When primarily osteolytic murine osteosarcoma tumor cells are injected and confined to the intramedullary space of the mouse femur, these tumor cells grow in a highly reproducible fashion as they proliferate, replacing the hematopoietic cells in the bone marrow [63,65]. Eventually, the entire marrow space is homogeneously filled with tumor cells and tumor-associated inflammatory/immune cells. In terms of bone remodeling, injection of osteosarcoma cells into the femur induces a dramatic proliferation and hypertrophy of osteoclasts at the tumor-bone interface, with significant bone destruction in both the proximal and distal heads of the femur (Fig. 1). In the osteosarcoma model, ongoing pain and movement-evoked pain-related behaviors increased in severity with time, and these pain-related behaviors correlated with the tumor growth and progressive tumor-induced bone destruction, mirroring what occurs in patients with primary or metastatic bone cancer. While sarcoma cells constituted the tumor used in the first bone cancer pain model we developed, we have since developed other bone cancer pain models using prostate, breast, melanoma, colon, and lung tumors, all of which provided insight into the similarities and differences by which different tumors drive bone cancer pain [62].

# Mechanisms Underlying Bone Cancer Pain

## Tumor- and Osteoclast-Induced Acidosis and Bone Cancer Pain

Reports from both animal studies and humans with bone cancer pain have suggested that osteoclasts (the cells that break down bone) play a significant role in cancer-induced bone loss [37] and that osteoclasts contribute to the etiology of bone cancer pain [40,73]. Osteoclasts are terminally differentiated, multinucleated, monocyte lineage cells that resorb bone by maintaining an extracellular microenvironment of acidic pH (4.0–5.0) at the osteoclast-mineralized bone interface [17]. Tumor-induced release of protons may be particularly important in the generation of bone cancer pain. Both osteolytic (bone-destroying) and osteoblastic (bone-forming) cancers are characterized by osteoclast proliferation and hypertrophy [19,26,29].

Bisphosphonates are a class of antiresorptive compounds that are pyrophosphate analogues which display high affinity for calcium ions, causing them to rapidly and avidly bind to the mineralized matrix of bone [19]. As osteoclasts resorb bone, they use endocytosis to clear the bone breakdown products from the osteoclast-bone interface (including the bisphosphonate that is bound to the mineralized bone). Bisphosphonates, once taken up by the osteoclasts, induce loss of function and ultimately apoptosis of the osteoclasts by impairing the synthesis of either adenosine triphosphate or cholesterol, both of which are necessary for osteoclast function and survival [19].

Animal and clinical studies of bone cancer have reported that the antiresorptive effects of bisphosphonate therapy simultaneously reduce bone cancer pain, tumor-induced bone destruction, and tumor growth within the bone [36,40,73]. Recent data also suggest that in addition to the antitumor effects that they produce by inhibiting the breakdown of mineralized bone, bisphosphonates may also destroy tumor cells growing in soft tissues [36]. This systemic tumoricidal effect of bisphosphonates is hypothesized to occur by reducing the circulating levels of vascular endothelial growth factor, which is an essential component of tumor angiogenesis [36]. Currently, clinical studies are being performed to determine the effect that bisphosphonates have on bone pain, tumor growth, and tumor metastasis in bone cancer [12].

Bisphosphonates are approved for, and are frequently used for, the reduction of tumor-induced bone destruction and bone cancer pain, but they do have unwanted side effects (including induction of arthralgias and osteonecrosis of the jaw) [19], and it has yet to be definitively shown that bisphosphonates increase the survival of patients with bone cancer. For this reason, other therapies targeting osteoclasts are already in mid- to late-stage clinical trials. These therapies hold significant promise for alleviating bone cancer pain and tumor-induced bone remodeling. One line of therapies attempts to block the binding of receptor activator for nuclear factor κB ligand (RANKL), which is an essential regulator of osteoclasts [37]. Studies in mice have shown that blockade of RANKL attenuates sarcoma-induced bone pain, bone remodeling, and tumor growth within the bone [29] (Figs. 1, 2). Recent clinical studies have shown that in humans with multiple myeloma or breast cancer metastasis to bone, denosumab (a fully humanized monoclonal antibody that inhibits RANKL) markedly reduces tumor-induced bone resorption and skeletal events (which include fracture and pain) [7]. Recently, a Phase III head-to-head trial evaluating denosumab versus zoledronic acid in the treatment of bone metastases in 2,049 patients with advanced breast cancer has been finalized. This clinical trial showed that denosumab significantly delayed the time to the first skeletal events (fracture, radiation to bone, surgery to bone, or spinal cord compression) and significantly reduced first and subsequent skeletal events as compared to zoledronic acid [1].

The finding that sensory neurons can be directly excited by protons or acids originating from cells such as osteoclasts in the bone has generated intense clinical interest in pain research [68]. Studies have shown that subsets of sensory neurons express different acid-sensing ion channels [32,49]. Two such channels expressed by nociceptors are transient receptor potential vanilloid-1 (TRPV1) [9,70] and acid-sensing ion channel-3 (ASIC-3) [4,49,68]. Both of these channels are sensitized and excited by a decrease in pH. The tumor stroma [24] and areas of the tumor that are necrotic typically exhibit lower extracellular pH than surrounding normal tissues. As inflammatory and immune cells invade the tumor stroma, these cells also release protons that generate a local acidosis. As tumor cells outgrow their vascular supply, tumor apoptosis that occurs in the tumor environment may also contribute to the development of an acidic environment.

Studies have shown that TRPV1 is expressed by a subset of sensory neuron fibers that innervate the mouse femur. In an in vivo model of bone cancer pain, acute or chronic administration of a TRPV1 antagonist or disruption of the TRPV1 gene significantly attenuated both ongoing

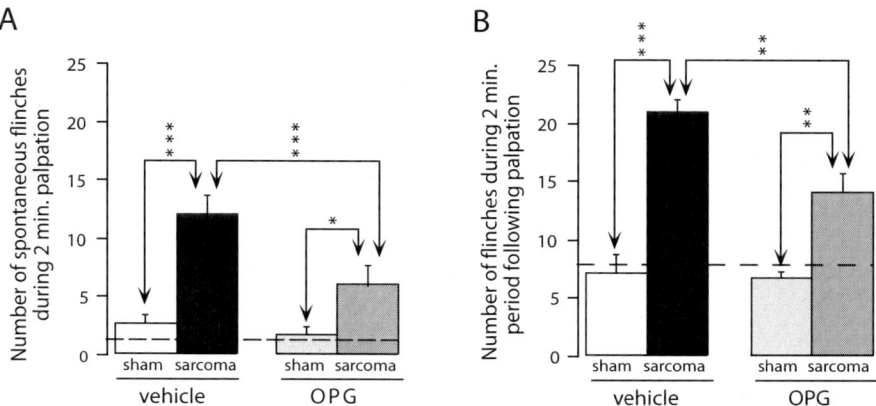

**Fig. 2.** Blockade of RANK/RANKL interactions attenuates both spontaneous and movement-evoked bone-cancer-related pain behaviors. (A) The number of spontaneous flinching behaviors in a 2-minute observation period and (B) the number of flinching behaviors in a 2-minute observation period after the completion of a normally nonnoxious palpation, 17 days after sham or sarcoma injection into the femora of mice that subsequently received vehicle or osteoprotegerin (OPG). Daily treatment with OPG significantly reduces spontaneous and movement-evoked nociceptive behaviors indicative of pain. Data represent mean ± standard error. Dashed lines, baseline values. * $P < 0.05$; ** $P < 0.01$; *** $P < 0.001$; one-way ANOVA and Fisher's protected least significant difference (brackets and downward arrows indicate groups being compared). Reprinted with permission of *Nature Medicine* from Honore et al. [28].

and movement-evoked nocifensive behaviors [22]. In addition, previous studies have shown that in a sarcoma model of bone cancer pain, administration of a TRPV1 antagonist retains its efficacy at early, middle, and late stages of tumor growth [22]. The ability of a TRPV1 antagonist to maintain its analgesic potency with disease progression is probably influenced by the fact that sensory nerve fibers innervating the tumor-bearing mouse femur maintain their expression of TRPV1 even as tumor growth and tumor-induced bone destruction progress. These results suggest that the TRPV1 channel plays a role in the integration of nociceptive signaling in a severe pain state and that antagonists of TRPV1 may be effective in attenuating difficult-to-treat mixed chronic pain states, such as that encountered in patients with bone cancer pain.

The discussion above has focused on osteoclast-mediated acidosis as a mechanism that drives bone cancer pain, yet both osteolytic and osteoblastic tumors reduce the mechanical strength and stability of the tumor-bearing bone so that normally innocuous mechanical stress can now produce distortion of the mechanosensitive sensory nerve fibers that innervate the bone. Previous results have shown that the pain associated with the fracture is significantly attenuated if the bone is stabilized and returned to its normal orientation [61]. Both bisphosphonates and molecules that sequester RANKL reduce the rate of tumor-induced bone remodeling and preserve the mechanical strength of bone. Preservation of the mechanical strength of bone should reduce movement-induced incident pain, which is probably driven in part by activation of normally silent mechanosensitive nociceptors that innervate the bone.

## Tumor-Derived Products in the Generation of Bone Cancer Pain

In most cancers the tumor mass is composed of tumor cells, as well as tumor stromal cells including macrophages, neutrophils, T-lymphocytes, fibroblasts, and endothelial cells. Tumor cells and/or tumor stromal cells have been shown to secrete a variety of factors that sensitize or directly excite primary afferent neurons, such as prostaglandins [21,47], tumor necrosis factor alpha [18,33,45,75], endothelins [16,46], interleukins IL-1 and IL-6 [18,51,74], epidermal growth factor [57], transforming growth factor-beta [56,60], platelet-derived growth factor [34,35,50,58], and nerve growth factor. Receptors for many of these factors are expressed by primary afferent neurons.

One important concept that has emerged over the past decade is that nerve growth factor (NGF), in addition to its ability to directly activate sensory neurons that express the TrkA receptor, modulates the expression and function of a wide variety of molecules and proteins expressed by sensory neurons that contain the TrkA or p75 receptor (Fig. 3). Some of these molecules and proteins include neurotransmitters (substance P and calcitonin gene-related peptide), bradykinin receptors, ion channels (TRPV1, ASIC-3, and sodium channels), transcription factors (ATF-3), and structural molecules (neurofilaments and the sodium channel anchoring molecule p11) [28,53] (Fig. 3). Additionally, NGF modulates the trafficking and insertion of sodium channels such as $Na_v1.8$ [23] and TRPV1 [31] in the sensory neurons and influences the expression profile of supporting cells in the dorsal root ganglia (DRG) and peripheral nerves, such as non-myelinating Schwann cells and macrophages [8,10]. Anti-NGF antibody therapy may be particularly effective in blocking bone cancer pain because NGF appears to be integrally involved in the upregulation, sensitization, and disinhibition of multiple neurotransmitters, ion channels, and receptors in the primary afferent nerve and DRG fibers that synergistically increase nociceptive signals originating from the tumor-bearing bone.

To test the hypothesis that an anti-NGF therapy would be efficacious in reducing bone cancer pain, we examined the analgesic efficacy of a murine anti-NGF monoclonal antibody in tumor-induced bone pain using the primarily osteolytic 2472 murine osteosarcoma cells, which express high levels of NGF, and the primarily osteoblastic canine ACE-1 prostate carcinoma cells, where NGF expression is undetectable (Fig. 4). In both of these models of tumor-induced bone cancer pain, we demonstrated that administration of an anti-NGF antibody was highly efficacious in reducing both early- and late-stage bone cancer pain-related behaviors; in fact, this reduction in pain-related behaviors was greater than that achieved with acute administration of 10 mg/kg of morphine sulfate [25,67]. These data suggest that therapeutic targeting of NGF or its cognate receptor TrkA may be useful in blocking bone cancer pain, whether or not the tumor that has metastasized to bone expresses NGF. Presumably, in the case where the tumor cells themselves do not express NGF, it is the tumor stromal cells (which comprise 2–60% of the total tumor mass) that are expressing and secreting NGF. Currently, a fully humanized monoclonal antibody to NGF known as tanezumab has been tested in human patients with osteoarthritis and has proven effective at reducing pain [64]. Human phase II clinical trials are being performed to evaluate tanezumab's effects at

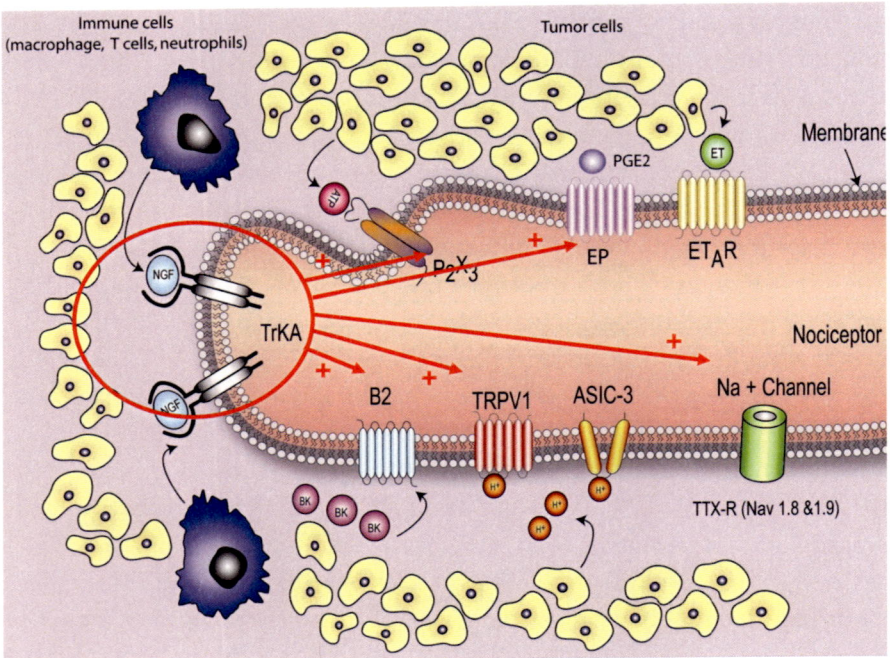

**Fig. 3.** Schematic showing factors in receptors or channels expressed by nociceptors that innervate the skeleton that drive bone cancer pain. A variety of cells (tumor cells; stromal cells, including inflammatory/immune cells; and osteoclasts) drive bone cancer pain. Nociceptors that innervate the bone use several different types of receptors to detect and transmit noxious stimuli that are produced by cancer cells (yellow), by tumor-associated immune cells (blue), or by other aspects of the tumor microenvironment. Multiple factors contribute to the pain associated with cancer. The transient receptor potential vanilloid receptor-1 (TRPV1) and acid-sensing ion channels (ASICs) detect extracellular protons produced by tumor-induced tissue damage or by abnormal osteoclast-mediated bone resorption. Tumor cells and associated inflammatory (immune) cells produce a variety of chemical mediators including prostaglandins (PGE$_2$), nerve growth factor (NGF), endothelins, bradykinin, and extracellular ATP. Several of these proinflammatory mediators have receptors on peripheral terminals and can directly activate or sensitize nociceptors. NGF and its cognate receptor TrkA may serve as a master regulator of bone cancer pain by modulating the sensitivity or increasing the expression of several receptors and ion channels contributing to increased excitability of nociceptors in the vicinity of the tumor.

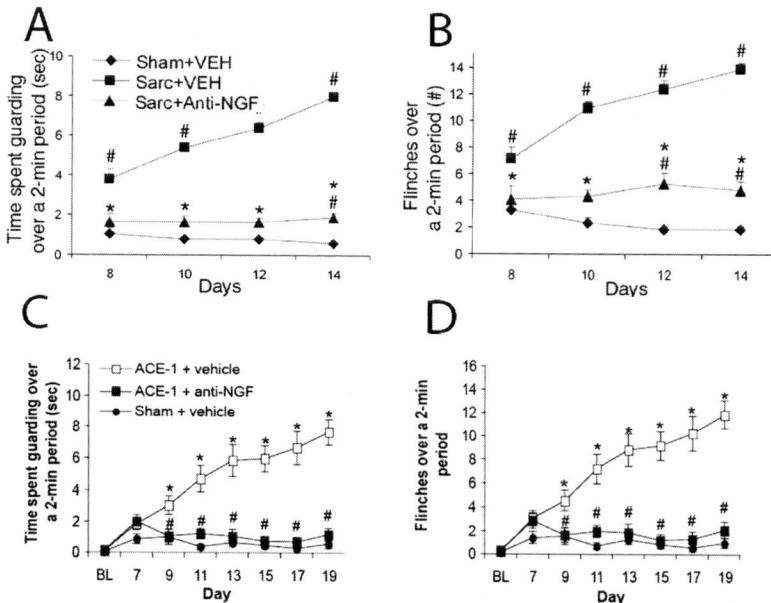

**Fig. 4.** Anti-nerve growth factor treatment attenuates spontaneous bone cancer pain in a model where the tumor cells do (mouse sarcoma cells) and do not (canine prostate cells) express NGF. Anti-NGF treatment (10 mg/kg, i.p., given on days 7, 12, and 17 post-tumor injection) attenuated ongoing bone cancer pain behavior on days 7 to 19 post-tumor injection. In these experiments, (A,B) mouse sarcoma cells or (C,D) canine prostate carcinoma (ACE-1) cells were injected into the femur of adult male mice. The time spent guarding and the number of spontaneous flinches of the affected limb over a 2-minute observation period were used as measures of ongoing pain. Anti-NGF treatment significantly reduced ongoing pain behaviors in tumor-injected mice as compared with (A,B) sarcoma + vehicle or (C,D) ACE-1 + vehicle. Whereas the mouse sarcoma cells express relatively high levels of NGF mRNA in vitro, ACE-1 cells in vitro express undetectable levels of NGF mRNA or protein, suggesting that NGF is released mainly from tumor-associated macrophages and immune cells. Bars represent mean ± standard error. * $P < 0.05$ versus sham + vehicle; # $P < 0.05$ versus ACE-1 + vehicle. Adapted with permission from Sevcik et al. [66] and Halvorson et al. [24].

reducing bone cancer pain in patients with advanced breast or prostate cancer [54,55].

## The Neuropathic Component of Bone Cancer Pain

Numerous studies have demonstrated that the periosteum is densely innervated by both sensory and sympathetic fibers [3,30,41]. Using a combination of minimal decalcification strategies and antigen amplification techniques, researchers have demonstrated that the bone marrow and mineralized bone also receive a significant innervation by both sensory and sympathetic nerve fibers [5,6,39,69]. Mineralized bone and periosteum are ultimately affected by fractures, ischemia, and the presence of tumor cells. Sensory fibers in any of these compartments may play a role in the generation and maintenance of bone cancer pain.

In examining the changes in the sensory innervation of bone induced by the osteolytic sarcoma cells, we observed sensory fibers at and within the leading edge of the tumor in the deep stromal regions of the tumor. Additionally, these sensory nerve fibers displayed a discontinuous and fragmented appearance, suggesting that following initial activation by the osteolytic tumor cells, the distal processes of the sensory fibers were ultimately injured by the invading tumor cells. In contrast, the sensory innervation of bone following injection of the primarily osteoblastic prostate cancer cells suggests that there is simultaneous injury and sprouting of sensory fibers in the bone [26].

In the sarcoma-injected animals, there was expression of activating transcription factor-3 (ATF-3) in the nucleus of sensory neurons that innervate the femur. ATF-3 is a member of the ATF/CREB (cyclic adenosine monophosphate response element-binding protein) family of transcription factors, which is not expressed at detectable levels in normal sensory neurons or in sensory neurons after peripheral inflammation, but is strongly expressed in sensory neurons following injury to peripheral nerves in neuropathic pain models [71]. It is likely that the expression of ATF-3 in sensory neurons of tumor-bearing animals is a result of the tumor-induced injury and destruction of the distal tips of the sensory and sympathetic nerve fibers that innervate the bone.

This tumor-induced injury of sensory nerve fibers in the sarcoma model was also accompanied by an increase in ongoing and movement-evoked pain behaviors, an upregulation of galanin by sensory neurons that innervate the tumor-bearing femur, upregulation of glial fibrillary acidic proteins, hypertrophy of satellite cells surrounding sensory neuron cell bodies within the ipsilateral DRG, and macrophage infiltration of the DRG ipsilateral to the tumor-bearing femur [52,67]. Similar neurochemical changes have been described following peripheral nerve injury and in other noncancerous neuropathic pain states [48]. Chronic treatment with gabapentin in the sarcoma model did not influence tumor growth, tumor-induced bone destruction, or the tumor-induced neurochemical reorganization that occurred in sensory neurons or the spinal cord, but it did attenuate both ongoing and movement-evoked bone cancer-related pain behaviors [52]. These results suggest that even when the tumor is confined within the bone, a component of bone cancer pain is due to tumor-induced injury to primary afferent nerve fibers that normally innervate the tumor-bearing bone.

# Conclusions

For the first time, animal models of cancer pain are now available that effectively mirror the clinical picture observed in humans with bone cancer pain. Information generated from these models has begun to provide insight into the mechanisms that generate and maintain bone cancer pain and to help target potential mechanism-based therapies to treat this chronic pain state. Interestingly, several therapies that attenuate bone cancer pain may also reduce tumor growth and tumor-induced bone remodeling. Thus, bisphosphonates are commonly used to treat bone cancer pain. Other therapies, including denosumab (anti-RANKL; Amgen), tanezumab (anti-NGF; Pfizer), and pregabalin (Pfizer) are in mid- to late-stage clinical trials. Successful development and clinical use of these therapies has the potential to improve the patient's functional status, quality of life, and survival.

# References

[1]    Amgen. Denosumab demonstrates superiority over Zometa(R) in pivotal phase 3 head-to-head trial in breast cancer patients with bone metastases. Amgen; 2009. Available at: http://www.amgen.com/media/media_pr_detail.jsp?year=2009&releaseID=1305355.
[2]    Arguello F, Baggs RB, Frantz CN. A murine model of experimental metastasis to bone and bone marrow. Cancer Res 1988;48:6876–81.
[3]    Asmus SE, Parsons S, Landis SC. Developmental changes in the transmitter properties of sympathetic neurons that innervate the periosteum. J Neurosci 2000;20:1495–504.
[4]    Bassilana F, Champigny G, Waldmann R, de Weille JR, Heurteaux C, Lazdunski M. The acid-sensitive ionic channel subunit ASIC and the mammalian degenerin MDEG form a heteromultimeric $H^+$-gated $Na^+$ channel with novel properties. J Biol Chem 1997;272:28819–22.
[5]    Bjurholm A, Kreicbergs A, Brodin E, Schultzberg M. Substance P- and CGRP-immunoreactive nerves in bone. Peptides 1988;9:165–71.
[6]    Bjurholm A, Kreicbergs A, Terenius L, Goldstein M, Schultzberg M. Neuropeptide Y-, tyrosine hydroxylase- and vasoactive intestinal polypeptide-immunoreactive nerves in bone and surrounding tissues. J Auton Nerv Syst 1988;25:119–25.

[7]   Body JJ, Facon T, Coleman RE, Lipton A, Geurs F, Fan M, Holloway D, Peterson MC, Bekker
      PJ. A study of the biological receptor activator of nuclear factor-kappaB ligand inhibitor, deno-
      sumab, in patients with multiple myeloma or bone metastases from breast cancer. Clin Cancer
      Res 2006;12:1221–8.
[8]   Brown A, Ricci MJ, Weaver LC. NGF message and protein distribution in the injured rat spinal
      cord. Exp Neurol 2004;188:115–27.
[9]   Caterina MJ, Leffler A, Malmberg AB, Martin WJ, Trafton J, Petersen-Zeitz KR, Koltzenburg
      M, Basbaum AI, Julius D. Impaired nociception and pain sensation in mice lacking the capsaicin
      receptor. Science 2000;288:306–13.
[10]  Chen ZL, Yu WM, Strickland S. Peripheral regeneration. Annu Rev Neurosci 2007;30:209–33.
[11]  Cherny N. New strategies in opioid therapy for cancer pain. J Oncol Manag 2000;9:8–15.
[12]  Coleman R, Gnant M. New results from the use of bisphosphonates in cancer patients. Curr
      Opin Support Palliat Care 2009;3:213–8.
[13]  Coleman RE. Clinical features of metastatic bone disease and risk of skeletal morbidity. Clin
      Cancer Res 2006;12:6243s–9s.
[14]  Coleman RE. Risks and benefits of bisphosphonates. Br J Cancer 2008;98:1736–40.
[15]  Coleman RE. Skeletal complications of malignancy. Cancer 1997;80(Suppl):1588–94.
[16]  Davar G. Endothelin-1 and metastatic cancer pain. Pain Med 2001;2:24–7.
[17]  Delaisse JM, Vaes G. Mechanism of mineral solubilization and matrix degradation in osteoclas-
      tic bone resorption. In: Rifkin BR, Gay CV, editors. Biology and physiology of the osteoclast. Ann
      Arbor: CRC; 1992. p. 289–314.
[18]  DeLeo JA, Yezierski RP. The role of neuroinflammation and neuroimmune activation in persis-
      tent pain. Pain 2001;90:1–6.
[19]  Drake MT, Clarke BL, Khosla S. Bisphosphonates: mechanism of action and role in clinical prac-
      tice. Mayo Clin Proc 2008;83:1032–45.
[20]  Dy SM, Asch SM, Naeim A, Sanati H, Walling A, Lorenz KA. Evidence-based standards for
      cancer pain management. J Clin Oncol 2008;26:3879–85.
[21]  Galasko CS. Diagnosis of skeletal metastases and assessment of response to treatment. Clin Or-
      thop Rel Res 1995;312:64–75.
[22]  Ghilardi JR, Rohrich H, Lindsay TH, Sevcik MA, Schwei MJ, Kubota K, Halvorson KG, Poblete
      J, Chaplan SR, Dubin AE, et al. Selective blockade of the capsaicin receptor TRPV1 attenuates
      bone cancer pain. J Neurosci 2005;25:3126–31.
[23]  Gould HJ 3rd, Gould TN, England JD, Paul D, Liu ZP, Levinson SR. A possible role for nerve
      growth factor in the augmentation of sodium channels in models of chronic pain. Brain Res
      2000;854:19–29.
[24]  Griffiths JR. Are cancer cells acidic? Br J Cancer 1991;64:425–7.
[25]  Halvorson KG, Kubota K, Sevcik MA, Lindsay TH, Sotillo JE, Ghilardi JR, Rosol TJ, Boustany
      L, Shelton DL, Mantyh PW. A blocking antibody to nerve growth factor attenuates skeletal pain
      induced by prostate tumor cells growing in bone. Cancer Res 2005;65:9426–35.
[26]  Halvorson KG, Sevcik MA, Ghilardi JR, Rosol TJ, Mantyh PW. Similarities and differences in
      tumor growth, skeletal remodeling and pain in an osteolytic and osteoblastic model of bone
      cancer. Clin J Pain 2006;22:587–600.
[27]  Harris JD. Management of expected and unexpected opioid-related side effects. Clin J Pain
      2008;24(Suppl 10):S8–S13.
[28]  Hefti FF, Rosenthal A, Walicke PA, Wyatt S, Vergara G, Shelton DL, Davies AM. Novel class of
      pain drugs based on antagonism of NGF. Trends Pharmacol Sci 2006;27:85–91.
[29]  Honore P, Luger NM, Sabino MA, Schwei MJ, Rogers SD, Mach DB, O'Keefe P F, Ramnaraine
      ML, Clohisy DR, Mantyh PW. Osteoprotegerin blocks bone cancer-induced skeletal destruc-
      tion, skeletal pain and pain-related neurochemical reorganization of the spinal cord. Nat Med
      2000;6:521–8.
[30]  Irie K, Hara-Irie F, Ozawa H, Yajima T. Calcitonin gene-related peptide (CGRP)-containing nerve
      fibers in bone tissue and their involvement in bone remodeling. Microsc Res Tech 2002;58:85–90.
[31]  Ji RR, Samad TA, Jin SX, Schmoll R, Woolf CJ. p38 MAPK activation by NGF in primary sensory
      neurons after inflammation increases TRPV1 levels and maintains heat hyperalgesia. Neuron
      2002;36:57–68.
[32]  Julius D, Basbaum AI. Molecular mechanisms of nociception. Nature 2001;413:203–10.
[33]  Khatami M. 'Yin and Yang' in inflammation: duality in innate immune cell function and tumori-
      genesis. Expert Opin Biol Ther 2008;8:1461–72.

[34] Kuhnert F, Tam BY, Sennino B, Gray JT, Yuan J, Jocson A, Nayak NR, Mulligan RC, McDonald DM, Kuo CJ. Soluble receptor-mediated selective inhibition of VEGFR and PDGFRbeta signaling during physiologic and tumor angiogenesis. Proc Natl Acad Sci USA 2008;105:10185–90.

[35] Lin SY, Yang J, Everett AD, Clevenger CV, Koneru M, Mishra PJ, Kamen B, Banerjee D, Glod J. The isolation of novel mesenchymal stromal cell chemotactic factors from the conditioned medium of tumor cells. Exp Cell Res 2008;314:3107–17.

[36] Lipton A. Emerging role of bisphosphonates in the clinic: antitumor activity and prevention of metastasis to bone. Cancer Treat Rev 2008;34(Suppl 1):S25–30.

[37] Lipton A. Future treatment of bone metastases. Clin Cancer Res 2006;12:6305s–8s.

[38] Lussier D, Huskey AG, Portenoy RK. Adjuvant analgesics in cancer pain management. Oncologist 2004;9:571–91.

[39] Mach DB, Rogers SD, Sabino MC, Luger NM, Schwei MJ, Pomonis JD, Keyser CP, Clohisy DR, Adams DJ, O'Leary P, Mantyh PW. Origins of skeletal pain: sensory and sympathetic innervation of the mouse femur. Neuroscience 2002;113:155–66.

[40] Mantyh PW. Cancer pain and its impact on diagnosis, survival and quality of life. Nat Rev Neurosci 2006;7:797–809.

[41] Martin CD, Jimenez-Andrade JM, Ghilardi JR, Mantyh PW. Organization of a unique net-like meshwork of CGRP+ sensory fibers in the mouse periosteum: implications for the generation and maintenance of bone fracture pain. Neurosci Lett 2007;427:148–52.

[42] Mercadante S. Malignant bone pain: pathophysiology and treatment. Pain 1997;69:1–18.

[43] Mercadante S, Fulfaro F. Management of painful bone metastases. Curr Opin Oncol 2007;19:308–14.

[44] Mercadante S, Villari P, Ferrera P, Casuccio A. Optimization of opioid therapy for preventing incident pain associated with bone metastases. J Pain Symptom Manage 2004;28:505–10.

[45] Nadler RB, Koch AE, Calhoun EA, Campbell PL, Pruden DL, Bennett CL, Yarnold PR, Schaeffer AJ. IL-1beta and TNF-alpha in prostatic secretions are indicators in the evaluation of men with chronic prostatitis. J Urol 2000;164:214–8.

[46] Nelson JB, Carducci MA. The role of endothelin-1 and endothelin receptor antagonists in prostate cancer. BJU Int 2000;85(Suppl 2):45–8.

[47] Nielsen OS, Munro AJ, Tannock IF. Bone metastases: pathophysiology and management policy. J Clin Oncol 1991;9:509–24.

[48] Obata K, Yamanaka H, Fukuoka T, Yi D, Tokunaga A, Hashimoto N, Yoshikawa H, Noguchi K. Contribution of injured and uninjured dorsal root ganglion neurons to pain behavior and the changes in gene expression following chronic constriction injury of the sciatic nerve in rats. Pain 2003;101:65–77.

[49] Olson TH, Riedl MS, Vulchanova L, Ortiz-Gonzalez XR, Elde R. An acid sensing ion channel (ASIC) localizes to small primary afferent neurons in rats. Neuroreport 1998;9:1109–13.

[50] Ono M. Molecular links between tumor angiogenesis and inflammation: inflammatory stimuli of macrophages and cancer cells as targets for therapeutic strategy. Cancer Sci 2008;99:1501–6.

[51] Opree A, Kress M. Involvement of the proinflammatory cytokines tumor necrosis factor-alpha, IL-1 beta, and IL-6 but not IL-8 in the development of heat hyperalgesia: effects on heat-evoked calcitonin gene-related peptide release from rat skin. J Neurosci 2000;20:6289–93.

[52] Peters CM, Ghilardi JR, Keyser CP, Kubota K, Lindsay TH, Luger NM, Mach DB, Schwei MJ, Sevcik MA, Mantyh PW. Tumor-induced injury of primary afferent sensory nerve fibers in bone cancer pain. Exp Neurol 2005;193:85–100.

[53] Pezet S, McMahon SB. Neurotrophins: mediators and modulators of pain. Annu Rev Neurosci 2006;29:507–38.

[54] Pfizer. Open label extension in cancer patients. NCT00830180. Available at: http://clinicaltrials.gov. Accessed January 2010.

[55] Pfizer. A study of tanezumab as add-on therapy to opioid medication in patients with pain due to cancer that has spread to bone. NCT00545129. Available at: http://clinicaltrials.gov. Accessed January 2010.

[56] Poon RT, Fan ST, Wong J. Clinical implications of circulating angiogenic factors in cancer patients. J Clin Oncol 2001;19:1207–25.

[57] Purow BW, Sundaresan TK, Burdick MJ, Kefas BA, Comeau LD, Hawkinson MP, Su Q, Kotliarov Y, Lee J, Zhang W, Fine HA. Notch-1 regulates transcription of the epidermal growth factor receptor through p53. Carcinogenesis 2008;29:918–25.

[58] Radinsky R. Growth factors and their receptors in metastasis. Semin Cancer Biol 1991;2:169–77.

[59]  Reid CM, Gooberman-Hill R, Hanks GW. Opioid analgesics for cancer pain: symptom control
      for the living or comfort for the dying? A qualitative study to investigate the factors influencing
      the decision to accept morphine for pain caused by cancer. Ann Oncol 2008;19:44–8.
[60]  Roman C, Saha D, Beauchamp R. TGF-beta and colorectal carcinogenesis. Microsc Res Tech
      2001;52:450–7.
[61]  Rubert C, Henshaw R, Malawer M. Orthopedic management of skeletal metastases. In: Body JJ,
      editor. Tumor bone disease and osteoporosis in cancer patients. New York: Marcel Dekker; 2000.
[62]  Sabino M, Luger N, Mach D, Rogers S, Schwei M, Feia K, Mantyh P. Different tumors in bone
      each give rise to a distinct pattern of skeletal destruction, bone cancer-related pain behaviors and
      neurochemical changes in the central nervous system. Int J Cancer 2003;104:550–8.
[63]  Sabino MA, Ghilardi JR, Jongen JL, Keyser CP, Luger NM, Mach DB, Peters CM, Rogers SD,
      Schwei MJ, de Felipe C, Mantyh PW. Simultaneous reduction in cancer pain, bone destruction,
      and tumor growth by selective inhibition of cyclooxygenase-2. Cancer Res. 2002;62:7343–9.
[64]  Schnitzer TJ, Lane NE, Smith MD, Brown MT. Efficacy and safety of tanezumab (PF04383119),
      an anti-nerve growth factor (NGF) antibody, for moderate to severe pain due to osteoarthritis
      (OA) of the knee: a randomized trial. Abstracts: 12th World Congress on Pain. Seattle: IASP;
      2008. PT 214.
[65]  Schwei MJ, Honore P, Rogers SD, Salak-Johnson JL, Finke MP, Ramnaraine ML, Clohisy DR,
      Mantyh PW. Neurochemical and cellular reorganization of the spinal cord in a murine model of
      bone cancer pain. J Neurosci 1999;19:10886–97.
[66]  Sevcik M, Jonas B, Lindsay T, Halvorson K, Ghilardi J, Kuskowski M, Mukherjee P, Maggio J,
      Mantyh P. Endogenous opioids inhibit early stage pancreatic pain in a mouse model of pancre-
      atic cancer. Gastroenterology 2006;131:900–10.
[67]  Sevcik MA, Ghilardi JR, Peters CM, Lindsay TH, Halvorson KG, Jonas BM, Kubota K, Kus-
      kowski MA, Boustany L, Shelton DL, Mantyh PW. Anti-NGF therapy profoundly reduces bone
      cancer pain and the accompanying increase in markers of peripheral and central sensitization.
      Pain 2005;115:128–41.
[68]  Sutherland S, Cook S, EW M. Chemical mediators of pain due to tissue damage and ischemia.
      Prog Brain Res 2000;129:21–38.
[69]  Tabarowski Z, Gibson-Berry K, Felten SY. Noradrenergic and peptidergic innervation of the
      mouse femur bone marrow. Acta Histochem 1996;98:453–7.
[70]  Tominaga M, Caterina MJ, Malmberg AB, Rosen TA, Gilbert H, Skinner K, Raumann BE, Bas-
      baum AI, Julius D. The cloned capsaicin receptor integrates multiple pain-producing stimuli.
      Neuron 1998;21:531–43.
[71]  Tsujino H, Kondo E, Fukuoka T, Dai Y, Tokunaga A, Miki K, Yonenobu K, Ochi T, Noguchi K.
      Activating transcription factor 3 (ATF3) induction by axotomy in sensory and motoneurons: a
      novel neuronal marker of nerve injury. Mol Cell Neurosci 2000;15:170–82.
[72]  van den Beuken-van Everdingen M, de Rijke J, Kessels A, Schouten H, van Kleef M, Patijn J.
      Prevalence of pain in patients with cancer: a systematic review of the past 40 years. Ann Oncol
      2007;18:1437–49.
[73]  von Moos R, Strasser F, Gillessen S, Zaugg K. Metastatic bone pain: treatment options with an
      emphasis on bisphosphonates. Support Care Cancer 2008;16:1105–15.
[74]  Watkins LR, Goehler LE, Relton J, Brewer MT, Maier SF. Mechanisms of tumor necrosis factor-
      alpha (TNF-alpha) hyperalgesia. Brain Res 1995;692:244–50.
[75]  Watkins LR, Maier SF. Implications of immune-to-brain communication for sickness and pain.
      Proc Natl Acad Sci USA 1999;96:7710–3.
[76]  Weber M, Huber C. Documentation of severe pain, opioid doses, and opioid-related side effects
      in outpatients with cancer: a retrospective study. J Pain Symptom Manage 1999;17:49–54.
[77]  Yoneda T, Sasaki A, Mundy GR. Osteolytic bone metastasis in breast cancer. Breast Cancer Res
      Treat 1994;32:73–84.

***Correspondence to:*** Patrick W. Mantyh, PhD, Department of Pharmacology, College of Medicine, University of Arizona, P.O. Box 245215, Tucson, AZ
85724, USA. Tel: 1-520-626-0742, fax: 1-520-626-4182; email: pmantyh@email.
arizona.edu.

# Part II

# Inflammation, Hyperalgesia, and Cancer Pain

# Cytokines and Cancer Pain

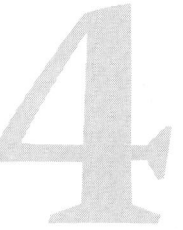

## Michaela Kress

*Department of Physiology, Innsbruck Medical University, Innsbruck, Austria*

At the advanced stages of cancer, 75–95% of patients experience cancer-related pain, including a local hypersensitivity (hyperalgesia or allodynia) to touch, warming, or cold (for review, see [72]). In addition, a transitory exacerbation of pain called breakthrough pain may occur, but estimates of the incidence of such pain vary widely in the literature [76,132].

## Animal Models of Cancer Pain

In recent years, several animal models have been developed to study bone cancer pain [114,146], skin cancer pain [109], and neuropathic cancer pain [119]. Among these, the bone cancer model in C3H mice has been most extensively used to study the contribution of particular proalgesic mediators in tumor-induced pain. Injection of fibrosarcoma cells into the mouse femur or calcaneous bone leads to cancer-associated pain with bone destruction by osteoclasts [114] and severe mechanical hypersensitivity of the respective limb [146]. The development of a tumor mass is accompanied by behavioral changes that closely resemble some aspects

*Cancer Pain: From Molecules to Suffering*
edited by Judith A. Paice, Rae F. Bell, Eija A. Kalso, and Olaitan A. Soyannwo
IASP Press, Seattle, © 2010

of human disease: animals show signs of tenderness, ongoing pain, and movement-evoked pain that are well correlated with the growth of the tumor and the degree of bone destruction [52,114]. Although nerve fibers have been found sprouting into the bone cancer tissue, we are only beginning to understand nociceptor function in cancer and metastasis, because it is very difficult to directly record from nociceptive afferents in this model. In bone cancer, 30% of fibers are spontaneously active, and heat activation thresholds are decreased by 3.5°C [19]. Similar changes are seen in a novel soft-tissue cancer model that allows investigators to study the mechanisms of nociceptors at a larger scale [24].

# Cancer and Cytokines

Progression of tumor growth leads to a variety of local changes, including chemotaxis of immune cells (macrophages, T cells, and dendritic cells) that coexist with the cancer cells and the production of mediators that are also found in inflamed tissue [3]. Several pro-inflammatory gene products have been identified that mediate a critical role in cancer cell proliferation, angiogenesis, invasion, and metastasis. Among these gene products are several members of the cytokine families including tumor necrosis factor (TNF) and members of its superfamily, the interleukins IL-1α, IL-1β, IL-6, IL-8, and IL-18, and the more recently discovered chemokines. The expression of all these genes is mainly regulated by the transcription factor nuclear factor (NF)-κB, which is constitutively active in most tumors and is induced by carcinogens (such as cigarette smoke), tumor promoters, carcinogenic viral proteins, chemotherapeutic agents, and gamma-irradiation [2,117]. In addition, plasma levels of inflammatory cytokines can change in response to cancer chemotherapy [100].

In general, cytokines are small proteins with a molecular mass lower than 30 kDa. Cytokines are produced on demand, have a short life span and therefore travel only over short distances. In vivo concentrations are in the range of a few picograms to nanograms per milliliter. Their binding is specific, and requires receptor molecules on the cell surface with binding constants between $10^{-12}$ and $10^{-10}$ M. Cytokines are a chemically diverse group of proteins which share common functions as regulators in the immune system. In addition to the classical interleukins and the chemotactic chemokines, growth factors such as neurotrophins or pro-kineticin 1 (also known as vascular endothelial growth factor, VEGF) or fibroblast growth factor (FGF) and colony-stimulating factors are considered cytokines because they exert pleiotropic actions and have regulatory functions in the immune system. Some cytokines or cytokine receptors are shed by metalloproteases, which therefore are closely related because they regulate cytokines and cytokine receptors in inflammation and cancer [2,55,108,140]. In spite of the redundancy and pleiotropy of the cytokine network, specific actions of individual cytokines and endogenous control mechanisms have been identified. Moreover, an increasing number of the classical proinflammatory cytokines—and more recently, chemokines (chemotactic cytokines)—have been found to be associated with cancer-related pain [46,124,150]. Besides acting as inflammatory mediators, cytokines may also specifically interact with neuronal receptors and ion channels to regulate neuronal excitability, sensitivity to external stimuli, and synaptic plasticity (Fig. 1; for review see also [111].)

## The Classical Proinflammatory Cytokines

### Tumor Necrosis Factor Alpha

Tumor necrosis factor alpha (TNF-$\alpha$) is generally accepted as the prototypic proinflammatory cytokine. It initiates the activation cascade of cytokines, chemokines, and growth factors in the inflammatory response. Histology of experimental tumors shows dedifferentiated carcinoma cells at various mitotic stages and a pronounced infiltration of the neoplastic tissue with macrophages and immune cells producing TNF-$\alpha$ [24,71,73]. Converging evidence points to a strong correlation between the number of macrophages, the level of TNF-$\alpha$ production, and the development of heat hyperalgesia in inflammatory and neuropathic animal models [57,127]. Moreover, an alleviation of heat hyperalgesia has been correlated with delayed recruitment of nonresident macrophages and with reduced levels of TNF-$\alpha$ expression or treatment with TNF-$\alpha$-neutralizing receptor bodies [127]. In animal models, injection of TNF induces mechanical and thermal hyperalgesia and nociceptor sensitization [24,27,98,153], and there is a clear link between TNF and the generation and maintenance of neuropathic pain [63,125,127,128,130,148]. TNF-$\alpha$ elicits neuronal discharge in dorsal root ganglion (DRG) neurons, and injured as well as neighboring uninjured afferent neurons exhibit increased sensitivity to this cytokine [110]. In bone cancer pain, TNF-α is generally accepted as a potent activator of osteoclasts, and injection of TNF-α induces mechanical hyperalgesia [63,147]. Therefore, it is not surprising that the TNF-α antagonist etanercept attenuates mechanical hypersensitivity in the bone cancer model [147], although a cellular mechanism for mechanical sensitization is not

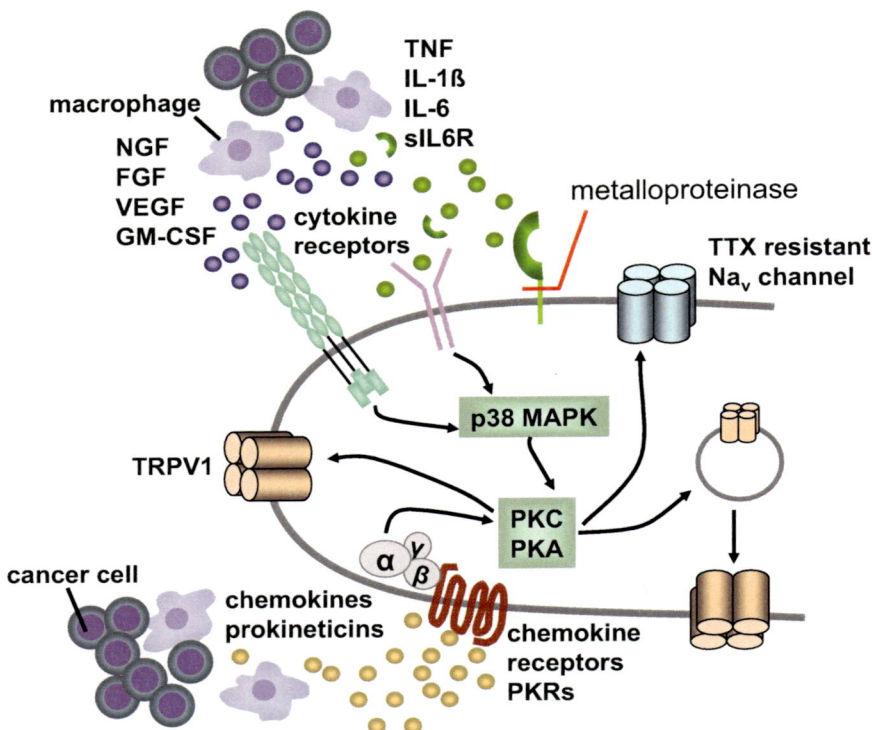

**Fig. 1.** Cytokines bind to specific membrane receptors to regulate nociceptive ion channels in cancer pain. Macrophages or cancer cells release cytokines, chemokines, or growth factors. Binding to membrane receptors or soluble receptors activates intracellular signaling cascades involving protein kinases, which phosphorylate ion channels and increase neuron excitability or sensitivity for natural stimuli. NGF: nerve growth factor, FGF: fibroblast growth factor: VEGF: vascular endothelial derived growth factor (prokineticin 1), GM-CSF: granulocyte macrophage colony-stimulating factor, TNF-α: tumor necrosis factor α, IL-1β: interleukin-1β, IL-6: interleukin-6, sIL-6R: soluble IL-6 receptor, TTX: tetrodotoxin, TRPV1: transient receptor potential vanilloid 1 receptor channel, PKR: prokineticin receptor, p38 MAPK: p38 mitogen- activated protein kinase, PKA: protein kinase A, PKC: protein kinase C.

yet known. More information is available regarding the cellular mechanisms of heat sensitization. However, few studies have addressed cancer-induced heat hyperalgesia.

In normal tissue, the sensation of heat pain occurs at a temperature of ~44°C. This finding correlates well with the activation threshold temperature of polymodal nociceptors and that of the nociceptor-specific heat transducer TRPV1 [22,138,139], a member of the transient receptor potential (TRP) family of ion channels [61]. The sensitivity of TRPV1 to heat and capsaicin depends on the phosphorylation status of the channel at intracellular serine/threonine or tyrosine sites [10,11,70,103]. In a melanoma model, tumor development was accompanied by signs of ongoing pain and heat hyperalgesia [109], and in the bone cancer model, TRPV1 was found to be upregulated in distinct subpopulations of DRG neurons [87]. In the same model, disruption of the TRPV1 gene or administration of a TRPV1 antagonist attenuates both ongoing and movement-evoked nocifensive behaviors that may occur as a consequence of tissue acidosis due to osteolytic activity and the activation of TRPV1 by low pH [44]. In addition, TNF seems to affect nociceptors directly, because sensitization of cutaneous nociceptors to heat also occurs in vitro at physiological pH, which largely excludes secondary effects [24,96].

TNF binds to TNF receptor 1 (TNFR1) and TNF receptor 2 (TNFR2) in the cell membrane. Whereas neuropathic pain largely seems to depend on TNFR1 [69,92,121,144], TNFR2 seems to be more relevant for the development of cancer-induced heat pain and hyperalgesia. However, cancer-induced mechanical hypersensitivity seems to be independent of TNF action [24].

Downstream of its receptors, TNF-α activates protein kinases, including mitogen-activated protein kinase (p38 MAPK) and protein kinase C (PKC) [141]. Heat hyperalgesia induced by TNF is mediated via p38 MAPK [59,78,112], and in cellular models, TNF-α induces a fast sensitization of responses both to heat and to the specific TRPV1 agonist capsaicin, which requires activation of p38 MAPK and PKC [24]. Although PKC phosphorylates TRPV1 at specific sites and regulates channel function [10,138], some of the phosphorylation sites at intracellular domains of the TRPV1 channel protein do not show a preference for PKC, PKA, or calmodulin kinase II (CaMKII) and could be possible targets for p38

MAPK phosphorylation. Besides regulating TRPV1 channel function on the cell membrane, TNF-$\alpha$ also upregulates TRPV1 expression [86]. Upregulation of TRPV1 was found in wild-type but not in TNFR2 knockout mice with experimental cancer [24]. Tumor-induced nociceptor sensitization to heat stimuli is largely prevented after neutralization of TNF-$\alpha$ with etanercept, suggesting that endogenous TNF-$\alpha$ plays a significant role in cancer pain [24]. Similarly, anti-TNF-$\alpha$ treatment of refractory pain in selected cancer patients significantly improves pain scores [136,137]. These findings suggest that TNF-$\alpha$ synthesized and released in tumor tissue induces heat hyperalgesia and pain by directly affecting nociceptors innervating the tumor area. Apart from the fact that TNF-$\alpha$ originating from the tumor itself is an important player in cancer pain, increasing evidence suggests that this cytokine may be of causative significance for pain resulting from cancer chemotherapies (for review see [152]). Mechanical allodynia and hyperalgesia induced by antimitotic paclitaxel was improved by the TNF antagonist and immune modulator thalidomide in an animal model [21]. Taken together, the existing data support the use of TNF-$\alpha$ antagonists in the treatment of cancer-related pain states. In particular, blockade of TNFR2 may open new avenues for pain management in cancer patients. There may be concerns regarding effects on cancer progression or severe inflammation due to immune suppression; however, this potential problem is currently controversial because biological activity of etanercept has also been reported in recurrent cancer.

### Interleukin-1β

More than any other cytokine family, the interleukin-1 (IL-1) family is closely linked to the innate immune response [32]. The IL-1 family consists of two major agonistic proteins, IL-1$\alpha$ and IL-1$\beta$, which are pleiotropic and mainly affect inflammation, immunity, and hemopoiesis. In their secreted form, IL-1$\alpha$ and IL-1$\beta$ bind to the same receptors and induce the same biological function but differ in their compartmentalization within the cell that produces them or the microenvironment. Thus, IL-1$\beta$ is solely active in its secreted form, whereas IL-1$\alpha$ is mainly active in cell-associated forms and is only rarely found as a secreted cytokine, in which case it is mainly produced by macrophages/monocytes (for review, see [6]). IL-1$\beta$ has been studied more than any other member of the IL-1 family because of its role in mediating autoimmune diseases. Major cellular sources for IL-1β in the context of pain include macrophages, glial cells, and both sympathetic and sensory neurons [25,40,150]. Inflammation associated with an adaptive immune response induces hyperalgesia that is mediated by an initial release of TNF-α, which triggers the subsequent release of IL-1β [29,33]; IL-1β then induces pain reflexes, perhaps due to a secondary increase in prostaglandins [115]. Inflammatory hyperalgesia can be prevented by experimental administration of endogenous IL-1 receptor antagonist (IL-1ra), and pain-associated behavior in mice with experimental neuropathy is reduced by neutralizing antibodies to IL-1 receptors [28,29,126].

IL-1 is abundant at tumor sites, being produced by cellular elements of the tumor microenvironment or by the malignant cells, and it affects not only various phases of the malignant process, such as carcinogenesis, tumor growth, and invasiveness, but also patterns of interactions between malignant cells and the host's immune system. Hence, the effects of the IL-1 molecules on the malignant process are complex (for review see [2,6]).

The peripheral pronociceptive actions of IL-1 are probably mediated by a complex signaling cascade and by secondary production of nitric oxide, bradykinin, or prostaglandins, which would explain the sensitization or excitation of nociceptors [35,41,42,58,98]. Expression of IL-1 receptor type I (IL-1RI) mRNA in sensory neurons suggests a possible direct influence of IL-1β on sensory processing [25,90]. IL-1β facilitates heat-evoked release of calcitonin gene-related peptide [96] and sensitizes heat-activated inward currents ($I_{heat}$) in sensory neurons via PKC and tyrosine kinases [90]. In addition, IL-1β acts in a p38 MAPK-dependent manner to increase the excitability of nociceptors by regulating tetrodotoxin-resistant voltage-gated sodium channels [12]. IL-1β induced pain hypersensitivity is largely reduced in mice carrying a null mutation for the voltage-gated sodium channel $Na_v1.9$ [4]. In addition, IL-1β-induced c-Src kinase activation was shown to regulate preprotachykinin gene expression in rat sensory ganglia and substance P secretion [56]. IL1-α and IL-1β both increased neuronal content of substance P. Interestingly, IL1-α was significantly more efficient than IL-1β in inducing substance P expression [122].

Based on its well-established role in tumor immunobiology and its involvement in inflammatory hyperalgesia, it is generally accepted that IL-1β plays a role in cancer pain. IL-1β levels are locally increased in osteosarcoma-bearing mice. To a certain extent, levels of IL-1βa in the spinal cord are also increased. Osteosarcoma-induced thermal and mechanical hyperalgesia is inhibited by high doses of systemic anakinra, a neutralizing anti-IL-1β antibody. This finding suggests that some hyperalgesic symptoms observed in the mouse model of bone cancer pain are mediated by peripheral IL-1β and may be inhibited by antagonists of type I IL-1 receptors [8]. Even the highest concentrations of anakinra were ineffective when administered intrathecally in this study. In contrast, IL-1β is reported to facilitate bone cancer pain in the rat by modulating the nociceptive system at spinal cord level: spinal IL-1β is upregulated and glutamate receptor phosphorylation is increased in rats with bone cancer. Rodents show a reduced mechanical hyperalgesia when treated with exogenous IL-1ra, the naturally occurring soluble IL-1 decoy receptor. In the spinal cord, the phosphorylation status of the NMDA-type glutamate receptor subunit NR1 is regulated by activation of IL-1RI localized in NR1-immunoreactive neurons [156]. Release of IL-1β from spinal microglia may contribute to the central sensitization associated with chronic pain states [47]. IL-1β enhances excitatory and reduces inhibitory spinal synaptic transmission and produces heat hyperalgesia after spinal injection [64]. In addition, data obtained from IL-1R knockout mice show that IL-1β signaling is required for the development of mechanical allodynia [66]. All of these data suggest that IL-β has a significant role in cancer pain and that inhibition of IL-1β signaling could be a relevant clinical strategy in the treatment of patients with cancer pain.

## *Interleukin-6*

Some tumors produce interleukin-6 [135], and elevations of serum IL-6 levels are found in up to 60% of patients with advanced stages of lung cancer [155]. IL-6, although it is involved in the generation of neuropathic pain states [7], may on the other hand protect against chemotherapy-induced neuropathies without impairing the antitumor activity of the antimitotic drugs [20]. The benefit of global neutralization of IL-6 signaling is still a matter of controversy. However, most experimental studies report proinflammatory and pronociceptive roles for IL-6 [31,93,99].

Apart from controlling immune cell interactions, IL-6 and its signal transducing receptor gp130 may account for the pain associated with inflammation, neuropathy, or cancer by directly regulating the sensitivity of pain-sensing neurons. IL-6 knockout mice show reduced thermal hyperalgesia after carrageenan inflammation or nerve constriction [80,154,157]. Antisera neutralizing endogenous IL-6 inhibit inflammatory hyperalgesia [36]. In neuropathic mice, nerve injury correlates well with upregulated IL-6 levels and with the development of thermal hyperalgesia and allodynia [31,80,94]. In most systems, including sympathetic neurons, the effects of IL-6 depend on the presence of the soluble IL-6 receptor (sIL-6R) [74]. After ligand binding, sIL-6R heteromerizes with the signal transducer molecule gp130, which is also utilized by other cytokines of the same family, such as leukemia-inhibitory factor [107,108,133]. The IL-6/sIL-6R complex or hyper-IL-6 (HIL-6), a fusion protein mimicking the effects of the IL-6/sIL-6R complex [37], can increase nociceptor responsiveness and induce thermal hypersensitivity [96,89,91]. The sensitization involved activation of the Janus tyrosine kinase (Jak) and PKC but no alteration in intracellular $Ca^{2+}$. Similar signaling pathways have been identified for IL-6 in promoting the regeneration of spinal axons [18,102]. In addition, IL-6 sensitizes unmyelinated nociceptors to mechanical stimuli [16], and a dual regulation by IL-6 and its soluble receptor sIL-6R has been reported [91]. Both in vitro and in vivo, the IL-6/gp130 ligand-receptor complex induces heat hypersensitivity, which is mediated by activation of PKC-δ via the adapter proteins Gab1/2 and phosphoinositide-3-kinase ($PI_3K$), and by subsequent regulation of TRPV1 [5]. Mice with a selective deletion of the signal transducer protein gp130 in neurons develop significantly reduced levels of inflammatory and tumor-induced pain independently of the degree of inflammation or tumor growth [5].

A pronociceptive effect of peripheral IL-6 is generally accepted, but the role of this cytokine in the central nervous system is still a matter of controversy. In vitro experiments showed that IL-6 induces central sensitization and hyperalgesia via synaptic mechanisms in superficial dorsal horn neurons by decreasing inhibitory synaptic transmission [64]. In contrast, intrathecal injection of IL-6 has been found to inhibit nociceptive transmission following neuropathy [38,39]. In addition, IL-6 upregulates μ-opioid receptor expression [15], which may at least partially explain the influence of cytokine genes on pain and response to analgesia in cancer patients. Individuals carrying the 174C/C IL-6 polymorphism suffer from increased pain severity and require an almost fivefold higher dose of opioids for cancer pain relief as compared with GG or GC genotypes [104]. Both the peripheral and central site of action of IL-6 may also be relevant to the side effects of cancer chemotherapy, which may increase plasma levels of IL-6 [100]. Increased levels of IL-6 have been correlated with sickness behavior in patients [145] and with treatment-associated symptoms such as pain and fatigue [149]. Currently, the launch of inhibitors of IL-6 or gp130 as a novel class of anti-inflammatory drugs has given rise to great hopes for the treatment of rheumatoid arthritis.

## Other Proinflammatory Cytokines

### Colony-Stimulating Factors

Although a number of candidate molecules have been associated with the generation of cancer pain, a mechanism-based understanding of tumor-induced heat hyperalgesia is not yet possible. For example, several types of non-hematopoietic tumors secrete hematopoietic colony-stimulating factors that act on myeloid cells and tumor cells (for review see [49]). Receptors and signaling mediators of granulocyte- and granulocyte-macrophage colony-stimulating factors (G-CSF and GM-CSF) are also found on sensory nerves, and GM-CSF sensitizes nerves to mechanical stimuli in vitro and in vivo. Inhibition of G-CSF and GM-CSF signaling in vivo reduces tumor growth and nerve remodeling and lessens bone cancer pain. G-CSF and GM-CSF are important in tumor-nerve interactions, and recent work suggests that their receptors on primary afferent nerve fibers constitute potential therapeutic targets in cancer pain [116].

### Chemokines

When tissue is invaded by immune cells, as in the case of cancer, chemokines are released as constituents of the resulting "inflammatory soup" [1]. Chemokines are small chemotactic cytokines of about 10 kD that are secreted in damaged tissue by leucocytes, and also by activated glial cells or neurons. More than 45 chemokines have been identified, and their classification is based on the presence and position of cysteine residues. The CC group has two cysteines, and in the CXC group the two cysteines are separated by one other amino acid. The CX3C chemokine CX3CL (also known as fractalkine), where the cysteines are separated by three other amino acid residues, is the only member of its class [158]. Chemokine actions are mediated by a family of seven-transmembrane domain G-protein-coupled receptors. Currently, 19 chemokine receptors have been identified. These receptors are expressed on a variety of cells, including immune cells, endothelial cells, and neurons (for review see [53,79,81,82]). Chemokines promote immune cell migration, induce astrocyte migration, and cause the proliferation of microglia regulating nociceptive transmission in the spinal dorsal horn (for review see [1]). In addition, chemokines such as CCL2 (monocyte chemoattractant protein 1, MCP-1), CCL5, or RANTES are highly expressed by breast cancer cells at primary tumor sites. The tumor-promoting role of CCL2 (MCP-1) is generally accepted [129]. This cytokine has been detected in microperfusates of experimental tumors [65] and is secreted by bone and sarcoma cells in experimental co-cultures of bone and sarcoma tissue. A synergistic interaction between the femur and the sarcoma results in enhanced secretion and expression of CCL2 and depends on the presence of the hematopoietic component of the bone as well as other bone cells [113]. CCL2 (and CXCL1) trigger calcitonin gene-related peptide release by exciting nociceptive neurons [101,131], and CCL2 induces mechanical hyperalgesia after intradermal injection [13]. In addition, CCL2 functions as a neuromodulator in neuropathic pain [13,62]. Therefore, it is very likely that it also contributes to chemical interactions between tumor tissue and sensory neurons to evoke cancer pain. The chemokine network activated at multiple levels of the peripheral and central nervous system has recently been identified as new target for pain relief [46]. Small-molecule antagonists for particular chemokine receptors may therefore not only be useful in acute and chronic inflammation [53,95] but may also be of relevance in cancer biology and pain therapy (for review see [46,123]).

## Growth Factors

A number of growth factors have been associated with the development of malignant tumors and metastasis. In most cases, we are just beginning to understand their role in cancer pain.

## Nerve Growth Factor

Nerve growth factor (NGF) was originally identified as an essential neuronal survival factor in the developing nervous system. In adults, NGF has a crucial role in generating pain and hyperalgesia. The expression of NGF is high in inflamed tissue, and anti-NGF treatment provides effective pain control in animal models of inflammatory pain (for review see [51]). Expression of NGF and its receptor is high in certain types of cancer and immune cells [30,34,142]. Recently, crosstalk between NGF and TNF-α has been associated with certain diseases, including cancer (for review see [134]). In animal models, neutralization of NGF improves bone cancer pain and reduces upregulation of biochemical markers of nociceptor activation, including the activating transcription factor ATF3, which is associated with nerve damage [48,118]. Several pharmaceutical companies have developed approaches to antagonize NGF, including agents that block NGF from binding to its receptors. NGF antagonism is expected to provide effective treatment for chronic pain states, including cancer pain [51,151]. More recently, other growth factors have also been found in cancer tissue.

Bone metastatic breast cancer cells secrete transforming growth factor beta (TGF-β), platelet-derived growth factor (PDGF), and insulin-like growth factor II (IGFII) and contribute to osteolytic lesions [77]. Bone cells are the major contributor of TGF-β and matrix metalloprotease MMP2 in experimental cocultures [113]. In particular, TGF-β has been associated with neuropathic pain after nerve injury [83]. Intrathecal injection of TGF-β produces tactile allodynia by affecting spinal microglia [75], suggesting a remote action on spinal nociceptive processing rather than a peripheral site of action. No direct association with cancer pain has been reported for this cytokine.

## Prokineticins

Prokineticins PK1 (VEGF) and PK2 (Bv8) are tissue-specific angiogenic factors that share certain aspects of cytokines: they are highly expressed by neutrophils and other inflammatory cells and play a role in immune-inflammatory responses. Prokineticin-like hyperalgesic activity was demonstrated in extracts of rat inflammatory granulocytes, and prokineticins seem to be new pronociceptive mediators in inflammatory tissues (for review see [85]). PK1 is significantly elevated in cancer patients [68], and it is secreted by islets and stellate cells in pancreatic cancer [60]. Nociceptors express prokineticin receptors PKR1 and PKR2 under the control of glial-derived neurotrophic factor (GDNF). The receptors for prokineticins are present in a fraction of peptidergic C-fiber neurons and in a fraction of myelinated A-fiber neurons. PKR-expressing neurons also express TRPV1. Bv8, an agonist at both PKR1 and PKR2, has recently been shown to sensitize TRPV1 channels [143]. Intraplantar injection of recombinant PK2 results in a strong and localized hyperalgesia with reduced thresholds to nociceptive stimuli. PK2 mobilizes calcium in dissociated DRG neurons, and mice lacking the PK2 gene display strong reduction in thermal and chemical nociception. However, PK2 mutant mice showed no difference in inflammatory response to capsaicin [54]. Mice lacking the PKR1 gene exhibit impaired Bv8-induced hyperalgesia, develop deficient responses to noxious heat, capsaicin, and protons, and show reduced thermal and mechanical hypersensitivity to paw inflammation, indicating a requirement for PKR1 signaling associated with activation and sensitization of primary afferent fibers [84]. Both PK1 and PK2 have been associated with the malignancy of prostate cancer and with neuroblastoma progression in humans [97]. However, their specific role in cancer pain has never been addressed in detail. This is also the case for several other growth factors, including fibroblast growth factor [9], which have pleiotropic effects and also regulate nociception and pain sensation [43].

## Metalloproteases

Lastly, a potential role will be addressed for the metalloproteases, which represent regulators of entire groups of cytokines and their signaling because they potentially affect receptor activation by shedding of membrane-bound receptor proteins or of target proteins relevant for nociceptor or immune cell function [14]. Matrix metalloproteases (MMPs) are a family of enzymes expressed by human malignant cells [45] that contribute to the degradation of the extracellular matrix. This process is generally accepted to facilitate tumor invasion, metastasis, and angiogenesis. MMP inhibitors are being developed in combination with chemotherapy to potentiate tumor cytotoxicity and to reduce the size and number of metastatic lesions (for review see [26,50]). Despite great initial hopes, the outcome of clinical trials with MMP inhibitors has been disappointing. More recent studies propose the disease-stage-dependent involvement of the metalloproteases MMP-1,-2,-3,-9,-13 and the enzymes ADAM-17 (TNF-converting enzyme, TACE) and ADAM-TS5 as major in vivo mediators of extracellular matrix degradation in inflammation. They represent promising therapeutic targets for treatment of osteoarthritic symptoms. More selective inhibitors are currently being developed (for review see [17]).

The MMPs are emerging as modulators of neuropathic pain [23,67,120]. Paclitaxel-induced painful peripheral neuropathy is a major dose-limiting factor. Recent studies show that macrophages accumulate in the DRG of paclitaxel-treated rats, and their activation is suggested to contribute to generation and development of the neuropathy. The upregulation of MMP-3 following macrophage activation in the DRG might be a significant event that could trigger a series of reactions leading to paclitaxel-induced peripheral neuropathic pain [88]. Therefore, MMP inhibitors could be potentially interesting for pain therapy induced by cancer and chemotherapy.

# Conclusion and Outlook

Severe symptoms persist in many cancer patients, even with the use of targeted therapies. Large individual variations in the responsiveness to treatment and in the severity of symptoms—including pain—have been assumed to result from either disease-related variables (stage of disease), clinical health status (performance status and comorbid conditions), or sociodemographic characteristics (age, sex, race, and marital status). We are only beginning to understand how genetic variations affect the experience of cancer-related symptoms and response to interventions. Cytokines are strongly linked to the symptoms and outcome of cancer [117], and there is significant evidence that polymorphisms in cytokine genes play a role in cancer pain. Cytokine gene variants (for example in the genes expressing TNF-α, IL-8, or IL-6) have been identified as markers for severe and debilitating symptoms associated with cancer or its treatment [105,106]. The long-term goal is to use this understanding of polymorphisms in cytokine genes and other genes to foster the development of targeted antitumor interventions that are the most effective and least toxic for patients surviving cancer. Understanding the molecular epidemiology of cancer-related symptoms offers the opportunity to identify specific genes involved in the cytokine network that could be used for a more personalized treatment of cancer pain. The first step toward a more mechanistic cancer pain therapy could be the use of antagonists or agonists at certain cytokine receptors, which might offer benefits for the patient not only by targeting tumor growth but in addition by relieving pain originating from cancer growth or cancer chemotherapy.

# References

[1]   Abbadie C. Chemokines, chemokine receptors and pain. Trends Immunol 2005;26:529–34.

[2]   Aggarwal BB, Shishodia S, Sandur SK, Pandey MK, Sethi G. Inflammation and cancer: how hot is the link? Biochem Pharmacol 2006;72:1605–21.

[3]   Alexander RB, Ponniah S, Hasday J, Hebel JR. Elevated levels of proinflammatory cytokines in the semen of patients with chronic prostatitis/chronic pelvic pain syndrome. Urology 1998;52:744–9.

[4]   Amaya F, Wang H, Costigan M, Allchorne AJ, Hatcher JP, Egerton J, Stean T, Morisset V, Grose D, Gunthorpe MJ, et al. The voltage-gated sodium channel Na,1.9 is an effector of peripheral inflammatory pain hypersensitivity. J Neurosci 2006;26:12852–60.

[5]   Andratsch M, Mair N, Constantin CE, Scherbakov N, Benetti C, Quarta S, Vogl C, Sailer CA, Üceyler N, Brockhaus J, et al. A key role for gp130 expressed on peripheral sensory nerves in pathological pain. J Neurosci 2009;29:13473–83.

[6]   Apte RN, Voronov E. Is interleukin-1 a good or bad 'guy' in tumor immunobiology and immunotherapy? Immunol Rev 2008;222:222–41.

[7]   Arruda JL, Colburn RW, Rickman AJ, Rutkowski MD, De Leo JA. Increase of interleukin-6 mRNA in the spinal cord following peripheral nerve injury in the rat: potential role of IL-6 in neuropathic pain. Brain Res Mol Brain Res 1998;62:228–35.

[8]   Baamonde A, Curto-Reyes V, Juárez L, Meana A, Hidalgo A, Menéndez L. Antihyperalgesic effects induced by the IL-1 receptor antagonist anakinra and increased IL-1beta levels in inflamed and osteosarcoma-bearing mice. Life Sci 2007;81:673–82.

[9]   Beenken A, Mohammadi M. The FGF family: biology, pathophysiology and therapy. Nat Rev Drug Discov 2009;8:235–53.

[10]  Bhave G, Hu HJ, Glauner KS, Zhu W, Wang H, Brasier DJ, Oxford GS, Gereau RW4. Protein kinase C phosphorylation sensitizes but does not activate the capsaicin receptor transient receptor potential vanilloid 1 (TRPV1). Proc Natl Acad Sci USA 2003;100:12480–5.

[11]  Bhave G, Zhu W, Wang H, Brasier DJ, Oxford GS, Gereau RW. cAMP-dependent protein kinase regulates desensitization of the capsaicin receptor (VR1) by direct phosphorylation. Neuron 2002;35:721–31.

[12]  Binshtok AM, Wang H, Zimmermann K, Amaya F, Vardeh D, Shi L, Brenner GJ, Ji RR, Bean BP, Woolf CJ, Samad TA. Nociceptors are interleukin-1beta sensors. J Neurosci 2008;28:14062–73.

[13]  Bogen O, Dina OA, Gear RW, Levine JD. Dependence of monocyte chemoattractant protein 1 induced hyperalgesia on the isolectin B4-binding protein versican. Neuroscience 2009;159:780–6.

[14]  Bonfil RD, Chinni S, Fridman R, Kim HR, Cher ML. Proteases, growth factors, chemokines, and the microenvironment in prostate cancer bone metastasis. Urol Oncol 2007;25:407–11.

[15]  Börner C, Kraus J, Schröder H, Ammer H, Höllt V. Transcriptional regulation of the human μ-opioid receptor gene by interleukin-6. Mol Pharmacol 2004;66:1719–26.

[16]  Brenn D, Richter F, Schaible HG. Sensitization of unmyelinated sensory fibers of the joint nerve to mechanical stimuli by interleukin-6 in the rat: an inflammatory mechanism of joint pain. Arthritis Rheum 2007;56:351–9.

[17]  Burrage PS, Brinckerhoff CE. Molecular targets in osteoarthritis: metalloproteinases and their inhibitors. Curr Drug Targets 2007;8:293–303.

[18]  Cafferty WBJ, Gardiner NJ, Das P, Qiu J, McMahon SB, Thompson SWN. Conditioning injury-induced spinal axon regeneration fails in interleukin-6 knock-out mice. J Neurosci 2004;24:4432–43.

[19]  Cain DM, Wacnik PW, Turner M, Wendelschafer-Crabb G, Kennedy WR, Wilcox GL, Simone DA. Functional interactions between tumor and peripheral nerve: changes in excitability and morphology of primary afferent fibers in a murine model of cancer pain. J Neurosci 2001;21:9367–76.

[20]  Callizot M, Andriambeloson E, Glass J, Revel M, Ferro P, Cirillo R, Vitte PA, Dreano M. Interleukin-6 protects against paclitaxel, cisplatin and vincristine-induced neuropathies without impairing chemotherapeutic activity. Cancer Chemother Pharmacol 2008;62:995–1007.

[21]  Cata JP, Weng HR, Dougherty PM. The effects of thalidomide and monocycline on taxol-induced hyperalgesia in rats. Brain Res 2008;1229:100–10.

[22]  Caterina MJ, Schumacher MA, Tominaga M, Rosen TA, Levine JD, Julius D. The capsaicin receptor: a heat-activated ion channel in the pain pathway. Nature 1997;389:816–24.

[23]  Chattopadhyay S, Myers RR, Janes J, Shubayev VI. Cytokine regulation of MMP-9 in peripheral glia: implications for pathological processes and pain in injured nerve. Brain Behav Immun 2007;21:561–8.

[24]  Constantin CE, Mair N, Sailer CA, Andratsch M, Xu ZZ, Blumer MJ, Scherbakov N, Davis JB, Bluethmann H, Ji RR, Kress M. Endogenous necrosis factor alpha (TNFalpha) requires TNF receptor type 2 to generate heat hyperalgesia in a mouse cancer model. J Neurosci 2008;28:5072–81.

[25]  Copray JC, Mantingh I, Brouwer N, Biber K, Kust BM, Liem RS, Huitinga I, Tilders FJ, Van Dam AM. Expression of interleukin-1beta in rat dorsal root ganglia. J Neuroimmunol 2001;118:203–11.

[26]  Coussens LM, Fingleton B, Matrisian LM. Matrix metalloproteinase inhibitors and cancer: trials and tribulations. Science 2002;295:2387–92.

[27]  Cunha FQ, Poole S, Lorenzetti BB, Ferreira SH. The pivotal role of tumour necrosis factor alpha in the development of inflammatory hyperalgesia. Br J Pharmacol 1992;107:660–4.

[28]  Cunha JM, Cunha FQ, Poole S, Ferreira SH. Cytokine-mediated inflammatory hyperalgesia limited by interleukin-1 receptor antagonist. Br J Pharmacol 2000;130:1418–24.

[29]  Cunha TM, Verri WA Jr, Valério DA, Guerrero AT, Noqueira LG, Vieira SM, Souza DG, Teixeira MM, Poole S, Ferreira SH, Cunha FQ. Role of cytokines in mediating mechanical hypernociception in a model of delayed-type hypersensitivity in mice. Eur J Pain 2008;12:1059–66.

[30]  Dang C, Zhang Y, Ma Q, Shimahara Y. Expression of nerve growth factor receptors is correlated with progression and prognosis of human pancreatic cancer. J Gastroenterol Hepatol 2006;232:90–8.

[31]  DeLeo JA, Colburn RW, Nichols M, Malhotra A. Interleukin-6-mediated hyperalgesia/allodynia and increased spinal IL-6 expression in a rat mononeuropathy model. J Interferon Cytokine Res 1996;16:695–700.

[32]  Dinarello CA. Immunological and inflammatory functions of the interleukin-1 family. Annu Rev Immunol 2009;27:519–50.

[33]  Dinarello CA, Cannon JG, Wolff S, Bernheim HA, Beutler B, Cerami A, Figari IS, Palladino MA Jr, O'Connor JV. Tumor necrosis factor (cachectin) is an endogenous pyrogen and induces production of interleukin 1. J Exp Med 1986;163:1433–50.

[34]  Dolle L, El Yazidi-Belkoura I, Andraenssens E, Nurcombe V, Hondermarck H. Nerve growth factor overexpression and autocrine loop in breast cancer cells. Oncogene 2003;22:5592–601.

[35]  Ferreira SH, Lorenzetti BB, Bristow AF, Poole S. Interleukin-1β as a potent hyperalgesic agent antagonized by a tripeptide analogue. Nature 1988;334:698–700.

[36]  Ferreira SH, Lorenzetti BB, Poole S. Bradykinin initiates cytokine-mediated inflammatory hyperalgesia. Br J Pharmacol 1993;110:1227–31.

[37]  Fischer A, Goldschmitt J, Peschel C, Brakenhoff JP, Kallen KJ, Wollmer A, Grotzinger J, Rose-John S. A bioactive designer cytokine for human haematopoietic progenitor cell expansion. Nat Biotechnol 1997;15:142–5.

[38]  Flatters SJ, Fox A, Dickenson AH. Spinal interleukin-6 (IL-6) inhibits nociceptive transmission following neuropathy. Brain Res 2003;984:54–62.

[39]  Flatters SJ, Fox AJ, Dickenson AH. Nerve injury alters the effects of interleukin-6 on nociceptive transmission in peripheral afferents. Eur J Pharmacol 2004;484:183–91.

[40]  Freidin M, Bennett MV, Kessler JA. Cultured sympathetic neurons synthesized and release the cytokine interleukin-1beta. Proc Nat Acad Sci USA 1992;89:10440–3.

[41] Fu LW, Longhurst JC. Interleukin-1beta sensitizes abdominal visceral afferents of cats to ischaemia and histamine. J Physiol 1999;521:249–60.

[42] Fukuoka H, Kawatani M, Hisamitsu T, Takeshige C. Cutaneous hyperalgesia induced by peripheral injection of interleukin-1beta in the rat. Brain Res 1994;657:133–40.

[43] Furushu M, Dupree JL, Bryant M, Bansal R. Disruption of fibroblast growth factor receptor signaling in nonmyelinating Schwann cells causes sensory axonal neuropathy and impairment of thermal pain sensitivity. J Neurosci 2009;29:1608–14.

[44] Ghilardi JR, Röhrich H, Lindsay TH, Sevcik MA, Schwei MJ, Kubota K, Halvorson KG, Poblete J, Chaplan SR, Dubin AE, et al. Selective blockade of the capsaicin receptor TRPV1 attenuates bone cancer pain. J Neurosci 2005;25:3126–31.

[45] Gorovetz M, Schwob O, Krimsky M, Yedgar S, Reich R. MMP production in human fibrosarcoma cells and their invasiveness are regulated by group IB secretory phospholipase A2 receptor-mediated activation of cytosolic phospholipase A2. Front Biosci 2008;13:1917–25.

[46] Gosselin RD, Dansereau MA, Pohl M, Kitabqi P, Beaudet N, Sarret P, Mélik Parsadaniantz S. Chemokine network in the nervous system: a new target for pain relief. Curr Med Chem 2008;15:2866–75.

[47] Gustafson-Vickers SL, Lu VB, Lai AY, Todd KG, Ballanyi K, Smith PA. Long-term actions of interleukin-1beta on delay and tonic firing neurons in rat superficial dorsal horn and their relevance to central sensitization. Mol Pain 2008;4:63.

[48] Halvorson KG, Kubota K, Sevcik MA, Lindsay TH, Sotillo JW, Ghilardi JR, Rosol TJ, Boustany L, Shelton DL, Mantyh PW. A blocking antibody to nerve growth factor attenuates skeletal pain induced by prostate tumor cells growing in bone. Cancer Res 2005;65:9426–35.

[49] Hamilton JA. Colony-stimulating factors in inflammation and autoimmunity. Nat Rev Immunol 2008;8:532–44.

[50] Heath EI, Grochow LB. Clinical potential of matrix metalloprotease inhibitors in cancer therapy. Drugs 2000;59:1043–55.

[51] Hefti FF, Rosenthal A, Walicke PA, Wyatt S, Vergara G, Shelton DL, Davies AM. Novel class of pain drugs based on antagonism of NGF. Trends Pharmacol Sci 2006;27:85–91.

[52] Honore P, Luger NM, Sabino MA, Schwei MJ, Rogers SD, Mach DB, O'Keefe PF, Ramnaraine ML, Clohisy DR, Mantyh PW. Osteoprotegerin blocks bone cancer-induced skeletal destruction, skeletal pain and pain-related neurochemical reorganization of the spinal cord. Nat Med 2000;6:521–8.

[53] Horuk R. Chemokine receptor antagonists: overcoming developmental hurdles. Nat Rev Drug Discov 2009;8:23–33.

[54] Hu WP, Zhang C, Li JD, Luo ZD, Amadesi S, Bunnett N, Zhou QY. Impaired pain sensation in mice lacking prokineticin 2. Mol Pain 2006;2:35–43.

[55] Huang SC, Sheu BC, Chang WC, Cheng CY, Wang PH, Lin S. Extracellular matrix proteases: cytokine regulation role in cancer and pregnancy. Front Biosci 2009;14:1571–88.

[56] Igwe OJ. c-Src kinase activation regulates preprotachykinin gene expression and substance P secretion in rat sensory ganglia. Eur J Neurosci 2003;18:1719–30.

[57] Inglis JJ, Nissim A, Lees DM, Hunt SP, Chernajovsky Y, Kidd BL. The differential contribution of tumour necrosis factor to thermal and mechanical hyperalgesia during chronic inflammation. Arthritis Res Ther 2005;7:R807–16.

[58] Inoue A, Ikoma K, Morioka N, Kumagai K, Hashimoto T, Hide I, Nakata Y. Interleukin-1β induces substance P release from primary afferent neurons through the cyclooxygenase system. J Neurochem 1999;73:2206–13.

[59] Ji R, Samad T, Jin S, Schmoll R, Woolf C. p38 MAPK activation by NGF in primary sensory neurons after inflammation increases TRPV1 levels and maintains heat hyperalgesia. Biophys J 2002;36:57–68.

[60] Jiang X, Abiatari I, Kong B, Erkan M, De Oliveira T, Giese NA, Michaelski CW, Friess H, Kleeff J. Pancreatic islet and stellate cells are the main sources of endocrine gland-derived vascular endothelial growth factor/prokineticin-1 in pancreatic cancer. Pancreatology 2009;9:165–72.

[61] Jordt SE, McKemy DD, Julius D. Lessons from peppers and peppermint: the molecular logic of thermosensation. Curr Opin Neurobiol 2003;13:487–92.

[62] Jung H, Toth PT, White FA, Miller RJ. Monocyte chemoattractant protein-1 functions as a neuromodulator in dorsal root ganglia neurons. J Neurochem 2008;104:254–63.

[63] Junger H, Sorkin LS. Nociceptive and inflammatory effects of subcutaneous TNFalpha. Pain 2000;85:145–51.

[64] Kawasaki Y, Zhang L, Cheng JK, Ji RR. Cytokine mechanisms of central sensitization: distinct and overlapping role of interleukin-1beta, interleukin-6, and tumor necrosis factor-alpha in regulating synaptic and neuronal activity in the superficial spinal cord. J Neurosci 2008;28:5189–94.

[65] Khasabova IA, Stucky CL, Harding-Rose C, Eikmeier L, Beitz AJ, Coicou LG, Hanson AE, Simone DA, Seybold VS. Chemical interactions between fibrosarcoma cancer cells and sensory neurons contribute to cancer pain. J Neurosci 2007;27:10289–98.

[66] Kleibeuker W, Gabay E, Kavelaars A, Zijlstra J, Wolf G, Ziv N, Yirmiya R, Shavit Y, Tal M, Heijnen CJ. IL-1 beta signaling is required for mechanical allodynia induced by nerve injury and for the ensuing reduction in spinal cord neuronal GRK2. Brain Behav Immun 2008;22:200–8.

[67] Kobayashi H, Chattopadhyay S, Kato K, Dolkas J, Kikuchi S, Myers RR, Shubayev VI. MMPs initiate Schwann cell-mediated MBP degradation and mechanical nociception after nerve damage. Mol Cell Neurosci 2008;39:619–27.

[68] Kraft A, Weindel K, Ochs A, Marth C, Zmija J, Schumacher P, Unger C, Marmé D, Gastl G. Vascular endothelial growth factor in the sera and effusions of patients with malignant and nonmalignant disease. Cancer 1999;85:178–87.

[69] Li Y, Ji A, Weihe E, Schäfer MK. Cell-specific expression and lipopolysaccharide-induced regulation of tumor necrosis factor alpha (TNFalpha) and TNF receptors in rat dorsal root ganglion. J Neurosci 2004;24:9623–31.

[70] Mandadi S, Tominaga T, Numazaki M, Murayama N, Saito N, Armati PJ, Roufogalis BD, Tominaga M. Increased sensitivity of desensitized TRPV1 by PMA occurs through PKCepsilon-mediated phosphorylation at S800. Pain 2006;123:106–16.

[71] Mantyh PW. Cancer pain and its impact on diagnosis, survival and quality of life. Nat Rev Neurosci 2006;7:797–809.

[72] Mantyh PW, Clohisy DR, Koltzenburg M, Hunt SP. Molecular mechanisms of cancer pain. Nat Rev Cancer 2002;2:201–9.

[73] Mantyh PW, Hunt SP. Mechanisms that generate and maintain bone cancer pain. Novartis Found Symp 2004;260:221–38.

[74] März P, Otten U, Rose-John S. Neural activities of IL-6-type cytokines often depend on soluble cytokine receptors. Eur J Neurosci 1999;11:2995–3004.

[75] Masuda J, Tsuda M, Tozaki-Saitoh H, Inoue K. Intrathecal delivery of PDGF produces tactile allodynia through its receptors in spinal microglia. Mol Pain 2009;11:23–32.

[76] Mercadante S, Radbruch L, Caraceni A, Cherny N, Kaasa S, Nauck F, Rimpanonti C, De Conno F; Steering Committee of the European Association for Palliative Care (EAPC) Research Network. Episodic (breakthrough) pain: consensus conference of an expert working group of the European Association for Palliative Care. Cancer 2002;94:832–9.

[77] Mercer RR, Mastro AM. Cytokines secreted by bone-metastatic breast cancer cells alter the expression pattern of f-actin and reduce focal adhesion plaques in osteoblasts through PI3K. Exp Cell Res 2005;310:270–81.

[78] Milligan ED, Twining C, Chacur M, Biedenkapp J, O'Connor K, Poole S, Tracey K, Martin D, Maier SF, Watkins LR. Spinal glia and proinflammatory cytokines mediate mirror-image neuropathic pain in rats. J Neurosci 2003;23:1026–40.

[79] Murdoch C, Finn A. Chemokine receptors and their role in inflammation and infectious diseases. Blood 2000;95:3032–43.

[80] Murphy PG, Ramer MS, Borthwick L, Gauldie J, Richardson PM, Bisby MA. Endogenous interleukin-6 contributes to hypersensitivity to cutaneous stimuli and changes in neuropeptides associated with chronic nerve constriction in mice. Eur J Neurosci 1999;11:2243–53.

[81] Murphy PM. International Union of Pharmacology. XXX. Update on chemokine receptor nomenclature. Pharmacol Rev 2002;54:227–9.

[82] Murphy PM, Baggiolini M, Charo IF, Hébert CA, Horuk R, Matsushima K, Miller LG, Oppenheim JJ, Power CA. International Union of Pharmacology. XXII. Nomenclature for chemokine receptors. Pharmacol Rev 2000;52:145–56.

[83] Narita M, Usui A, Narita M, Niikura K, Nozaki H, Khotib J, Nabumo Y, Yajima Y, Suzuki T. Protease-activated receptor-1 and platelet-derived growth factor in spinal cord neurons are implicated in neuropathic pain after nerve injury. J Neurosci 2005;25:10000–9.

[84] Negri L, Lattanzi R, Giannini E, Colucci M, Margheriti F, Melchiorri P, Vellani V, Tian H, DeFelice M, Porreca F. Impaired nociception and inflammatory pain sensation in mice lacking the prokineticin receptor PKR1: focus on interaction between PKR1 and the capsaicin receptor TRPV1 in pain behavior. J Neurosci 2006;26:6716–27.

[85] Negri L, Lattanzi R, Giannini E, Melchiorri P. Modulators of pain: bv8 and prokineticins. Curr Neuropharmacol 2006;4:215.

[86] Nicol GD, Lopshire JC, Pafford CM. Tumor necrosis factor enhances the capsaicin sensitivity of rat sensory neurons. J Neurosci 1997;17:975–82.

[87] Niiyama Y, Kawamata T, Yamamoto J, Omote K, Namiki A. Bone cancer increases transient receptor potential vanilloid subfamily 1 expression within distinct subpopulations of dorsal root ganglion neurons. Neuroscience 2007;148:560–72.

[88] Nishida K, Kuchiiwa S, Oiso S, Futagawa T, Masuda S, Takeda Y, Yamada K. Up-regulation of matrix metalloproteinase-3 in the dorsal root ganglion of rats with paclitaxel-induced neuropathy. Cancer Sci 2008;99:1618–25.

[89] Obreja O, Biasio W, Andratsch M, Lips KS, Rathee PK, Ludwig A, Rose-John S, Kress M. Fast modulation of heat-activated ionic current by proinflammatory interleukin 6 in rat sensory neurons. Brain 2005;128:1634–41.

[90. Obreja O, Rathee PK, Lips S, Distler C, Kress M. IL-1β potentiates heat-activated currents in rat sensory neurons: involvement of IL-1RI, tyrosine kinase and protein kinase C. FASEB J 2002;16:1497–1503.

[91] Obreja O, Schmelz M, Poole S, Kress M. Interleukin-6 in combination with its soluble IL-6 receptor sensitizes rat skin nociceptors to heat, in vivo. Pain 2002;96:57–62.

[92] Ohtori S, Takahashi K, Moriya H, Myers RR. TNF-alpha and TNF-alpha receptor type 1 upregulation in glia and neurons after peripheral nerve injury: studies in murine DRG and spinal cord. Spine 2004;29:1082–8.

[93] Oka T, Oka K, Hosoi M, Hori T. Intracerebroventricular injection of interleukin-6 induces thermal hyperalgesia in rats. Brain Res 1995;692:123–8.

[94] Okamoto K, Martin DP, Schmelzer JD, Mitsui Y, Low PA. Pro- and anti-inflammatory cytokine expression in rat sciatic nerve chronic constriction injury model of neuropathic pain. Exp Neurol 2001;169:386–91.

[95] Onuffer JJ, Horuk R. Chemokines, chemokine receptors and small-molecule antagonists: recent developments. Trends Pharmacol Sci 2002;23:459–67.

[96] Oprée A, Kress M. Involvement of the proinflammatory cytokines tumor necrosis factor-α, IL-1β, and IL-6 but not IL-8 in the development of heat hyperalgesia: effects on heat-evoked calcitonin gene-related peptide release from rat skin. J Neurosci 2000;20:6289–93.

[97] Pasquali D, Rossi V, Staibano S, De Rosa G, Chieffi P, Prezioso D, Mirone V, Mascolo M, Tramontano D, Bellastella A, Sinisi AA. The endocrine-gland-derived vascular endothelial growth factor (EG-VEGF)/prokineticin 1 and 2 and receptor expression in human prostate: up-regulation of EG-VEGF/prokineticin 1 with malignancy. Endocrinology 2006;147:4245–51.

[98] Perkins MN, Kelly D. Interleukin-1 beta induced-desArg9bradykinin-mediated thermal hyperalgesia in the rat. Neuropharmacology 1994;33:657–60.

[99] Poole S, Cunha FQ, Selkirk S, Lorenzetti BB, Ferreira SH. Cytokine-mediated inflammatory hyperalgesia limited by interleukin-10. Br J Pharmacol 1995;115:684–8.

[100] Pusztai L, Mendoza TR, Reuben JM, Martinez MM, Willey JS, Lara K, Syed A, Fritsche HA, Bruera E, Booser D, et al. Changes in plasma levels of inflammatory cytokines in response to paclitaxel chemotherapy. Cytokine 2004;25:94–102.

[101] Qin X, Wan Y, Wang X. CCL2 and CXCL1 trigger calcitonin gene-related peptide release by exciting primary nociceptive neurons. J Neurosci Res 2005;82:51–62.

[102] Qiu J, Cafferty WBJ, McMahon SB, Thompson SWN. Conditioning injury-induced spinal axon regeneration requires signal transducer and activator of transcription 3 activation. J Neurosci 2005;25:1645–53.

[103] Rathee PK, Distler C, Obreja O, Neuhuber W, Wang GK, Wang SY, Nau C, Kress M. PKA/AKAP/VR-1 module: A common link of Gs-mediated signaling to thermal hyperalgesia. J Neurosci 2002;22:4740–5.

[104] Reyes-Gibby CC, El Osta B, Spitz MR, Parsons H, Kurzrock R, Wu X, Shete S, Bruera E. The influence of tumor necrosis factor-alpha G/A and IL-6−174 G/C on pain and analgesia response in lung cancer patients receiving supportive care. Cancer Epidemiol Biomarkers Prev 2008;17:3262–7.

[105] Reyes-Gibby CC, Spitz M, Wu X, Merriman K, Etzel C, Bruera E, Kurzrock R, Shete S. Cytokine genes and pain severity in lung cancer: exploring the influence of TNF-alpha-308 G/A IL6-174G/C and IL8-251T/A. Cancer Epidemiol Biomarkers Prev 2007;16:2745–51.

[106] Reyes-Gibby CC, Wu X, Spitz M, Kurzrock R, Fisch M, Bruera E, Shete S. Molecular epidemiology, cancer-related symptoms, and cytokines pathway. Lancet Oncol 2008;9:777–85.

[107] Rose-John S, Heinrich P. Soluble receptors for cytokines and growth factors: generation and biological function. Biochem J 1994;300:281–90.

[108] Rose-John S, Mitsuyama K, Matsumoto S, Thaiss WM, Scheller J. Interleukin-6 trans-signaling and colonic cancer associated with inflammatory bowel disease. Curr Pharm Des 2009;15:2095–103.

[109] Sasamura T, Nakamura S, Iida Y, Fujii H, Murata J, Saiki I, Nojima H, Kuraishi Y. Morphine analgesia suppresses tumor growth and metastasis in a mouse model of cancer pain produced by orthotopic tumor inoculation. Eur J Pharmacol 2002;441:185–91.

[110] Schäfers M, Lee DH, Brors D, Yaksh TL, Sorkin LS. Increased sensitivity of injured and adjacent uninjured rat primary sensory neurons to exogenous tumor necrosis factor-alpha after spinal nerve ligation. J Neurosci 2003;23:3028–38.

[111] Schäfers M, Sorkin LS. Effect of cytokines on neuronal excitability. Neurosci Lett 2008;437:188–93.

[112] Schäfers M, Svensson CI, Sommer C, Sorkin LS. Tumor necrosis factor-alpha induces mechanical allodynia after spinal nerve ligation by activation of p38 MAPK in primary sensory neurons. J Neurosci 2003;23:2517–21.

[113] Schiller KR, Zillhardt MR, Alley J, Borjesson DL, Beitz AJ, Mauro LJ. Secretion of MCP-1 and other paracrine factors in a novel tumor-bone coculture model. BMC Cancer 2009;9:45.

[114] Schwei MJ, Honoré P, Rogers SD, Salak-Johnson JL, Finke MP, Ramnaraine ML, Clohisy DR, Mantyh CR. Neurochemical and cellular reorganization of the spinal cord in a murine model of bone cancer pain. J Neurosci 1999;19:10886–97.

[115] Schweizer A, Feige U, Fontana A, Müller K, Dinarello CA. Interleukin-1 enhances pain reflexes. Mediation through increased prostaglandin $E_2$ levels. Agents Actions 1988;25:246–51.

[116] Schweizerhof M, Stösser S, Kurejova M, Njoo C, Gangadharan V, Agarwal N, Schmelz M, Bali KK, Michalski CW, Brugger S, et al. Hematopoietic colony-stimulating factors mediate tumor-nerve interactions and bone cancer pain. Nat Med 2009;15:802–7.

[117] Seruga B, Zhang H, Bernstein LJ, Tannock IF. Cytokines and their relationship to the symptoms and outcome of cancer. Nat Rev Cancer 2008;8:887–99.

[118] Sevcik MA, Ghilardi JR, Peters CA, Lindsay TH, Halvorson KG, Jonas BM, Kubota K, Kuskowski MA, Boustany L, Shelton DL, Mantyh PW. Anti-NGF therapy profoundly reduces bone cancer pain and the accompanying increase in markers of peripheral and central sensitization. Pain 2005;115:128–41.

[119] Shimoyama M, Tanaka K, Hasue F, Shimoyama N. A mouse model of neuropathic cancer pain. Pain 2002;99:167–74.

[120] Shubayev VI, Angert M, Dolkas J, Campana WM, Palenscar K, Myers RR. TNF-alpha-induced MMP-9 promotes macrophage recruitment into injured peripheral nerve. Mol Cell Neurosci 2006;31:407–15.

[121] Shubayev VI, Myers RR. Upregulation and interaction of TNFalpha and gelatinases A and B in painful peripheral nerve injury. Brain Res 2000;855:83–9.

[122] Skoff AM, Zhao C, Adler JE. Interleukin-1alpha regulates substance P expression and release in adult sensory neurons. Exp Neurol 2009;217:395–400.

[123] Slettenaar VI, Wilson JL. The chemokine network: a target in cancer biology? Adv Drug Deliv Rev 2006;58:962–74.

[124] Sommer C, Kress M. Recent findings on how proinflammatory cytokines cause pain: peripheral mechanisms in inflammatory and neuropathic hyperalgesia. Neurosci Lett 2004;361:184–7.

[125] Sommer C, Lindenlaub T, Teuteberg P, Schäfers M, Hartung T, Toyka K. Anti-TNF-neutralizing antibodies reduce pain-related behavior in two different mouse models of painful mononeuropathy. Brain Res 2001;913:86–9.

[126] Sommer C, Petrausch S, Lindenlaub T, Toyka K. Neutralizing antibodies to interleukin 1-receptor reduce pain associated behavior in mice with experimental neuropathy. Neurosci Lett 1999;270:25–8.

[127] Sommer C, Schäfers M. Painful mononeuropathy in C57BL/Wld mice with delayed Wallerian degeneration: differential effects of cytokine production and nerve regeneration on thermal and mechanical hypersensitivity. Bain Res 1998;784:154–62.

[128] Sommer C, Schäfers M, Marziniak M, Toyka KV. Etanercept reduces hyperalgesia in experimental painful neuropathy. J Periph Nerv Syst 2001;6:67–72.

[129] Soria G, Ben-Baruch A. The inflammatory chemokines CCL2 and CCL5 in breast cancer. Cancer Lett 2008;267:271–85.

[130] Sorkin LS, Xiao WH, Wagner R, Myers RR. Tumor necrosis factor-alpha induces ectopic activity in nociceptive primary afferent fibres. Neuroscience 1997;81:255–63.

[131] Sun JH, Yang B, Donnelly DF, Ma C, LaMotte RH. MCP-1 enhances excitability of nociceptive neurons in chronically compressed dorsal root ganglia. J Neurophysiol 2006;96:2189–99.

[132] Svendsen KB, Andersen S, Arnason S, Arnér S, Breivik H, Heiskanen T, Kalso E, Kongsgaard UE, Sjögren P, Strang P, et al. Breakthrough pain in malignant and non-malignant diseases: a review of prevalence, characteristics and mechanisms. Eur J Pain 2005;9:195–206.

[133] Taga T, Hibi M, Hirata Y, Yamasaki K, Yasukawa K, Matsuda T, Hirano T, Kishimoto T. Interleukin-6 triggers the association of its receptor with a possible signal transducer, gp130. Cell 1989;58:573–81.

[134] Takei Y, Laskey R. Interpreting crosstalk between TNF-alpha and NGF: potential implications for disease. Trends Mol Med 2008;14:381–8.

[135] Takeuchi E, Ito M, Mori M, Yamaguchi T, Nakagawa M, Yokota S, Nishikawa H, Sakuma-Mochizuki J, Hayashi S, Ogura T. Lung cancer producing interleukin-6. Intern Med 1996;35:212–4.

[136] Tobinick EL. Targeted etanercept for treatment-refractory pain due to bone metastasis: two case reports. Clin Ther 2003;25:2279–88.

[137] Tobinick EL, Davoodifar S. Efficacy of etanercept delivered by perispinal administration for chronic back and/or neck disc-related pain: a study of clinical observations in 143 patients. Curr Med Res Opin 2004;20:1075–85.

[138] Tominaga M, Caterina MJ, Malmberg AB, Rosen TA, Gilbert H, Skinner K, Raumann BE, Basbaum AI, Julius D. The cloned capsaicin receptor integrates multiple pain-producing stimuli. Neuron 1998;21:531–43.

[139] Tominaga M, Tominaga T. Structure and function of TRPV1. Pflugers Arch 2005;451:143–50.

[140] Van Lint P, Libert C. Chemokine and cytokine processing by matrix metalloproteinases and its effect on leukocyte migration and inflammation. J Leukoc Biol 2007;82:1375–81.

[141] Vandenabeele P, Declercq W, Beyaert R, Fiers W. Two tumour necrosis factor receptors: structure and function. Trends Cell Biol 1995;5:392–9.

[142] Vega JA, Garcia-Suarez O, Hannestad J, Perez-Perez M, Germana A. Neurotrophins and the immune system. J Anat 2003;203:1–19.

[143] Vellani V, Colucci M, Lattanzi R, Giannini E, Negri L, Melchiorri P, McNaughton PA. Sensitization of transient receptor potential vanilloid 1 by the prokineticin receptor agonist Bv8. J Neurosci 2006;26:5109–16.

[144] Vogel C, Lindenlaub T, Tiegs G, Toyka KV, Sommer C. Pain-related behavior in TNF-receptor deficient mice. In: Devor M, Rowbotham MC, Wiesenfeld-Hallin Z. Proceedings of the 9th World Congress on Pain, Progress in pain research and management, Vol. 16. Seattle, IASP Press; 2000. p. 249–57.

[145] Vollmer-Conna U, Fazou C, Cameron B, Li H, Brennan C, Luck L, Davenport T, Wakefield D, Hickie I, Lloyd A. Production of pro-inflammatory cytokines correlates with the symptoms of acute sickness behaviour in humans. Psychol Med 2004;34:1289–97.

[146] Wacnik PW, Eikmeier LJ, Ruggles TR, Ramnaraine ML, Walcheck BK, Beitz AJ, Wilcox GL. Functional interactions between tumor and peripheral nerve: morphology, algogen identification, and behavioral characterization of a new murine model of cancer pain. J Neurosci 2001;21:9355–66.

[147] Wacnik PW, Eikmeier LJ, Simone DA, Wilcox GL, Beitz AJ. Nociceptive characteristics of tumor necrosis factor-alpha in naive and tumor-bearing mice. Neuroscience 2005;132:479–91.

[148] Wagner R, Myers RR. Endoneurial injection of TNF-alpha produces neuropathic pain behaviors. Neuroreport 1997;7:2897–2901.

[149] Wang XS, Williams LA, Cleeland CS, Mobley GM, Reuben JM, Lee BN, Giralt SA. Serum interleukin-6 predicts the development of multiple symptoms at nadir of allogeneic hematopoietic stem cell transplantation. Cancer 2008;113:2102–9.

[150] Watkins LR, Maier SF. Cytokines and pain. Basel: Birkhäuser; 1999.

[151] Watson JJ, Allen SJ, Dawbarn D. Targeting nerve growth factor in pain: what is the therapeutic potential. BioDrugs 2008;22:349–59.

[152] Wood LJ, Nail LM, Gilster A, Winters KA, Elsea CR. Cancer chemotherapy-related symptoms: evidence to suggest a role for proinflammatory cytokines. Oncol Nurs Forum 2006;33:535–42.

[153] Woolf CJ, Allchorne A, Safieh-Garabedian B, Poole S. Cytokines, nerve growth factor and inflammatory hyperalgesia: the contribution of tumor necrosis factor alpha. Br J Pharmacol 1997;121:417–24.

[154] Xu XJ, Hao JX, Andell-Jonsson S, Poli V, Bartfai T, Wiesenfeld-Hallin Z. Nociceptive responses in interleukin-6-deficient mice to peripheral inflammation and peripheral nerve section. Cytokine 1997;9:1028–33.

[155] Yamaguchi T, Yamamoto Y, Yokota S, Nakagawa M, Ito M, Ogura T. Involvement of interleukin-6 in the elevation of plasma fibrinogen levels in lung cancer patients. Jpn J Clin Oncol 1998;28:740–4.

[156] Zhang RX, Liu B, Wang L, Ren K, Qiao J-T, Berman BM, Lao L. Interleukin 1β facilitates bone cancer pain in rats by enhancing NMDA receptor NR-1 subunit phosphorylation. Neuroscience 2008;154:1533–8.

[157] Zhong J, Dietzel DI, Wahle P, Kopf M, Heumann R. Sensory impairments and delayed regeneration of sensory axons in interleukin-6-deficient mice. J Neurosci 1999;19:4305–13.

[158] Zlotnik A, Yoshie O. Chemokines: a new classification system and their role in immunity. Immunity 2000;12:121–7.

***Correspondence to:*** Michaela Kress, Dr. med., Department of Physiology, Medical University Innsbruck, Fritz Pregl Str. 3, Innsbruck 6020, Austria. Email: michaela.kress@i-med.ac.at.

# General Inflammatory Reaction and Cachexia in Cancer: Implications for Hyperalgesia

**Marie T. Fallon,[a] Lesley Colvin,[b] and Barry J.A. Laird[a]**

[a]*Institute of Genetics and Molecular Medicine, University of Edinburgh, Edinburgh, United Kingdom;* [b]*Department of Clinical Neurosciences, Western General Hospital, Edinburgh, United Kingdom*

Cancer is associated with many symptoms, both physical (e.g. pain and nausea) and psychological (e.g. distress and depression). Pain is the most common symptom in cancer, with some studies reporting that approximately 90% of patients have pain [3]. Some cancer sequelae, such as changes in weight, are more subtle in their presentation than cancer pain. Weight gain or loss are frequently regarded as good and bad signs, respectively, in patients with cancer. Loss of weight (principally the loss of lean tissue) results in the development of cancer cachexia, which is almost always associated with disease progression and functional decline. Thus, patients with advanced cancer have a complex mix of symptoms imposed on an ever-worsening background of disease progression. Systemic inflammation triggered by the tumor is thought to be a key mechanism of cancer pain that can have varied and complex influences on symptom development. Although the role of systemic inflammation in cancer development and symptomatology has been debated for decades, a recent resurgence in research in this area has led to a greater understanding of this complex process. This chapter will discuss systemic inflammation in cancer and, in particular, its role in cachexia and pain.

# The Relationship between Inflammation and Cancer

Cancer has been known to be associated with inflammation for the last 200 years. Initial anecdotal observations that cancer was related to sites of inflammation have been substantiated by both preclinical and clinical studies. Epidemiological studies have demonstrated that inflammatory conditions are risk factors for certain tumor types, including pancreatic cancer (chronic pancreatitis), gastric cancer (*Helicobacter pylori* infection), and colon cancer (inflammatory bowel disease) [28,31,47]. Systemic inflammation has been implicated in oncogenic mutations and is observed in experimental animal models of tumor development [30]. Targeting systemic inflammation through various therapies has been shown to reduce cancer risk and cancer metastases [30].

It is now widely accepted that cancer and inflammation are inextricably linked. Two pathways have been described to show how inflammation and cancer development are connected [1,30]. (1) The *extrinsic pathway* is mediated by inflammation and maintained by proinflammatory cytokines. This pathway creates a microenvironment of inflammation, promoting carcinogenesis, tumor invasion, and metastasis, which may explain why certain inflammatory conditions favor tumor development. (2) In the *intrinsic pathway,* potential tumor cells have inherent genetic alterations (oncogenes), which, when activated, produce inflammation in the microenvironment and may be the reason why some malignancies develop when there are no obvious predisposing factors. The resulting inflammation favors tumor development.

It is unlikely that these pathways work in isolation; instead, it is probably a combination of these pathways that ultimately results in cancer [30]. In cancer-related inflammation, the immune system acts both as a defense against cancer and as a tumor promoter. Whereas the normal function of the immune system is to protect the body from disease, tumor cells recruit the inherent inflammatory mediators and use them as fuel, feeding cancer development [6].

# Cancer Cachexia and Inflammation

Cancer cachexia has been described as a "multi-factorial syndrome that ranges from early weight loss to a state of severe incapacity incompatible with life" [14]. Most cancer patients lose weight due to a combination of decreased intake of food (anorexia) and abnormal metabolism. Anorexia alone can be treated by managing exacerbating factors such as nausea and using nutritional supplements as appropriate; however, management of the abnormal metabolism that exists in cancer is more complex. The cause of the abnormality is not clear, but it is unlikely that it is due to a single mechanism. Instead, it probably results from a variety of complex interactions between the host and the tumor.

Systemic inflammation is clearly implicated in the development and maintenance of cancer, and its role in cachexia has also been substantiated. In animal models, proinflammatory cytokine activity has been associated with the development of cancer cachexia [49]. It is clear, therefore, that systemic inflammation is associated with the initial stages of cancer development, cancer progression, and the associated sequelae, including cachexia.

# Systemic Inflammation as a Prognostic Indicator

Systemic inflammation in cancer may be due to a variety of mechanisms, either tumor driven or related to an altered immune response within the host. A strong correlation between systemic inflammation and survival has long been identified (Fig. 1) [35]. As CRP decreases, so does overall survival. In recent years, systemic inflammation has also been examined as a possible prognostic indicator in cancer [33].

Systemic inflammation can be assessed by testing serum levels of C-reactive protein (CRP). CRP is an acute-phase plasma protein, manufactured in the liver [19,41]. CRP concentrations rise dramatically during inflammation and remain elevated as long as the underlying inflammatory process remains active. The half-life of CRP is 19 hours, and levels only remain elevated if there is an ongoing stimulus for production, usually underlying inflammation or malignancy [52].

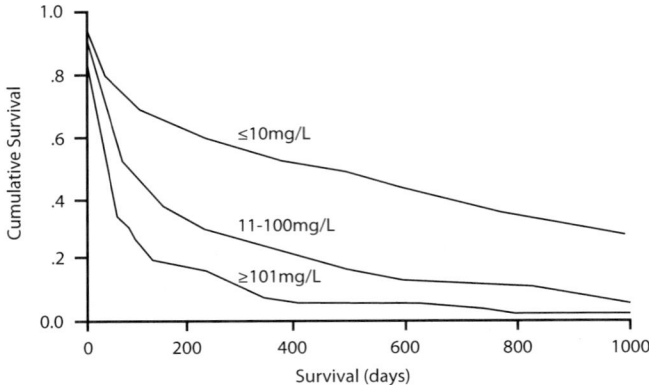

**Fig. 1.** Relationship between serum C-reactive protein (CRP, measured in milligrams per liter) and survival in patients with cancer, according to an analysis of 772 cancer patients by McMillan et al. [35].

CRP has been used as a general marker of systemic inflammation in both hormone-dependent and hormone-independent cancer [7,13,39]. It is directly related to other proinflammatory mediators. On its own, CRP is a useful prognostic factor in gastrointestinal and some urinary cancers [7,22,34]. The combination of CRP with other biomarkers, such as albumin, has also been examined as a prognostic indicator. Anecdotal evidence has associated lower albumin levels with a poor prognosis; in cancer cachexia, albumin is frequently low. These two biomarkers—CRP and albumin—have been combined as a prognostic indicator in the Glasgow Prognostic Score (GPS) [16]. Elevated CRP (>10 mg/L) and hypoalbuminemia (<35 g/L) are each allocated a score of 1. If both are abnormal, a combined score of 2 is assigned; if only one is abnormal, a score of 1 is assigned; and if both are normal the score is 0; therefore, the higher the score, the poorer the prognosis. The GPS has also been shown to be independent of the tumor stage [33]. This finding underlines the importance of inflammation and hypoalbuminemia in cancer progression.

The inclusion of CRP as a crucial component of the GPS highlights the complex role that systemic inflammation plays in cancer. Systemic inflammation is integral to tumor initiation and development; the fact that it is also associated adversely with prognosis supports the need to target inflammation per se, in addition to prescribing standard tumoricidal therapy as a means of treating symptoms (both tumoricidal therapy and anti-inflammatory therapy may reduce symptoms).

# Interleukin-6 and Inflammation

Cytokines are proteins released by cells of the immune system. Their function is to facilitate intercellular interactions and communication. Interleukin-6 (IL-6) is a proinflammatory cytokine that has multiple roles and is essential to the normal functioning of the immune system. It is a critical mediator of inflammation and of the proinflammatory cytokine response [24]. IL-6 is present in many cells, although the main sources are monocytes and macrophages (in acute inflammation) and T cells (in chronic inflammation) [37]. When production of IL-6 is dysregulated, an inflammatory cascade can result, which can lead to the development of chronic inflammatory conditions, either benign (e.g., rheumatoid arthritis) or malignant (e.g., multiple myeloma) [37].

The role of IL-6 in cancer development has been examined in animal models. Knockout mice (genetically engineered to lack IL-6) are less likely to develop tumors than mice with increased levels of IL-6 [17]. IL-6 activates signal transducer and activator of transcription 3 (STAT3), which blocks cell death during inflammation, causing cells to be maintained in toxic inflammatory microenvironments. This effect can result in these cells growing without regulation, ultimately causing cancer [23].

Studies in cancer patients have shown that IL-6 is independently associated with CRP and that CRP is a useful surrogate measure of IL-6 [32,44].

# Cancer Pain and Inflammation

Pain and inflammation have been associated anecdotally for centuries. The four key components of inflammation were first described as *calor* (heat), *dolor* (pain), *rubor* (redness), and *tumor* (swelling). The observation that pain is associated with inflammation has been substantiated by clinical experience and, more recently, by basic scientific evidence. The relationship between pain and inflammation—both highly prevalent in cancer—is of great interest.

Systemic inflammation, mediated by a proinflammatory cytokine drive, has been associated with pain in animal and human models [58]. IL-6 is a useful marker of systemic inflammation and has been shown to be elevated in various pain states in animal models. Administration of IL-6 in rodents produces allodynia and thermal hyperalgesia [9]. In IL-6 knockout mice, physiological pain mechanisms are affected, resulting in a diminished pain response [43]. In animal models of inflammatory pain, IL-6 concentrations are increased [61].

IL-6 is only one of many proinflammatory cytokines. It is unlikely that these cytokines act in isolation, and any painful effects that they have are likely to be produced by a combined response. Recent work has demonstrated that genetic polymorphisms in interleukin-8 (IL-8) are predictors for severe pain [46]. Other proinflammatory cytokines—including interleukin 1β and tumor necrosis factor-alpha (TNF-α)—are also involved in systemic inflammation [63].

The proinflammatory cytokine response, as well as the disruption of the normal balance between pro- and anti-inflammatory cytokines associated with pain, may provide therapeutic opportunities [63]. In animal models, proinflammatory cytokines are able to diminish analgesia previously provided by opioids in both acute and chronic pain states [25]. As mentioned above, controlled studies have shown that IL-6 knockout mice have a delayed development of pain [43]. Such an intervention is unlikely to be appropriate in humans, although this basic science work clearly illustrates the important role IL-6 plays in the development of pain. Recently, the role of IL-6 in cancer pain has been substantiated; cancer patients with polymorphisms in IL-6 have greater pain severity [45].

Work recently undertaken has shown that CRP correlates with pain in a cohort of cachexic cancer patients [27]. The demographics of this cohort are shown in Table I. CRP levels were measured in a subgroup of patients, and the correlation between pain and CRP is shown in Table II. This evidence further supports the role of IL-6 in pain mediation (given that CRP is a surrogate measure of IL-6) and, in turn, underlines the potential impact that targeting this cytokine may have on the treatment of pain. The role of the IL-6 receptor antibody in cancer pain modulation remains unsubstantiated thus far, although pilot work has shown that inhibitors of TNF-α are effective in neuropathic pain of nonmalignant origin [20].

Table I
Demographics of 654 patients included in a
study of pain, depression, and fatigue as a
symptom cluster in advanced cancer

| Variable | No. Patients |
|---|---|
| *Sex* | |
| Male | 423 |
| Female | 231 |
| *Type of Cancer* | |
| Upper gastrointestinal | 183 |
| Pancreatic | 181 |
| Lower gastrointestinal | 79 |
| Lung | 205 |
| Unclassified gastrointestinal | 6 |

*Source:* Laird et al. [27].

In addition to targeting the proinflammatory response, it may be appropriate to address levels of anti-inflammatory cytokines. In patients with chronic pain, decreased levels of anti-inflammatory cytokines have been demonstrated [51]. Increasing the relative concentrations of anti-inflammatory cytokines (e.g., IL-4 and IL-10) may serve to reduce the proinflammatory cytokine-driven inflammation that exists in pain states.

Systemic inflammation is clearly part of the complex pain jigsaw. As cancer progresses, patients tend to experience more pain, and while, in a simplistic way, this may be due to an increase in the symptom burden, it may also be due to other mechanisms such as systemic inflammation. Pain is related in some degree to the underlying activity of proinflammatory cytokines, particularly IL-6. Most of the pertinent research has been done

Table II
Relationship between pain and C-reactive protein (CRP)
in patients with cancer ($n$ = 449)

| | | CRP |
|---|---|---|
| Pain | Pearson correlation | 0.126–0.163* |
| | Significance (2-tailed) | 0.032–0.032 |

*Source:* Laird et al. [27].
* Pain is positively correlated with CRP in a subgroup of patients.

in non-cancer pain, but it would seem unlikely that cancer pain behaves differently, particularly when systemic inflammation is present. Inflammation, and in particular proinflammatory cytokine activity, may be an area where cancer pain therapy should be targeted.

Currently the mainstay of cancer pain therapy is opioid analgesia. Opioids bind to mu, delta, and kappa receptors; however, opioids also have an anti-inflammatory action [55]. In the inflammation pathway, opioid receptors are present at multiple sites, and when activated, they partially inhibit the inflammatory cascade. Other drugs that can have anti-inflammatory and analgesic benefits are nonsteroidal anti-inflammatory drugs (NSAIDs) and corticosteroids. Despite our detailed understanding of their pharmacology, the rationale for the use of NSAIDs and corticosteroids in some pain states remains unclear. The role of such drugs in cancer pain in general has been supported; however, in some specific pain states their use is not advocated [12]. Recent evidence-based guidelines do not advise the use of NSAIDs in the management of neuropathic pain [15], but some basic science work and human studies do support their use for this indication [53]. It would seem reasonable that, as the importance of the inflammatory pathway in pain mediation becomes increasingly established, anti-inflammatory drugs are likely to have an important role. Definitive studies supporting the use of NSAIDs and corticosteroids in specific pain syndromes are awaited.

# Hyperalgesia and Inflammation

Hyperalgesia is not solely a descriptive term but is more accurately regarded as pain facilitation resulting in an exaggerated pain response. Allodynia (an exaggerated response to a normally non-painful stimulus) is a component of hyperalgesia; however, it may not be regarded as painful in the normal way [58]. As described in detail above, proinflammatory cytokines such as IL-6 are a key component of systemic inflammation. Animal models clearly demonstrate that pain is one of the end products of the inflammatory cascade.

Animal models have demonstrated that administration of the proinflammatory cytokine interleukin-1 (IL-1) results in hyperalgesia [29,40].

This evidence is supported by further work using other proinflammatory cytokines such as IL-6 [9]. The administration of anti-inflammatory cytokines can also reduce hyperalgesic states, substantiating the role of inflammation in hyperalgesia [42].

The relationship between proinflammatory cytokines (such as IL-6) and modification of pain processing within the spinal cord is also of interest. It has been established that the perception of pain is affected by altered mechanisms in the spinal cord that occur in chronic pain states. One such mechanism is glial activation. Glia, the supporting cells within the spinal cord, are important in pain perception. When chronic pain states exist, glia become activated, resulting in the release of chemicals that can amplify pain [59]. Of these chemicals, IL-6 and other proinflammatory cytokines seem the most critical components in the amplification of pain observed following glial activation [60]. Aside from promoting cytokine release, glial activation facilitates other agents, including nitric oxide and arachidonic acid, that have a proven role in hyperalgesia [36]. The plasticity within the central nervous system allows for adaptation of pain processing and may result in hyperalgesia. Changes in neurotransmitters, receptors, and intracellular signaling cascades all occur with inflammation and are likely to be major facilitators of the hyperalgesic pain state.

# Symptom Clusters and Their Relation to Systemic Inflammation

Symptoms are the physical and psychological manifestations of the underlying cancer and may be modulated by tumoricidal therapy. Cancer symptoms, however, rarely exist in isolation, and patients with advanced cancer have a median of 11 symptoms (range 1–27) [56]. Because so many symptoms often coexist in cancer patients, it has been postulated that common symptoms may be related. In recent years, the concept of "symptom clusters" in cancer patients has emerged. A symptom cluster has been defined as "three or more concurrent symptoms that are related to each other" [10]. The coexistence of several symptoms is insufficient for them to be labeled as a cluster [11]. To be classified as a cluster, symptoms must be related to one another and occur concurrently.

Due to the large number of potential cancer-related symptoms, the number of different symptom clusters is vast. Several symptom clusters have been described, which vary in the number of symptoms in the cluster (ranging from two to five symptoms) and in their focus (e.g., gastrointestinal or psychological). There is also a great deal of overlap between symptom clusters in that a given symptom may be present in more than one cluster [4,5,57]. No consensus on specific symptom cluster types has been reached.

Pain, depression, and fatigue are highly prevalent in cancer patients and often coexist [2,18,21,48]. The possibility that these symptoms form an important symptom cluster was addressed by the National Cancer Institute in its State-of-the-Science Conference [38]. Experts concluded that there is insufficient evidence to support the concept of a symptom cluster of pain, depression, and fatigue, but that more research is required. It has also been argued that research into symptom clusters should be driven theoretically.

Pain, depression, and fatigue may be related through a common underlying pathophysiological mechanism such as systemic inflammation. Systemic inflammation in cancer is thought to be a proinflammatory host-tumor interaction that may depend partly on constitutive proinflammatory cytokine release by tumor cells, but may also relate to a pre-existing proinflammatory tendency in the host (e.g., due to comorbidity or genetic factors). Systemic inflammation has been related to anorexia, fatigue, hypermetabolism, weight loss, and shortened survival in a range of types of cancer. The inflammatory response, therefore, may be a common physiological pathway for a symptom cluster of pain, depression, and fatigue in cancer patients.

In animal models, the administration of inflammatory agents and proinflammatory cytokines results in "cytokine-induced sickness behavior" [8,26]. These behavioral changes are comparable to the combination of pain, depression, and fatigue in humans [58,62]. In humans, the response to infection results in increased production of proinflammatory cytokines (IL-1, IL-6, and TNF-$\alpha$). The effects of these proinflammatory cytokines correlate with clinical symptoms that mirror the animal models of sickness behavior [54]. These symptoms appear to be similar to those seen in cancer patients, but this topic requires further evaluation.

Recent work has examined the correlated symptoms of pain, depression, and fatigue in cancer patients [27]. This study assessed a cohort of 654 patients, as shown in Table I. Cluster analysis was conducted on data from these patients, and CRP was used as a biomarker of systemic inflammation in cancer. The study supported a symptom cluster of pain, depression, and fatigue in cancer patients (Fig. 2). Systemic inflammation as a possible underlying mechanism for these symptoms was not demonstrated, perhaps because CRP, while it is a sensitive marker of inflammation, is not specific and may be affected by other variables [50].

Systemic inflammation seems plausible as one possible mechanism for the symptom cluster of pain, depression, and fatigue. Work in nonmalignant disease in humans would support cytokine-induced sickness behavior as a possible biological basis for the symptom cluster of pain, depression, and fatigue, but there is insufficient evidence to support the same conclusion in cancer patients. This lack of evidence may be due to insufficiently sensitive measures of the proinflammatory drive that fail to show a biological basis for symptom clusters.

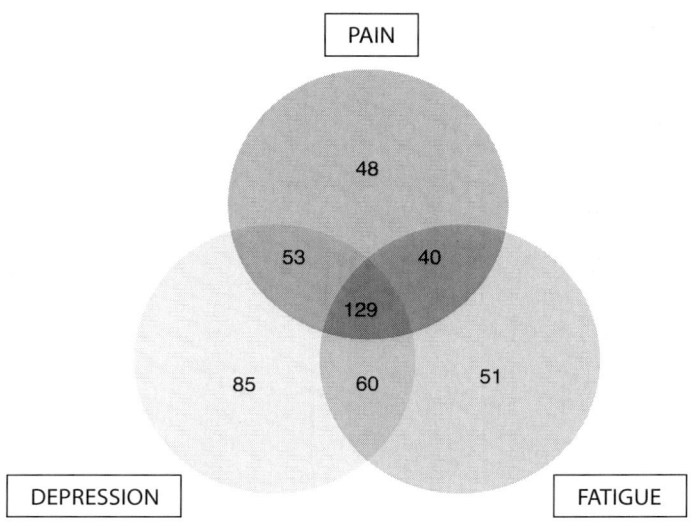

**Fig. 2.** Venn diagram showing a symptom cluster of pain, depression, and fatigue in 654 cancer patients assessed by Laird et al. [27]; 188 patients had no symptoms.

# Conclusion

The clear link between inflammation and cancer has implications at many levels. Some chronic inflammatory conditions are predisposing factors for the development of certain types of cancer, and basic science work has highlighted the importance of the extrinsic pathway in this process. Trials have shown that anti-inflammatory medications reduce the prevalence of cancer [30]. The intrinsic pathway, in which an altered microenvironment can result in the development of neoplasia, seems equally important. These pathways do not act in isolation; instead, each plays a part in the development and progression of cancer.

Systemic inflammation is a useful prognostic indicator in cancer. Biomarkers such as CRP provide an indication of cancer prognosis, which illustrates that ongoing systemic inflammation in cancer adversely affects outcome.

It is clear that systemic inflammation is linked to cancer and also to pain (Fig. 3). Pain has been linked to systemic inflammation in animal models, in human models of noncancer pain, and more recently in cancer pain. It is reasonable to conclude that the inflammation that exists in the cancer state is not only responsible for tumor growth, but may also

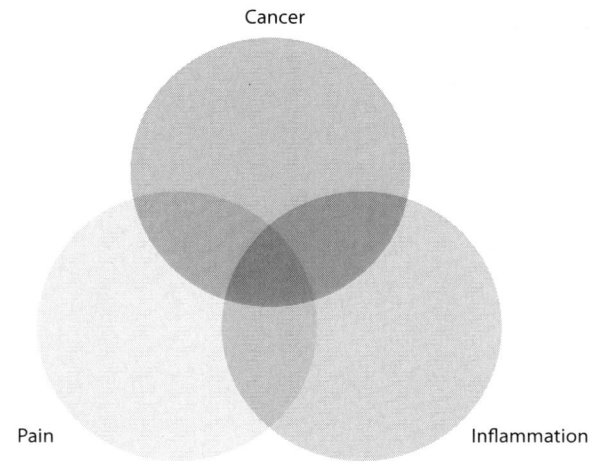

***Fig. 3.*** The triad of cancer, pain, and inflammation.

be linked to the development of symptoms such as pain and cachexia. This common underlying pathophysiological mechanism of systemic inflammation would seem a suitable therapeutic target. Cancer prevention, prevention of disease progression, and symptom control are often approached independently. A new strategy is needed in which symptom control and tumoricidal therapy are integrated with treatment of systemic inflammation, unifying the approach to cancer treatment.

Research on inflammation in cancer has been limited to certain tumor groups. Systemic inflammation that exists in gastrointestinal cancer and pancreatic cancer may not be as pertinent a feature in other tumor sites. Further work is needed to examine systemic inflammation as a cause and effect of other tumors. This work may lead to different approaches to tumoricidal management and symptom control.

Our knowledge of cytokines and systemic inflammation is improving but remains limited. Cytokines can be either pro- or anti-inflammatory, and their role in the immune system is complex. Our understanding of systemic inflammation in cancer and the role of individual cytokines needs to be improved, to allow the development of therapies that counteract tumor-supporting inflammation. These inflammation-targeted therapies may reduce cancer sequelae such as cachexia and pain. There is clearly a potential critical link between systemic inflammation, pain, and depression. This important area is worthy of further clinical research.

# References

[1]   Allavena P, Garlanda C, Borrello MG, Sica A, Mantovani A. Pathways connecting inflammation and cancer. Curr Opin Genet Dev 2008;18:3–10.
[2]   Bower JE, Ganz PA, Desmond KA, Rowland JH, Meyerowitz BE, Belin TR. Fatigue in breast cancer survivors: occurrence, correlates, and impact on quality of life. J Clin Oncol 2000;18:743–53.
[3]   Caraceni A, Portenoy RK. An international survey of cancer pain characteristics and syndromes. IASP Task Force on Cancer Pain. International Association for the Study of Pain. Pain 1999;82:263–74.
[4]   Chen ML, Lin CC. Cancer symptom clusters: a validation study. J Pain Symptom Manage 2007;34:590–9.
[5]   Chow E, Fan G, Hadi S, Wong J, Kirou-Mauro A, Filipczak L. Symptom clusters in cancer patients with brain metastases. Clin Oncol 2008;20:76–82.
[6]   Coussens LM, Werb Z. Inflammation and cancer. Nature 2002;420:860–7.
[7]   Crumley AB, McMillan DC, McKernan M, McDonald AC, Stuart RC. Evaluation of an inflammation-based prognostic score in patients with inoperable gastro-oesophageal cancer. Br J Cancer 2006;94:637–41.
[8]   Dantzer R. Cytokine-induced sickness behaviour: a neuroimmune response to activation of innate immunity. Eur J Pharmacol 2004;500:399–411.

[9]   DeLeo JA, Colburn RW, Nichols M, Malhotra A. Interleukin-6-mediated hyperalgesia/allodynia and increased spinal IL-6 expression in a rat mononeuropathy model. J Interferon Cytokine Res 1996;16:695–700.

[10]  Dodd M, Miaskowski C, Paul S. Symptom clusters and their effect on the functional status of patients with cancer. Oncol Nurs Forum 2001;28:465–70.

[11]  Dodd MJ, Miaskowski C, Lee KA. Occurrence of symptom clusters. J Natl Cancer Inst Monogr 2004;32:76–8.

[12]  Eisenberg E, Berkey CS, Carr DB, Mosteller F, Chalmers TC. Efficacy and safety of nonsteroidal antiinflammatory drugs for cancer pain: a meta-analysis. J Clin Oncol 1994;12:2756–65.

[13]  Falconer JS, Fearon KC, Ross JA, Elton R, Wigmore SJ, Garden OJ, Carter DC. Acute-phase protein response and survival duration of patients with pancreatic cancer. Cancer 1995;75:2077–82.

[14]  Fearon KC. Cancer cachexia: developing multimodal therapy for a multidimensional problem. Eur J Cancer 2008;44:1124–32.

[15]  Finnerup NB, Otto M, McQuay HJ, Jensen TS, Sindrup SH. Algorithm for neuropathic pain treatment: an evidence based proposal. Pain 2005;118:289–305.

[16]  Forrest LM, McMillan DC, McArdle CS, Angerson WJ, Dunlop DJ. Comparison of an inflammation-based prognostic score (GPS) with performance status (ECOG) in patients receiving platinum-based chemotherapy for inoperable non-small-cell lung cancer. Br J Cancer 2004;90:1704–6.

[17]  Gado K, Silva S, Paloczi K, Domjan G, Falus A. Mouse plasmacytoma: an experimental model of human multiple myeloma. Haematologica 2001;86:227–36.

[18]  Gaston-Johansson F, Fall-Dickson JM, Bakos AB, Kennedy MJ. Fatigue, pain, and depression in pre-autotransplant breast cancer patients. Cancer Pract 1999;7:240–7.

[19]  Gaw A, Cowan R, O'Reilly D, Stewart M, Shepherd J. Clinical biochemistry. New York: Churchill Livingstone; 1995.

[20]  Genevay S, Stingelin S, Gabay C. Efficacy of etanercept in the treatment of acute, severe sciatica: a pilot study. Ann Rheum Dis 2004;63:1120–3.

[21]  Glover J, Dibble SL, Dodd MJ, Miaskowski C. Mood states of oncology outpatients: does pain make a difference? J Pain Symptom Manage 1995;10:120–8.

[22]  Hilmy M, Bartlett JM, Underwood MA, McMillan DC. The relationship between the systemic inflammatory response and survival in patients with transitional cell carcinoma of the urinary bladder. Br J Cancer 2005;92:625–7.

[23]  Hodge DR, Hurt EM, Farrar WL. The role of IL-6 and STAT3 in inflammation and cancer. Eur J Cancer 2005;41:2502–12.

[24]  Hodge DR, Peng B, Cherry JC, Hurt EM, Fox SD, Kelley JA, Munroe DJ, Farrar WL. Interleukin 6 supports the maintenance of p53 tumor suppressor gene promoter methylation. Cancer Res 2005;65:4673–82.

[25]  Hutchinson MR, Coats BD, Lewis SS, Zhang Y, Sprunger DB, Rezvani N, Baker EM, Jekich BM, Wieseler JL, Somogyi AA, et al. Proinflammatory cytokines oppose opioid-induced acute and chronic analgesia. Brain Behav Immun 2008;22:1178–89.

[26]  Konsman JP, Parnet P, Dantzer R. Cytokine-induced sickness behaviour: mechanisms and implications. Trends Neurosci 2002;25:154–9.

[27]  Laird BJ, Scott AC, Colvin LA, McKeon A, Murray G, Fearon KCH, Fallon MT. Pain, depression and fatigue as a symptom cluster in advanced cancer. Proceedings of the EAPC Research Forum: Conference Abstracts; 2009.

[28]  Macarthur M, Hold GL, El-Omar EM. Inflammation and cancer II. Role of chronic inflammation and cytokine gene polymorphisms in the pathogenesis of gastrointestinal malignancy. Am J Physiol Gastrointest Liver Physiol 2004;286:G515–20.

[29]  Maier SF, Wiertelak EP, Martin D, Watkins LR. Interleukin-1 mediates the behavioral hyperalgesia produced by lithium chloride and endotoxin. Brain Res 1993;623:321–4.

[30]  Mantovani A, Allavena P, Sica A, Balkwill F. Cancer-related inflammation. Nature 2008;454:436–44.

[31]  McKay CJ, Glen P, McMillan DC. Chronic inflammation and pancreatic cancer. Best Pract Res Clin Gastroenterol 2008;22:65–73.

[32]  McKeown DJ, Brown DJ, Kelly A, Wallace AM, McMillan DC. The relationship between circulating concentrations of C-reactive protein, inflammatory cytokines and cytokine receptors in patients with non-small-cell lung cancer. Br J Cancer 2004;91:1993–5.

[33]  McMillan DC. Systemic inflammation, nutritional status and survival in patients with cancer. Curr Opin Clin Nutr Metab Care 2009;12:223–6.

[34] McMillan DC, Canna K, McArdle CS. Systemic inflammatory response predicts survival following curative resection of colorectal cancer. Br J Surg 2003;90:215–9.

[35] McMillan DC, Elahi MM, Sattar N, Angerson WJ, Johnstone J, McArdle CS. Measurement of the systemic inflammatory response predicts cancer-specific and non-cancer survival in patients with cancer. Nutr Cancer 2001;41:64–9.

[36] Meller ST, Gebhart GF. Spinal mediators of hyperalgesia. Drugs 1994;47(Suppl 5):10–20.

[37] Naugler WE, Karin M. The wolf in sheep's clothing: the role of interleukin-6 in immunity, inflammation and cancer. Trends Mol Med 2008;14:109–19.

[38] NIH. NIH State-of-the-Science Statement on symptom management in cancer: pain, depression, and fatigue. NIH Consens State Sci Statements 2002;19:1–29.

[39] O'Gorman P, McMillan DC, McArdle CS. Impact of weight loss, appetite, and the inflammatory response on quality of life in gastrointestinal cancer patients. Nutr Cancer 1998;32:76–80.

[40] Oka T, Aou S, Hori T. Intracerebroventricular injection of interleukin-1 beta induces hyperalgesia in rats. Brain Res 1993;624:61–8.

[41] Pepys MB, Hirschfield GM. C-reactive protein: a critical update. J Clin Invest 2003;111:1805–12.

[42] Poole S, Cunha FQ, Selkirk S, Lorenzetti BB, Ferreira SH. Cytokine-mediated inflammatory hyperalgesia limited by interleukin-10. Br J Pharmacol 1995;115:684–8.

[43] Ramer MS, Murphy PG, Richardson PM, Bisby MA. Spinal nerve lesion-induced mechanoallodynia and adrenergic sprouting in sensory ganglia are attenuated in interleukin-6 knockout mice. Pain 1998;78:115–21.

[44] Ramsey S, Lamb GW, Aitchison M, McMillan DC. The longitudinal relationship between circulating concentrations of C-reactive protein, interleukin-6 and interleukin-10 in patients undergoing resection for renal cancer. Br J Cancer 2006;95:1076–80.

[45] Reyes-Gibby CC, El Osta B, Spitz MR, Parsons H, Kurzrock R, Wu X, Shete S, Bruera E. The influence of tumor necrosis factor-alpha-308 G/A and IL-6 -174 G/C on pain and analgesia response in lung cancer patients receiving supportive care. Cancer Epidemiol Biomarkers Prev 2008;17:3262–7.

[46] Reyes-Gibby CC, Shete S, Yennurajalingam S, Frazier M, Bruera E, Kurzrock R, Crane CH, Abbruzzese J, Evans D, Spitz MR. Genetic and nongenetic covariates of pain severity in patients with adenocarcinoma of the pancreas: assessing the influence of cytokine genes. J Pain Symptom Manage 2009;38:894–902.

[47] Santiago C, Pagan B, Isidro AA, Appleyard CB. Prolonged chronic inflammation progresses to dysplasia in a novel rat model of colitis-associated colon cancer. Cancer Res 2007;67:10766–73.

[48] Smets EM, Visser MR, Willems-Groot AF, Garssen B, Schuster-Uitterhoeve AL, de Haes JC. Fatigue and radiotherapy: (B) experience in patients 9 months following treatment. Br J Cancer 1998;78:907–12.

[49] Strassmann G, Fong M, Freter CE, Windsor S, D'Alessandro F, Nordan RP. Suramin interferes with interleukin-6 receptor binding in vitro and inhibits colon-26-mediated experimental cancer cachexia in vivo. J Clin Invest 1993;92:2152–9.

[50] Tsilidis KK, Branchini C, Guallar E, Helzlsouer KJ, Erlinger TP, Platz EA. C-reactive protein and colorectal cancer risk: a systematic review of prospective studies. Int J Cancer 2008;123:1133–40.

[51] Uceyler N, Valenza R, Stock M, Schedel R, Sprotte G, Sommer C. Reduced levels of antiinflammatory cytokines in patients with chronic widespread pain. Arthritis Rheum 2006;54:2656–64.

[52] Vigushin DM, Pepys MB, Hawkins PN. Metabolic and scintigraphic studies of radioiodinated human C-reactive protein in health and disease. J Clin Invest 1993;91:1351–7.

[53] Vo T, Rice AS, Dworkin RH. Non-steroidal anti-inflammatory drugs for neuropathic pain: how do we explain continued widespread use? Pain 2009;143:169–71.

[54] Vollmer-Conna U, Fazou C, Cameron B, Li H, Brennan C, Luck L, Davenport T, Wakefield D, Hickie I, Lloyd A. Production of pro-inflammatory cytokines correlates with the symptoms of acute sickness behaviour in humans. Psychol Med 2004;34:1289–97.

[55] Walker JS. Anti-inflammatory effects of opioids. Adv Exp Med Biol 2003;521:148–60.

[56] Walsh D, Donnelly S, Rybicki L. The symptoms of advanced cancer: relationship to age, gender, and performance status in 1,000 patients. Support Care Cancer 2000;8:175–9.

[57] Wang SY, Tsai CM, Chen BC, Lin CH, Lin CC. Symptom clusters and relationships to symptom interference with daily life in Taiwanese lung cancer patients. J Pain Symptom Manage 2008;35:258–66.

[58] Watkins LR, Maier SF. The pain of being sick: implications of immune-to-brain communication for understanding pain. Annu Rev Psychol 2000;51:29–57.

[59]  Watkins LR, Milligan ED, Maier SF. Glial proinflammatory cytokines mediate exaggerated pain states: implications for clinical pain. Adv Exp Med Biol 2003;521:1–21.
[60]  Wieseler-Frank J, Maier SF, Watkins LR. Glial activation and pathological pain. Neurochem Int 2004;45:389–95.
[61]  Xie WR, Deng H, Li H, Bowen TL, Strong JA, Zhang JM. Robust increase of cutaneous sensitivity, cytokine production and sympathetic sprouting in rats with localized inflammatory irritation of the spinal ganglia. Neuroscience 2006;142:809–22.
[62]  Yirmiya R. Endotoxin produces a depressive-like episode in rats. Brain Res 1996;711:163–74.
[63]  Zhang JM, An J. Cytokines, inflammation, and pain. Int Anesthesiol Clin 2007;45:27–37.

*Correspondence to:* Prof. Marie T. Fallon, Institute of Genetics and Molecular Medicine, University of Edinburgh, Edinburgh Cancer Research Centre (CR UK Building), Western General Hospital, Crewe Road, Edinburgh EH4 2XR, United Kingdom. Email: marie.fallon@ed.ac.uk.

# Opioid-Induced Hyperalgesia and Cancer Pain: Effects on Tumor Growth and Disease Progression

6

Tamara King, Frank Porreca, and Todd W. Vanderah

*Department of Pharmacology, University of Arizona, Tucson, Arizona, USA*

## Cancer Pain Management

Opioids are the primary, and most effective, treatment for cancer-induced pain. Pain is the first symptom of cancer in 20–50% of all cancer patients, and 75–90% of advanced or terminal cancer patients must cope with chronic pain syndromes related to chemotherapy, failed treatment, tumor progression, and associated pathology in tumor-bearing tissue [3,54]. Current treatment for cancer patients with bone cancer pain follows the World Health Organization's ladder approach for pain relief [10,75]. This approach recommends adjusting the strength and potency of the analgesic according to pain intensity, with nonsteroidal anti-inflammatory drugs (NSAIDs) primarily used to treat mild to moderate pain, and opioids, with or without coanalgesics/adjuvant analgesics, used to treat moderate to severe pain. In patients with advanced cancer, pain is described as moderate to severe in approximately 40–50% and very severe or excruciating in 25–30% of patients [14]. Cancer pain is multifaceted, with varying degrees of intensity and frequency, and occurs at multiple anatomical locations, with multiple pain descriptors, such as nociceptive and neuropathic, suggesting the likelihood of different underlying mechanisms driving these components of pain [42]. The most commonly diagnosed cancers—lung, prostate, and breast cancers—often metastasize to bone, and in advanced states, they are associated with bone remodeling and eventual bone fracture that contributes to incapacitating pain and limited or total loss of daily activity [2,42]. Pain limits daily activity in 41% of patients reporting mild to moderate pain and in 94% of patients reporting moderate to severe pain, leading to greatly diminished quality of life [14]. Advances in cancer therapies have significantly improved survival of patients with cancer, including those with bone metastases. However, these patients still experience pain that can be severe and unpredictable and can greatly limit daily activity [10,20,42]. Effective treatments that can be given over long periods of time with tolerable side effects are thus essential for maintaining quality of life. Currently available treatments, including opioids, while necessary and important in the treatment of cancer pain, unfortunately also often severely and negatively affect quality of life.

Numerous barriers limit effective treatment of cancer pain with opioids [10]. In some cases, viewpoints related to opioid use held by physicians, patients, and patients' families provide impediments to effective pain control [10]. Such concerns often include fears of physical dependence and addiction. Additionally, opioid administration, particularly at high doses, can be associated with severe, sometimes debilitating side effects, including somnolence, mental confusion, and especially constipation [6]. Some patients develop analgesic tolerance to opioids, in which greater doses of the opioids are required to produce effective pain management [10,60]. Multiple factors may contribute to dose escalation in cancer patients, including changes in endogenous opioid function, disease progression, and development of opioid-induced hyperalgesia (OIH) [11,49,60]. Surprisingly, relatively little is known regarding the long-term neural consequences of prolonged opioid treatment for chronic pain [11]. Preclinical studies indicate that long-term opioid exposure may induce cellular changes in opioid signaling [31], neurochemical changes that may result in enhanced pain signaling [31,53], and effects on cancer growth, metastases [19,67], and cancer-induced pathology [32]. These changes suggest maladaptive activity of opioids that could manifest clinically.

# Long-Term Opioid Administration and Hyperalgesia

Successful opioid treatment of any duration depends on achieving a favorable balance between analgesia and adverse effects [3,62]. Importantly, there is great interindividual variability in opioid effects. Even for patients with a similar type or severity of pain, the effective opioid dose as well as the relative toxicity ratios may vary greatly [3,62]. Critical for effective management of cancer pain is appropriate knowledge of analgesic (primarily opioid) pharmacology with respect to dosing, timing, alternative routes of administration (such as oral, transdermal, transmucosal, subcutaneous, epidural, and intrathecal), and converting from intravenous to oral therapies [3,62]. The American Pain Society proposes several important considerations for appropriate pain management, including: (1) the source/type of the patient's pain; (2) the patient's age, general health, and comorbidities; (3) the potential for medication-related adverse effects; (4) potential drug interactions; (5) comorbidities that may be relieved by nonanalgesic effects of the medications (e.g., sleep disturbances, depression, or anxiety); (6) comorbidities that may be exacerbated by the nonanalgesic effects of the medications (e.g., hypertension, ulceration, renal impairment, or cognitive impairment); (7) costs associated with therapy; (8) potential risks for medication abuse; and (9) risks of overdose [3]. Of note, it is suggested that although no single opioid is optimal for all patients, an optimal opioid can generally be found for each patient [62].

Morphine is the most frequently used opioid for treatment of moderate to severe cancer pain [48], with other opioids increasingly being used. Although opioids have good efficacy with acute treatment, it has been argued that analgesic efficacy for chronic pain conditions, although initially good, is not always sustained during continuous and long-term treatment (months to years) [4,62]. Importantly, the chronic nature of cancer pain often requires prolonged opioid administration through controlled-release tablets, repeated bolus injections, or transdermal patches [1,21,74]. Decreased analgesic efficacy could arise from multiple mechanisms, including receptor desensitization, OIH, and subtle and intermittent episodes of withdrawal, as well as psychological factors [4,60]. Mechanisms of opioid tolerance are described by Inturrisi and Gregus in

Chapter 7, and pharmacological strategies to reduce or reverse tolerance are discussed by Kalso in Chapter 9. Increased doses of opioids may result in the advancement of the disease, resulting in greater pain and therefore requiring more opioids [4,11,12,50]. Clinical studies have reported that opioids acutely administered via different routes of administration (transdermal, oral, intrathecal, or intravenous) can unexpectedly produce hyperalgesia and allodynia, particularly during rapid opioid dose escalation [49]. Recent clinical studies have indicated that OIH also occurs in humans with chronic opioid exposure. Interpretation of these studies is complicated by numerous factors. For example, subjects already may have been chronically exposed to opioids, precluding the establishment of a firm causal relationship between opioid use and the development of OIH, and subjects with chronic pain may have unique properties that could confound pain measurements [4,11,12].

These limitations highlight the difficulty in well-controlled prospective studies on long-term opioid exposure. Recently, Chu et al. conducted a prospective study on the development of OIH in opioid-naive chronic pain patients [12]. In this study, patients with chronic low back pain were measured for cold and heat pain thresholds prior to and 1 month into oral morphine therapy. Experimental pain threshold and pain tolerance were significantly decreased after 1 month of morphine therapy, indicating development of OIH [12]. A corresponding decrease in the potency of remifentanil-induced analgesia was also observed 1 month into oral morphine therapy [12]. Although the sample was small, the study presents a potential methodology for controlled clinical experiments to determine (1) the time course and magnitude of opioid tolerance and hyperalgesia in patients treated with opioids for chronic pain; (2) the likelihood of these sequelae; (3) the degree to which tolerance and hyperalgesia limit the utility of opioids for treatment of chronic pain; and (4) what cotherapies diminish OIH and analgesic tolerance.

Preclinical studies have begun to examine potential mechanisms underlying OIH, reporting hypersensitivity across a number of stimulus modalities as well as neuroplastic adaptations (Table I; for reviews see [4,53,60]). Structurally distinct opioids, including nonpeptidic agonists (e.g., morphine, oxymorphone, and fentanyl) as well as peptides acting at $\mu$-opioid receptors (e.g., the enkephalin DAMGO) have been shown to produce hyperalgesia [53]. Many studies have demonstrated that sustained opioid administration for several days induces neuroplastic adaptations, including enhanced signaling by primary afferent fibers, spinal sensitization, and activation of descending pain facilitatory pathways that promote pain (Fig. 1) (for reviews see [31,43,44,53]). Several groups have demonstrated that sustained morphine upregulates pronociceptive

Table I

Summary of pain behaviors and neuroplastic changes induced by (A) inflammation injury, (B) opioid infusion (uninjured), (C) cancer-induced bone pain (sarcoma), and (D) cancer-induced bone pain with opioid infusion

| Preclinical Behavioral and Neuroplastic Changes | A | B | C | D |
|---|---|---|---|---|
| *Behavioral Measures of Pain* | | | | |
| Tactile allodynia | X | X | X | ↑ |
| Spontaneous pain behaviors | X | ? | X | ↑ |
| Thermal hyperalgesia | X | X | – | ? |
| Mechanical hyperalgesia | X | X | ? | ? |
| Capsaicin hyperalgesia | ↑ | ↑ | ? | ? |
| *Peripheral Changes* | | | | |
| Plasma extravasation | ↑ | ↑ | ? | ? |
| p-p38 MAPK (DRG expression) | ↑ | ↑ | ↑ | ? |
| TRPV1 channels in peripheral tissue | ↑ | ↑ | ↑ | ? |
| CGRP and SP expression in DRG | ↑ | ↑ | – | ↑ |
| ATF3 expression in DRG (marker for neuronal damage) | – | – | ↑ | ↑↑ |
| *Spinal Cord Changes* | | | | |
| CGRP and SP content in spinal cord | ↑ | ↑ | – | ? |
| CGRP and SP release in spinal cord | ↑ | ↑ | ? | ? |
| NK1-receptor internalization in deep dorsal horn | ↑ | ↑ | ↑ | ? |
| Dynorphin content in spinal cord | ↑ | ↑ | ↑ | ? |
| Wide-dynamic-range (WDR) neuronal activity | ↑ | ↑ | ↑ | ? |
| Touch-evoked FOS | ↑ | ↑ | ? | ? |
| Proinflammatory cytokines | ↑ | ↑ | ↑ | ? |
| *Descending Pain Facilitation (RVM)* | ↑ | ↑ | ? | ? |

*Note:* X indicates behaviors reported in the literature, ↑ indicates an increase in the measure, – indicates no change, and ? indicates that there are no known reports on this measure. ATF3, activating transcription factor 3; CGRP, calcitonin gene-related peptide; DRG, dorsal root ganglion; MAPK, mitogen-activated kinases; NK1, neurokinin 1; RVM, rostral ventral medulla; SP, substance P; TRPV1, transient receptor potential vanilloid 1.

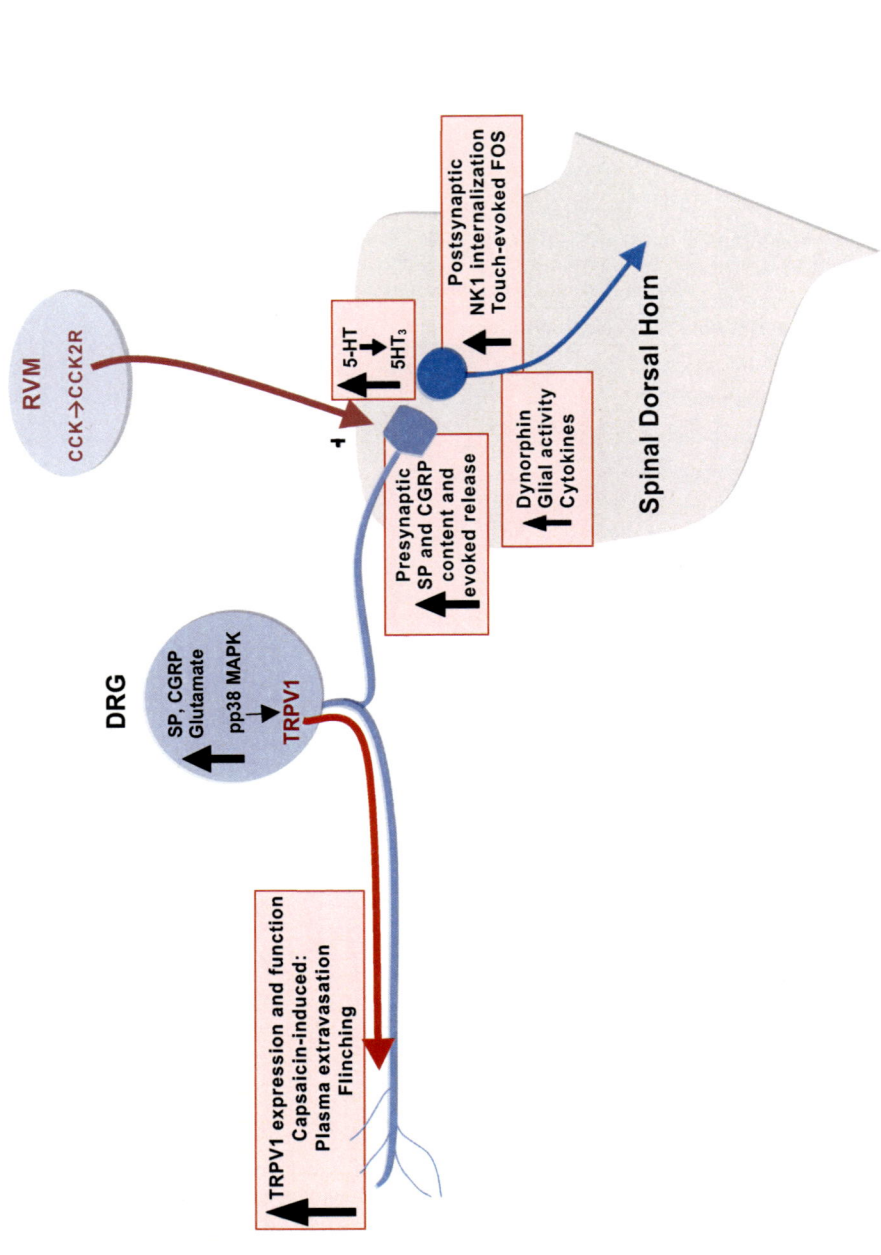

neurotransmitters within the primary afferent fibers, including substance P, calcitonin gene-related peptide (CGRP) and glutamate [18,30,45,55,56]. Moreover, there is a corresponding increase in evoked signaling by nociceptors. Capsaicin-evoked release of substance P and CGRP was increased in isolated spinal cord from rats treated with morphine infusion across 6–7 days [18,30]. In addition, morphine infusion across 6 days increased noxious mechanical stimulation-induced neurokinin-1 (NK1) receptor internalization within the deep laminae of the spinal dorsal horn, indicating enhanced signaling by excitatory neurotransmitters in morphine-treated rats [30]. Subsequent research has indicated that enhanced signaling might be mediated, in part, by enhanced transient receptor potential vanilloid 1 (TRPV1) receptor function [9,72]. Sustained morphine infusion in rats significantly upregulates TRPV1 expression in primary afferent fibers, which results in selective trafficking to the peripheral terminal of the afferent fiber (Fig. 1) [9,72]. A corresponding enhanced TRPV1 function in the periphery was observed with enhanced capsaicin-induced pain behaviors and plasma extravasation [72]. Although sustained morphine does not appear to increase TRPV1 expression within the spinal dorsal horn, enhanced capsaicin-evoked release of excitatory neurotransmitters in isolated dorsal horn sections indicates enhanced TRPV1 receptor function within the spinal cord as well.

Additional potential mechanisms implicated in morphine-induced sensitization of primary afferent fibers include activation of mitogen-activated protein kinases (MAPKs). Sustained morphine

**Fig. 1.** Neuroplastic changes proposed to underlie opioid-induced hyperalgesia and allodynia. Sustained opioid exposure upregulates TRVP1 expression in a p38 mitogen-activated protein kinase (MAPK)-dependent manner that corresponds to increased TRPV1 function in the periphery. Increased expression of the excitatory neuropeptides, calcitonin gene-related peptide (CGRP) and substance P, has been demonstrated within the dorsal root ganglion (DRG) and spinal dorsal horn, with increased capsaicin-evoked release of the peptides reported within the spinal cord. This may correspond to increased NK1-receptor internalization within deep dorsal horn neurons. Prolonged opioid infusion increases glial activity and upregulates pronociceptive cytokines, such as interleukin-1β (IL-1β). Reports of touch-evoked FOS indicate that opioids induce spinal sensitization. Spinal administration of a 5-HT$_3$-receptor antagonist has been demonstrated to block opioid-induced hyperalgesia. In addition, opioid infusion produces upregulation of dynorphin content, which has been demonstrated to be dependent on descending pain facilitatory pathways from the rostral ventromedial medulla (RVM). These pain-facilitatory pathways mediate opioid-induced hyperalgesia. Cholecystokinin-2 (CCK2) receptors mediate descending facilitation from the RVM.

exposure was demonstrated to increase phosphorylation of MAPKs including p38 MAPK, extracellular signal-regulated kinases (ERK), and c-jun N-terminal kinases (JNK) within neurons in the dorsal root ganglia (DRG) [9,38]. Moreover, intrathecal administration of p38 MAPK, ERK, or JNK inhibitors reduced sustained morphine-induced thermal hyperalgesia and blocked the morphine-induced upregulation of TRPV1 receptors [9]. Administration of a MAP/ERK inhibitor (MEK1) attenuated the morphine-induced increase in phosphorylated ERK (pERK) and phosphorylated cAMP-responsive element binding protein (pCREB) as well as morphine-induced increased expression of CGRP and substance P in cultured neonatal DRG neurons [38]. It is likely that morphine-induced enhanced function of MAP kinases and TRPV1 and corresponding enhanced content and evoked release of excitatory neurotransmitters from primary afferent fibers in the spinal dorsal horn contribute to sustained morphine-enhanced evoked signaling within the spinal cord and to OIH.

Within the spinal cord, sustained morphine has been demonstrated to: (1) upregulate excitatory neurotransmitters in primary afferent fiber terminals [18,30,45]; (2) increase evoked release of excitatory neurotransmitters within the spinal cord [18,30]; (3) upregulate spinal dynorphin levels, promoting enhanced input from afferent nociceptors [18]; and (4) produce glial activation and expression of multiple chemokines and cytokines [24,26]. Moreover, sustained morphine induces spinal sensitization, as indicated by increased excitability in neurons of the deep dorsal horn [66] as well as increased touch-evoked FOS in morphine-treated rats [73]. Enhanced signaling within the spinal cord may be a critical component in the ascending pathway that ultimately results in the recruitment of descending pain modulatory systems. Studies have demonstrated that sustained morphine-induced enhanced pain depends on activation of a spinal-supraspinal-spinal loop proposed to mediate enhanced pain in injury models [73]. Ablation of NK1-receptor-expressing neurons within the spinal cord prevented sustained morphine-induced thermal and mechanical hypersensitivity as well as sustained morphine-induced upregulation of spinal dynorphin and enhanced touch-evoked FOS [73]. In addition, spinal administration of ondansetron, a serotonin 5-HT$_3$-receptor antagonist, blocked sustained morphine-induced hypersensitivity [73]. These data indicate that ablation of the NK1-receptor-expressing cells within the spinal cord probably eliminates morphine-induced activation of the ascending limb of a spinal-bulbospinal loop that engages descending facilitation, ultimately engaging the 5-HT$_3$ receptor [73].

Several studies have demonstrated that sustained morphine infusion activates descending pain facilitation from the rostral ventromedial medulla (RVM) which is required for expression of OIH in rodents [46,71,76]. Sustained morphine has been demonstrated to increase the proportion of ON cells, purported pain facilitation cells, within the RVM [46]. Inactivation of descending pain facilitatory pathways blocked OIH and neuroplastic changes observed at the spinal cord. Administration of lidocaine into the RVM or lesion of the dorsolateral funiculus (DLF) blocked upregulation of spinal dynorphin and enhanced evoked release of excitatory neurotransmitters [71]. Further research implicates a role for cholecystokinin (CCK) acting on CCK2 receptors in OIH [76]. Sustained morphine produced a fivefold increase in basal CCK levels within the RVM. Further, administration of a CCK2 receptor antagonist into the RVM blocked OIH [76]. These studies suggest that sustained morphine enhances endogenous CCK activity in the RVM that may drive descending pain facilitatory mechanisms to exacerbate and maintain spinal nociceptive sensitivity.

# Prolonged Opioid Administration and Cancer-Induced Bone Pain

The above studies on OIH have focused on opioid-induced pronociceptive changes in uninjured animals. However, the effects of prolonged, sustained opioid administration in the presence of a persistent pain state, such as cancer-induced bone pain, have only recently been examined [57]. Single bolus injections of morphine were shown to effectively block behavioral measures of cancer-induced bone pain [36]. Similar efficacy was observed with daily bolus morphine injections, with no tolerance to morphine's antinociceptive effects [70]. In contrast, sustained delivery of morphine through osmotic minipumps, designed to maintain stable blood plasma levels across 7 days [17], enhanced cancer-induced pain in a murine model of sarcoma-induced bone pain [32]. Moreover, sustained morphine infusion increased apparent expression of excitatory neurotransmitters (substance P and CGRP) in primary afferent fibers, suggesting a potential for enhanced nociceptive signaling in the morphine-treated animals [32]. In addition, sustained morphine administration surprisingly enhanced sarcoma-induced bone loss and fracture, as well as expression of activating transcription factor 3 (ATF3) in cell bodies of primary afferent fibers, a marker of neuronal damage [32]. These data indicate that the sustained morphine infusion may result in "add-on" mechanisms of pain beyond those engaged by the sarcoma alone [32]. In addition, sustained morphine infusion accelerated sarcoma-induced bone loss and doubled the incidence of sarcoma-induced fracture [32], which most likely contributes to the enhanced pain observed in the sarcoma-treated mice with morphine infusion. Of note, both the enhanced cancer-induced bone pain and bone loss were dose dependent, and both were reversed by coadministration of naloxone. These data indicate that sustained morphine enhancement of sarcoma-induced pain occurs through morphine's interaction with the opioid receptors [32].

The fact that morphine-induced enhanced sarcoma-induced bone pain is dose dependent and naloxone reversible suggests that these effects are mediated through morphine interaction with the opioid receptors, yet others have reported instances in which OIH occurs in the absence of $\mu$-, $\delta$-, and $\kappa$-opioid receptors [28] or in the presence of the opioid receptor antagonist naltrexone [27]. Moreover, others have proposed that opioids cause direct glial activation through toll-like receptors, a class of pattern recognition receptors [23]. Opioid agonists have been demonstrated to activate glia, and this activation is blocked by the opioid-receptor-inactive (+)-naloxone, which is proposed to block toll-like receptor 4 (TLR4) receptor activation [23]. Blockade of glial function, as well as of proinflammatory cytokines within the spinal cord, has been suggested to block OIH as well as opioid-induced analgesic tolerance in rats [24,26]. As both the opioid-receptor-active and -inactive naloxone enantiomers have been shown to effectively block activity at these receptors, it is possible that the blockade of the enhanced sarcoma-induced pain by the opioid antagonist naloxone is mediated through blockade of opioid actions at TLR4. In such a case, administration of (+)-naloxone in conjunction with an opioid agonist may enhance opioid analgesia and diminish the incidence of OIH; however, such possibilities require further investigation.

While many cancer patients respond well to opioids for pain management [47,78], these preclinical data raise the possibility that prolonged opioid administration might produce unintended deleterious actions in some patients and thus may require supplemental pain medication to overcome both opioid- and cancer-induced hyperalgesia and pain. Whether indications from the mouse osteosarcoma model may be generalized clinically remains to be established. It is important to note that many factors are likely to influence the effects of prolonged opioid exposure on cancer-induced pain, including the specific opioid administered, the type of metastasis, whether osteolytic or osteoblastic lesions are observed, and the route, dose, and schedule of opioid administration [3,52,59,69,70]. Moreover, there is a significant genetic basis for OIH that may underlie the significant individual variability reported in opioid response [29,51].

# Sustained Opioids: Effects on Tumor Growth and Bone Loss

Sustained morphine exposure has also been suggested to alter cancer growth. However, there are conflicting results as to whether morphine enhances or inhibits tumor cell proliferation. Several studies have shown that morphine inhibits tumor cell proliferation [39,40,64,65,68,77]. Others have found that morphine promotes tumor cell proliferation as well as metastasis and mortality [16,19,25,61]. The discrepancies between these results may be due to a number of factors, including testing different cell lines, using different doses of morphine, and having different durations of morphine exposure across experiments [19,67]. Xenograft studies in which human MCF-7 breast cancer cells were implanted (subcutaneously) in the mouse demonstrated that daily bolus administration of morphine (30 mg/kg) inhibits growth through 20 days of administration [68]. In contrast, the same treatment failed to alter the growth of human colon cancer cells [68]. Others reported that long-term treatment with bolus injection of morphine (0.714 mg/kg/day on days 1–15; 1.43 mg/kg/day from day 16 on) enhanced the growth of the same line of human MCF-7 breast cancer cells, with significant differences between the morphine-treated and saline-treated (control) groups emerging 28 days into treatment [19]. Importantly, this enhanced growth was accompanied by increased tumor neovascularization, indicating that the prolonged morphine treatment might promote tumor growth by stimulating tumor angiogenesis [19]. These experiments indicate (1) that the dose of morphine is important in modulating tumor growth and (2) that potential increases in tumor growth occur following very long-term treatment with morphine, with changes observed after weeks of morphine treatment. Moreover, the effects of morphine on tumor growth appear to differ depending on the cell line treated.

It is unknown whether these effects will generalize to other cancers or to opioids other than morphine. There is a clear need for increased understanding of the neurobiological consequences of prolonged opioid exposure in chronic pain conditions. Such an understanding may allow improvements in the use of opioids and enhance the effective management of patients with chronic cancer pain. The debilitating side effects of opioids and chronic opioid treatment required in most patients with bone metastases, together with the increase in survival time of prostate cancer patients with bone metastases, emphasize the need for better pain management options.

# Morphine and the Tumor Microenvironment

Another important factor that must be considered regarding the effect of long-term treatment with opioids on disease progression is the impact of opioids on the tumor microenvironment. Sustained morphine administration for 1 week was found to enhance pain and accelerate bone loss and fracture without altering tumor growth within the bone [32]. These data suggest that the enhanced sarcoma-induced bone loss observed in the morphine-infused mice may be due to alterations in bone resorption. Bone resorption and rebuilding take place continuously for bone maintenance and repair and are mediated by osteoclast (resorption) and osteoblast (building) activity [7,8]. Several studies have shown that osteolytic cancers, such as the sarcoma cell line used in these studies, upregulate osteoclasts within the bone, resulting in bone loss [22,32,35,58]. Morphine infusion significantly increased sarcoma-induced upregulation of osteoclasts, which most likely mediates the morphine-induced acceleration of the sarcoma-induced bone loss and fracture [32]. The mechanism by which morphine enhances osteoclastogenesis and consequent bone loss is unknown.

A potential mechanism by which morphine may enhance pain as well as bone loss is by upregulation of growth factors and other agents within the periphery and the central nervous system. Sustained morphine upregulates many factors that modulate pain, enhances neovascularization, which may contribute to tumor growth, and increases osteoclastogenesis, which may contribute to enhanced bone resorption associated with osteolytic bone metastases. For example, sustained morphine increased IL-1β within the bone microenvironment in sarcoma-treated mice [32]. Interleukin 1 (IL-1) is a proinflammatory cytokine that plays an important role in osteoclastogenesis through direct mechanisms such as stimulating differentiation of osteoclast precursors, as well as indirect mechanisms such as increasing expression of RANKL (receptor activator of nuclear factor κB ligand), which plays a critical role in osteoclast maturation, activation, and survival [5,13,15]. Moreover, IL-1β has been implicated in enhanced pain through sensitization of primary afferent fibers (peripheral sensitization) [63]. Importantly, sustained systemic administration of morphine has been demonstrated to upregulate IL-1β within the spinal cord and the lumbosacral cerebrospinal fluid [26]. Blockade of IL-1β within the spinal cord blocked OIH [26], supporting the idea that pronociceptive changes occur at multiple levels of the pain-processing pathway with systemic morphine infusion and may contribute to enhanced cancer-induced bone pain in mice treated with sustained morphine infusion.

Few studies have examined the effects of prolonged opioid exposure on primary or metastatic tumors within clinically relevant microenvironments such as the breast, prostate, or bone. Preclinical studies report conflicting findings on the effects of prolonged opioid administration on cancer-induced pain, tumor growth, and tumor-associated pathology. These conflicting reports may arise from differences in the site of tumor and associated differences in the microenvironment, the dose or route of opioid administration, the time course of opioid administration, and the tumor cell line used in the study. Reports of adverse effects of prolonged morphine administration in some studies highlight the need for a better understanding of the effects of prolonged opioid exposure on cancer-induced pain as well as on other aspects of disease progression, including tumor growth, metastases, and tumor-associated pathology. It should be emphasized that opioids are necessary and appropriate for the treatment of cancer pain. Observations described above highlight a need to better understand potential adverse effects of opioids that may lead to improved treatment options, including the use of adjunct therapies that might diminish the adverse effects of opioids and enhance their pain-alleviating effects.

# Potential Benefits of Coanalgesics on Opioid-Induced Hyperalgesia and Tumor Growth

Coanalgesics are drugs administered in conjunction with NSAIDs and opioids that may enhance the analgesic activity of these compounds. Coanalgesics typically have independent analgesic activity in certain pain states, such as neuropathic pain, or may counteract some of the adverse side effects associated with NSAIDs or opioids [3]. Several preclinical studies indicate that combination therapies may prove beneficial in improving the analgesic efficacy of opioids as well as diminishing adverse side effects and disease progression. Coadministration of selective cyclooxygenase-2 (COX-2) inhibitors with morphine has been demonstrated to diminish tumor growth in vitro as well as in vivo. Moreover, COX-2 inhibitors were demonstrated to block morphine-induced enhanced tumor growth, angiogenesis, and metastases in preclinical studies [16,58]. Others have demonstrated that COX-2 inhibitors block the development of OIH [33]. Moreover, coadministration of COX inhibitors with morphine provided synergistic antiallodynic effects in a rat model of neuropathic pain [34]. Given that neuropathic pain is a recognized component of cancer-induced bone pain [41], coadministration of COX inhibitors may prove a useful strategy for effective pain management that limits the adverse side effects of opioids.

Clinically, coanalgesics consist of a diverse range of drug classes, including anticonvulsants (e.g., gabapentin, pregabalin), antidepressants (e.g., tricyclic agents, selective serotonin reuptake inhibitors, and serotonin norepinephrine reuptake inhibitors), N-methyl-D aspartate

(NMDA) receptor antagonists (e.g., ketamine), corticosteroids, skeletal muscle relaxants, local anesthetics, and $\alpha_2$-adrenergic agonists (e.g., clonidine) [3]. Coanalgesics are frequently administered with opioids in efforts to diminish the dose required for effective pain management and reduce adverse effects [37]. The American Pain Society states that the proper use of coanalgesics is critical to successful pain management, and depends on evaluation of risks (adverse effects and drug interactions) versus benefits (improved pain relief, sleep, and quality of life) [3]. Moreover, the use of coanalgesics that target neuropathic pain may be particularly important because opioid use for treatment of neuropathic pain may require higher doses, and neuropathic pain occurs in 40–50% of patients with cancer pain [41]. Overall, multimodal therapy for pain management is recommended [3], for several reasons. First, coadministration of adjuvants that block adverse effects such as nausea, constipation, and OIH will improve pain management and decrease adverse side effects, improving the patient's quality of life. Second, combination pharmacotherapy is often better than an opioid alone due to multiple mechanisms of action, particularly given the multifaceted aspect of cancer pain, which includes neuropathic, inflammatory, and mechanical qualities [3,42]. Therefore, such therapy can be expected to decrease opioid demand. In combination with these traditional analgesics, patients also receive therapies designed to diminish tumor burden (e.g., radiation therapy) or bone remodeling (e.g., bisphosphonates) [3]. As stated above, issues of potential interactions between analgesics and nonanalgesic medications must be taken into account to optimize disease treatment and pain management in cancer patients [3].

# Conclusion

Opioids are the most effective and most appropriate treatment for moderate to severe cancer-induced pain, and they remain the appropriate front-line treatment for cancer pain patients. However, care must be taken to closely monitor patients for potential adverse effects of opioids, including opioid-induced hyperalgesia. Within the clinic, alternatives such as cotherapies and opioid rotation must be considered and used appropriately to minimize opioid-induced adverse side effects and to maintain the analgesic efficacy of opioid treatment (see Chapter 8 by Vissers et al.). Focusing on the impact of the disease as well as that of the therapeutic strategies becomes particularly important as chemotherapeutic treatments advance and extend the lifespan of patients. Important advances are increasing the therapeutic options for patients with metastatic bone pain. New drugs, such as anti-nerve growth factor (NGF) antibodies are currently undergoing clinical trials for cancer-induced bone pain. In addition, preclinical studies indicate that coadministration of agents such as COX inhibitors, NK1 antagonists, or 5-HT$_3$ antagonists along with opioids may be considered as adjuncts in ameliorating the necessary doses of opioids and their side effects, including hyperalgesia and analgesic tolerance, thus increasing the therapeutic potential of the opioids in these patients.

Recent studies highlight our limited knowledge on the effects of long-term opioid treatment on cancer-induced pain and disease progression. Advances in cancer therapies have led to increased survival time in patients, including those with bone metastases. Such increased survival times require prolonged pain management, leading in some cases to adverse medication-induced side effects. Clinical studies on the benefits of coadministration of currently available agents—COX inhibitors, NK1 antagonists, 5-HT$_3$ antagonists, anti-tumor necrosis factor (TNF) drugs, and anti-IL-6 agents—and compounds currently in clinical trials (e.g., anti-NGF drugs) are critical. Especially important are not only measures of the impact of the combined therapies on disease progression, but also measures of pain at rest, instances and severity of breakthrough pain, and overall quality of life in these patients (alertness, mobility, and so on). Preclinical studies are needed to determine potential new targets for long-term treatment of cancer-induced pain. Moreover, preclinical studies must be performed to determine potential opioid-sparing effects of currently available and newly developed compounds, if well-controlled studies cannot be performed within the clinic due to technical and ethical considerations. Such studies on the effects of prolonged opioid exposure on pain processing and disease progression, as well as potential combination therapies diminishing or eliminating side effects associated with prolonged opioid therapy, will provide important insights as to potential improvements in prolonged pain management in cancer patients with chronic tumor-induced pain.

# References

[1] Allan L, Hays H, Jensen N-H, de Waroux BLP, Bolt M, Donald R, Kalso E. Randomised cross-over trial of transdermal fentanyl and sustained release oral morphine for treating chronic non-cancer. BMJ 2001;322:1154–8.

[2] American Cancer Society. Cancer facts and figures 2008. Atlanta: American Cancer Society; 2008.

[3] American Pain Society. Principles of analgesic use in the treatment of acute pain and cancer pain. Glenview: American Pain Society; 2008.

[4] Angst MS, Clark JD. Opioid-induced hyperalgesia: a qualitative systematic review. Anesthesiology 2006;104:570–87.

[5] Blair HC, Robinson LJ, Zaidi M. Osteoclast signalling pathways. Biochem Biophys Res Commun 2005;328:728–38.

[6] Blum RH, Novetsky D, Shasha D, Fleishman S. The multidisciplinary approach to bone metastases. Oncology (Huntingt) 2003;17:845–57.

[7] Boyce BF, Hughes DE, Wright KR, Xing L, Dai A. Recent advances in bone biology provide insight into the pathogenesis of bone diseases. Lab Invest 1999;79:83–94.

[8] Boyce BF, Xing L, Shakespeare W, Wang Y, Dalgarno D, Iuliucci J, Sawyer T. Regulation of bone remodeling and emerging breakthrough drugs for osteoporosis and osteolytic bone metastases. Kidney Int Suppl 2003;85:2–5.

[9] Chen Y, Geis C, Sommer C. Activation of TRPV1 contributes to morphine tolerance: involvement of the mitogen-activated protein kinase signaling pathway. J Neurosci 2008;28:5836–45.

[10] Christo PJ, Mazloomdoost D. Cancer pain and analgesia. Ann NY Acad Sci 2008;1138:278–98.

[11] Chu LF, Angst MS, Clark D. Opioid-induced hyperalgesia in humans: molecular mechanisms and clinical considerations. Clin J Pain 2008;24:479–96.

[12] Chu LF, Clark DJ, Angst MS. Opioid tolerance and hyperalgesia in chronic pain patients after one month of oral morphine therapy: a preliminary prospective study. J Pain 2006;7:43–8.

[13] Clohisy DR, Mantyh PW. Bone cancer pain. Cancer 2003;97(3 Suppl):866–73.

[14] Coyle N, Adelhardt J, Foley KM, Portenoy RK. Character of terminal illness in the advanced cancer patient: pain and other symptoms during the last four weeks of life. J Pain SymptomManage 1990;5:83–93.

[15] Dougall WC, Chaisson M. The RANK/RANKL/OPG triad in cancer-induced bone diseases. Cancer Metastasis Rev 2006;25:541–9.

[16] Farooqui M, Li Y, Rogers T, Poonawala T, Griffin RJ, Song CW, Gupta K. COX-2 inhibitor celecoxib prevents chronic morphine-induced promotion of angiogenesis, tumour growth, metastasis and mortality, without compromising analgesia. Br J Cancer 2007;97:1523–31.

[17] Feng P, Rahim RT, Cowan A, Liu-Chen L-Y, Peng X, Gaughan J, Meissler JJJ, Adler MW, Eisenstein TK. Effects of mu, kappa or delta opioids administered by pellet or pump on oral Salmonella infection and gastrointestinal transit. Eur J Pharmacol 2006;534:250–7.

[18] Gardell LR, Wang R, Burgess SE, Ossipov MH, Vanderah TW, Malan TP Jr, Lai J, Porreca F. Sustained morphine exposure induces a spinal dynorphin-dependent enhancement of excitatory transmitter release from primary afferent fibers. J Neurosci 2002;22:6747–55.

[19] Gupta K, Kshirsagar S, Chang L, Schwartz R, Law PY, Yee D, Hebbel RP. Morphine stimulates angiogenesis by activating proangiogenic and survival-promoting signaling and promotes breast tumor growth. Cancer Res 2002;62:4491–8.

[20] Halvorson KG, Sevcik MA, Ghilardi JR, Rosol TJ, Mantyh PW. Similarities and differences in tumor growth, skeletal remodeling and pain in an osteolytic and osteoblastic model of bone cancer. Clin J Pain 2006;22:587–600.

[21] Heiskanen T, Kalso E. Controlled-release oxycodone and morphine in cancer related pain. Pain 1997;73:37–45.

[22] Honore P, Luger NM, Sabino MA, Schwei MJ, Rogers SD, Mach DB, O'Keefe P F, Ramnaraine ML, Clohisy DR, Mantyh PW. Osteoprotegerin blocks bone cancer-induced skeletal destruction, skeletal pain and pain-related neurochemical reorganization of the spinal cord. Nat Med 2000;6:521–8.

[23] Hutchinson MR, Bland ST, Johnson KW, Rice KC, Maier SF, Watkins LR. Opioid-induced glial activation: mechanisms of activation and implications for opioid analgesia, dependence, and reward. Scientific World Journal 2007;7:98–111.

[24] Hutchinson MR, Coats BD, Lewis SS, Zhang Y, Sprunger DB, Rezvani N, Baker EM, Jekich BM, Wieseler JL, Somogyi AA, et al. Proinflammatory cytokines oppose opioid-induced acute and chronic analgesia. Brain Behav Immun 2008;22:1178–89.

[25] Ishikawa M, Tanno K, Kamo A, Takayanagi Y, Sasaki K. Enhancement of tumor growth by morphine and its possible mechanism in mice. Biol Pharm Bull 1993;16:762–6.

[26] Johnston IN, Milligan ED, Wieseler-Frank J, Frank MG, Zapata V, Campisi J, Langer S, Martin D, Green P, Fleshner M, et al. A role for proinflammatory cytokines and fractalkine in analgesia, tolerance, and subsequent pain facilitation induced by chronic intrathecal morphine. J Neurosci 2004;24(33):7353–65.

[27] Juni A, Klein G, Kest B. Morphine hyperalgesia in mice is unrelated to opioid activity, analgesia, or tolerance: evidence for multiple diverse hyperalgesic systems. Brain Res 2006;1070:35–44.

[28] Juni A, Klein G, Pintar JE, Kest B. Nociception increases during opioid infusion in opioid receptor triple knock-out mice. Neuroscience 2007;147:439–44.

[29] Kest B, Hopkins E, Palmese CA, Adler M, Mogil JS. Genetic variation in morphine analgesic tolerance: a survey of 11 inbred mouse strains. Pharmacol Biochem Behav 2002;73:821–8.

[30] King T, Gardell LR, Wang R, Vardanyan A, Ossipov MH, Malan TP Jr, Vanderah TW, Hunt SP, Hruby VJ, Lai J, Porreca F. Role of NK-1 neurotransmission in opioid-induced hyperalgesia. Pain 2005;116:276–88.

[31] King T, Ossipov MH, Vanderah TW, Porreca F, Lai J. Is paradoxical pain induced by sustained opioid exposure an underlying mechanism of opioid antinociceptive tolerance? Neurosignals 2005;14:194–205.

[32] King T, Vardanyan A, Majuta L, Melemedjian O, Nagle R, Cress AE, Vanderah TW, Lai J, Porreca F. Morphine treatment accelerates sarcoma-induced bone pain, bone loss, and spontaneous fracture in a murine model of bone cancer. Pain 2007;132:154–68.

[33] Koetzner L, Hua XY, Lai J, Porreca F, Yaksh T. Nonopioid actions of intrathecal dynorphin evoke spinal excitatory amino acid and prostaglandin E2 release mediated by cyclooxygenase-1 and -2. J Neurosci 2004;24:1451–8.

[34] Lashbrook JM, Ossipov MH, Hunter JC, Raffa RB, Tallarida RJ, Porreca F. Synergistic antiallodynic effects of spinal morphine with ketorolac and selective COX1- and COX2-inhibitors in nerve-injured rats. Pain 1999;82:65–72.

[35] Luger NM, Honore P, Sabino MA, Schwei MJ, Rogers SD, Mach DB, Clohisy DR, Mantyh PW. Osteoprotegerin diminishes advanced bone cancer pain. Cancer Res 2001;61:4038–47.

[36] Luger NM, Sabino MAC, Schwei MJ, Mach DB, Pomonis JD, Keyser CP, Rathbun M, Clohisy DR, Honore P, Yaksh TL, Mantyh PW. Efficacy of systemic morphine suggests a fundamental difference in the mechanisms that generate bone cancer vs. inflammatory pain. Pain 2002;99:397–406.

[37] Lussier D, Huskey AG, Portenoy RK. Adjuvant analgesics in cancer pain management. Oncologist 2004;9:571–91.

[38] Ma W, Zheng W-H, Powell K, Jhamandas K, Quirion R. Chronic morphine exposure increases the phosphorylation of MAP kinases and the transcription factor CREB in dorsal root ganglion neurons: an in vitro and in vivo study. Eur J Neurosci 2001;14:1091–104.

[39] Maneckjee R, Minna JD. Opioid and nicotine receptors affect growth regulation of human lung cancer cell lines. Proc Natl Acad Sci USA 1990;87:3294–8.

[40] Maneckjee R, Minna JD. Opioids induce while nicotine suppresses apoptosis in human lung cancer cells. Cell Growth Differ 1994;5:1033–40.

[41] Manfredi PL, Gonzales GR, Sady R, Chandler S, Payne R. Neuropathic pain in patients with cancer. J Palliat Care 2003;19:115–8.

[42] Mantyh PW, Clohisy DR, Koltzenburg M, Hunt SP. Molecular mechanisms of cancer pain. Nat Rev Cancer 2002;2:201–9.

[43] Mao J. Opioid-induced abnormal pain sensitivity: implications in clinical opioid therapy. Pain 2002;100:213–7.

[44] Mao J, Mayer DJ. Spinal cord neuroplasticity following repeated opioid exposure and its relation to pathological pain. Ann NY Acad Sci 2001;933:175–84.

[45] Menard DP, van Rossum D, Kar S, St Pierre S, Sutak M, Jhamandas K, Quirion R. A calcitonin gene-related peptide receptor antagonist prevents the development of tolerance to spinal morphine analgesia. J Neurosci 1996;16:2342–51.

[46] Meng ID, Harasawa I. Chronic morphine exposure increases the proportion of on-cells in the rostral ventromedial medulla in rats. Life Sci 2007;80:1915–20.

[47] Mercadante S. Opioid rotation for cancer pain: rationale and clinical aspects. Cancer 1999;86:1856–66.
[48] Mercadante S, Arcuri E, Ferrera P, Villari P, Mangione S. Alternative treatments of break-through pain in patients receiving spinal analgesics for cancer pain. J Pain Symptom Manage 2005;30:485–91.
[49] Mercadante S, Ferrera P, Villari P, Arcuri E. Hyperalgesia: an emerging iatrogenic syndrome. J Pain Symptom Manage 2003;26:769–75.
[50] Mercadante S, Portenoy RK. Opioid poorly-responsive cancer pain. Part 1: clinical considerations. J Pain Symptom Manage 2001;21:144–50.
[51] Mogil JS, Ritchie J, Smith SB, Strasburg K, Kaplan L, Wallace MR, Romberg RR, Bijl H, Sarton EY, Fillingim RB, Dahan A. Melanocortin-1 receptor gene variants affect pain and mu-opioid analgesia in mice and humans. J Med Genet 2005;42:583–7.
[52] Ossipov MH, Lai J, King T, Vanderah TW, Malan TP Jr, Hruby VJ, Porreca F. Antinociceptive and nociceptive actions of opioids. J Neurobiol 2004;61:126–48.
[53] Ossipov MH, Lai J, King T, Vanderah TW, Porreca F. Underlying mechanisms of pronociceptive consequences of prolonged morphine exposure. Biopolymers 2005;80:319–24.
[54] Portenoy RK, Lesage P. Management of cancer pain. Lancet 1999;353:1695–700.
[55] Powell KJ, Ma W, Sutak M, Doods H, Quirion R, Jhamandas K. Blockade and reversal of spinal morphine tolerance by peptide and non-peptide calcitonin gene-related peptide receptor antagonists. Br J Pharmacol 2000;131:875–84.
[56] Powell KJ, Quirion R, Jhamandas K. Inhibition of neurokinin-1-substance P receptor and prostanoid activity prevents and reverses the development of morphine tolerance in vivo and the morphine-induced increase in CGRP expression in cultured dorsal root ganglion neurons. Eur J Neurosci 2003;18:1572–83.
[57] Raghavendra V, Rutkowski MD, DeLeo JA. The role of spinal neuroimmune activation in morphine tolerance/hyperalgesia in neuropathic and sham-operated rats. J Neurosci 2002;22:9980–9.
[58] Sabino MA, Ghilardi JR, Jongen JL, Keyser CP, Luger NM, Mach DB, Peters CM, Rogers SD, Schwei MJ, de Felipe C, Mantyh PW. Simultaneous reduction in cancer pain, bone destruction, and tumor growth by selective inhibition of cyclooxygenase-2. Cancer Res 2002;62:7343–9.
[59] Sacerdote P, Limiroli E, Gaspani L. Experimental evidence for immunomodulatory effects of opioids. Adv Exp Med Biol 2003;521:106–16.
[60] Silverman SM. Opioid induced hyperalgesia: clinical implications for the pain practitioner. Pain Physician 2009;12:679–84.
[61] Simon RH, Arbo TE. Morphine increases metastatic tumor growth. Brain Res Bull 1986;16:363–7.
[62] Slatkin NE. Opioid switching and rotation in primary care: implementation and clinical utility. Curr Med Res Opin 2009;25:2133–50.
[63] Sommer C, Kress M. Recent findings on how proinflammatory cytokines cause pain: peripheral mechanisms in inflammatory and neuropathic hyperalgesia. Neurosci Lett 2004;361:184–7.
[64] Sueoka E, Sueoka N, Kai Y, Okabe S, Suganuma M, Kanematsu K, Yamamoto T, Fujiki H. Anti-cancer activity of morphine and its synthetic derivative, KT-90, mediated through apoptosis and inhibition of NF-kappaB activation. Biochem Biophys Res Commun 1998;252:566–70.
[65] Sueoka N, Sueoka E, Okabe S, Fujiki H. Anti-cancer effects of morphine through inhibition of tumour necrosis factor-alpha release and mRNA expression. Carcinogenesis 1996;17:2337–41.
[66] Suzuki R, Porreca F, Dickenson AH. Evidence for spinal dorsal horn hyperexcitability in rats following sustained morphine exposure. Neurosci Lett 2006;407:156–61.
[67] Tegeder I, Geisslinger G. Opioids as modulators of cell death and survival--unraveling mechanisms and revealing new indications. Pharmacol Rev 2004;56:351–69.
[68] Tegeder I, Grosch S, Schmidtko A, Haussler A, Schmidt H, Niederberger E, Scholich K, Geisslinger G. G-protein-independent G1 cell cycle block and apoptosis with morphine in adenocarcinoma cells: involvement of p53 phosphorylation. Cancer Res 2003;63:1846–52.
[69] Tegeder I, Meier S, Burian M, Schmidt H, Geisslinger G, Lotsch J. Peripheral opioid analgesia in experimental human pain models. Brain 2003;126:1092–1102.
[70] Urch CE, Donovan-Rodriguez T, Gordon-Williams R, Bee LA, Dickenson AH. Efficacy of chronic morphine in a rat model of cancer-induced bone pain: behavior and in dorsal horn pathophysiology. J Pain 2005;6:837–45.
[71] Vanderah TW, Suenaga NM, Ossipov MH, Malan TP Jr, Lai J, Porreca F. Tonic descending facilitation from the rostral ventromedial medulla mediates opioid-induced abnormal pain and antinociceptive tolerance. J Neurosci 2001;21:279–86.

[72] Vardanyan A, Wang R, Vanderah TW, Ossipov MH, Lai J, Porreca F, King T. TRPV1 receptor in expression of opioid-induced hyperalgesia. J Pain 2009;10:243–52.
[73] Vera-Portocarrero LP, Zhang ET, King T, Ossipov MH, Vanderah TW, Lai J, Porreca F. Spinal NK-1 receptor expressing neurons mediate opioid-induced hyperalgesia and antinociceptive tolerance via activation of descending pathways. Pain 2007;129:35–45.
[74] Warfield CA. Controlled-release morphine tablets in patients with chronic cancer pain: a narrative review of controlled clinical trials. Cancer 1998;82:2299–306.
[75] World Health Organization. Cancer pain relief and palliative care: technical report series. Geneva: World Health Organization; 1986.
[76] Xie JY, Herman DS, Stiller CO, Gardell LR, Ossipov MH, Lai J, Porreca F, Vanderah TW. Cholecystokinin in the rostral ventromedial medulla mediates opioid-induced hyperalgesia and antinociceptive tolerance. J Neurosci 2005;25:409–16.
[77] Zagon IS, McLaughlin PJ. Opioids and differentiation in human cancer cells. Neuropeptides 2005;39:495–505.
[78] Zech DF, Grond S, Lynch J, Hertel D, Lehmann KA. Validation of World Health Organization Guidelines for cancer pain relief: a 10-year prospective study. Pain 1995;63:65–76.

***Correspondence to:*** Tamara King, PhD, Department of Pharmacology, University of Arizona, P.O. Box 245050, Tucson, AZ 85724-5050, USA. Email: kingt@email.arizona.edu.

# Part III

# Opioid Tolerance

# Mechanisms of Opioid Tolerance

## Charles E. Inturrisi[a,b] and Ann M. Gregus[a]

*aDepartment of Pharmacology, Weill Cornell Medical College, New York, New York, USA;*
*bPain and Palliative Care Service, Memorial Sloan-Kettering Cancer Center, New York,*
*New York, USA*

# Opioid Tolerance and Cross-Tolerance

The clinical utility of opioids for pain management can be limited significantly by the development of analgesic tolerance that can occur in many patients receiving long-term therapy [31,44]. In addition to analgesic tolerance, some meaningful degree of tolerance also develops to opioid-induced respiratory depression, sedation, and nausea with chronic administration. In contrast, significant tolerance does not appear to develop to the constipating effects of opioids. The cellular mechanisms responsible for the very limited tolerance to the constipating effects of opioids are not understood. Electrophysiological studies found that excitatory myenteric neurons from morphine-tolerant animals require increased morphine concentrations to produce the same inhibition of firing compared to naive tissues. However, neither mu-opioid-receptor (MOP) function nor signaling mechanisms are impaired in morphine-tolerant myenteric tissues [57]. In addition, persistent occupation of MOP causes a sustained hyperpolarization of myenteric neurons, which may explain

*Cancer Pain: From Molecules to Suffering*
edited by Judith A. Paice, Rae F. Bell, Eija A. Kalso, and Olaitan A. Soyannwo
IASP Press, Seattle, © 2010

the powerful contractions of gastrointestinal smooth muscle that are seen with opioid withdrawal [57].

Opioid tolerance is defined as a reduction in response to the same dose of an opioid after repeated exposure or when increasingly high doses must be administered to obtain the effects observed with the original dose. In pharmacological terms, tolerance is the reduction of analgesic potency, which may be illustrated quantitatively by a rightward shift in the dose-response curve for analgesia and an increase in the $ED_{50}$, or median effective dose [21,28]. In a small controlled trial, Houde found that cancer patients who received morphine for pain each day, as required, for 1 week, the morphine dose-response curve was shifted to the right so that 15 mg of morphine provided the same pain relief as 10 mg on day 1 [21]. Thus, tolerance can be defined in terms of the magnitude of the change in response and the temporal onset of this change.

In more general terms, a decrease in the effectiveness of a drug as a result of repeated administration may be the result of the development of associative tolerance or pharmacological (nonassociative) tolerance. Preclinical studies showing that the analgesic effects of morphine can be environmentally dependent have led to the conclusion that the tolerance observed in these paradigms is not entirely pharmacologically based but may include a conditioned or associative component. For some classically conditioned behaviors, the conditioned responses are compensatory or opposite to the unconditioned responses, as is the case with associative tolerance (see Bespalov et al. [6] for a review). Pharmacological (nonassociative) tolerance can be the result of changes in drug disposition, usually as a consequence of the induction of drug biotransformation reactions that decrease the effective concentrations of the drug of interest. This type of tolerance is designated pharmacokinetic tolerance. Alternatively, tolerance can result from a neuronal adaptation that decreases the response to the presence of constant or increasing concentrations of drug, an adaptation known as pharmacodynamic tolerance. Tolerance to opioids is predominantly of the pharmacodynamic type.

In the tolerant state, analgesia may be restored by increasing the dose and/or frequency of administration of the opioid, but this approach can exacerbate adverse effects typically observed with therapeutic doses (e.g., sedation and constipation) and may initiate adverse effects such as multifocal myoclonus that manifest at higher doses [8]. Clinically, tolerance may be observed as an increase in opioid requirements so that consideration must be given to factors in the clinical situation that can result in a decrease in opioid analgesia and/or dose escalation. In addition to pharmacodynamic tolerance, resulting in a loss of opioid potency, other factors such as progression of disease (e.g., malignancy, arthritic changes, nerve damage), the effects of treatment (e.g., chemotherapy or radiation), psychological factors (e.g., depression, anxiety), addiction and/or diversion, and opioid-induced hyperalgesia can contribute to or be the primary cause of dose escalation [13].

In patients with pain it is difficult to separate a change in the pain stimulus (worsening pain) from the development of tolerance. Clearly, in patients whose opioid dose must be rapidly escalated to provide analgesia, the contribution of progression of disease must be evaluated. Thus, in some patients, tolerance may be a primary driving force for analgesic dose escalation or it may develop secondary to the escalation of the opioid to manage an increase in pain.

Often the first sign of the development of opioid analgesic tolerance is a decrease in the duration of pain relief so that while some analgesia occurs at the time of the peak response, the duration of effective analgesia is appreciably diminished. There are no prospective randomized controlled trials on the rate of development of tolerance with chronic opioid administration. Some observational studies report a pattern of relatively rapid dose escalation lasting several weeks to a few months, followed by a period of up to 3 years in which doses increase at a slower rate. In advanced cancer patients, progression of metastatic disease with increasing severity of pain was the major factor in escalation of opioid dose [34]. However, many patients—particularly those with noncancer pain—discontinue chronic opioid therapy due to adverse effects, which clearly limits the generality of these observations [13].

It is essential that the term "tolerance" be distinguished from the terms "opioid physical dependence" and "opioid addiction." Opioid physical dependence refers to an altered physiological state produced by repeated administration that necessitates the continued administration of the opioid to prevent the appearance of a stereotypical syndrome, the withdrawal or abstinence syndrome, that is characteristic for the particular opioid. In contrast, opioid addiction is a behavioral pattern of use, characterized by overwhelming involvement with the use of an opioid (compulsive use), the securing of a supply, continued use despite harm, and a high tendency to relapse after withdrawal.

Cross-tolerance refers to the fact that tolerance to the effects of one opioid confers tolerance to another opioid. Cross-tolerance is readily demonstrated in animal studies [47]. In a small controlled study in cancer patients with pain, Houde et al. [21,28] measured tolerance and cross-tolerance between morphine and metopon (methyldihydromorphinone, a semisynthetic analogue of morphine) (Fig. 1). He found that at the start of the study, the analgesic potency ratio of metopon to morphine was 2.0; i.e., metopon was twice as potent as morphine (Fig. 1). Next, these patients received morphine on demand for the next week. On day 8 the analgesic potency ratio again was determined. The metopon to morphine ratio had increased to 2.6 (Fig. 1). Houde also did the converse experiment and found that if metopon was given on demand

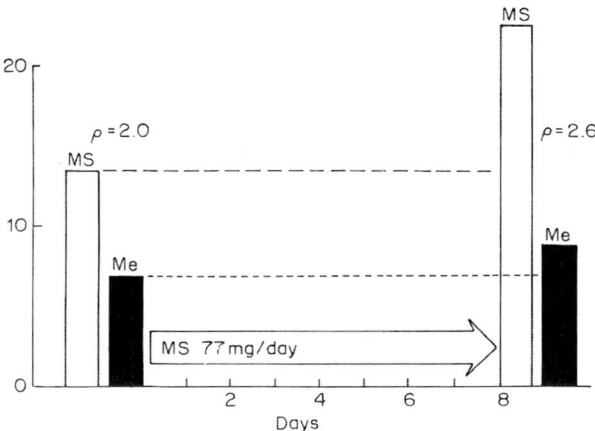

**Fig. 1.** Tolerance and apparent cross-tolerance to morphine, plotted in terms of equianalgesic doses of morphine sulfate (MS, open bars) and metopon (Me, filled bars). Cancer patients were given morphine as required for pain in the interval between the first equianalgesic dose estimation (left plot) and after second determination (right plot). The patients received an average of daily dosage of 77 mg of morphine per day for 8 days (chronic administration). The relative potency estimates are indicated by rho ($\rho$). Initially metopon was twice as potent as morphine ($\rho$ = 2.0). By day 8 the relative potency of morphine had decreased so that metopon was now 2.6 times more potent than morphine ($\rho$ = 2.6). From [21], with permission from the publisher.

for 1 week instead of morphine, cross-tolerance to morphine was less than the analgesic tolerance to metopon [28]. Houde concluded that these results were observed because the tolerance to repeated morphine, which all the patients had been receiving (Fig. 1), was greater than the cross-tolerance to "challenge" doses of metopon. Further, he suggested that while some cross-tolerance was observed among μ-opioids such as morphine and metopon, it was partial or "incomplete." This observation, together with clinical anecdotal observations with other μ-opioids, is the basis for the use of opioid switching or rotation in pain management. Thus, as tolerance or limiting adverse effects develop to the analgesic effects, a patient is switched from one mu opioid to another with the expectation that incomplete cross-tolerance will allow the use of a lower dose of the new opioid. Since the adverse effects of opioids are dose-related, switching can allow more flexibility in dosing and open a wider therapeutic window between analgesia and adverse effects. However, switching from one opioid to another requires an estimate of the equianalgesic dose conversion ratio, which has led to confusion and controversy [12,32,48].

One pharmacological explanation for incomplete cross-tolerance suggests that the dose-response curves of μ-opioids may not be parallel. The consequence of nonparallel analgesic dose-response curves is that the equianalgesic dose ratio will change as the dose of opioid is increased (i.e., as you move up the dose-response curve). Thus, for example, in Fig. 2 the dose ratio of drug A to B is 1:2 at the low end of the curve (10 mg of A is equianalgesic to 20 mg of B). If the dose response curves remain parallel as the dose required to produce analgesia to B is increased (presumably due to the development of tolerance), then the 1:2 equianalgesic dose conversion ratio would be correct at all doses shown (compare curve A with dotted line curve for B). However, if the dose-response curve for B (dashed line) is not parallel to A (in this case as a result of the more rapid development of tolerance to B than to A), then the initial equianalgesic dose conversion ratio of 1:2 is not correct as the dose of B is increased. In this example, the dose ratio of A to B is 1:5 in mid-range (20 mg of A is equianalgesic to 100 mg of B) and 1:10 at the higher end of the dose-response curve (compare the curve for A with the dashed curve for B). If the development of tolerance to drug

B necessitated switching to drug A, then the equianalgesic dose ratio would depend on where on the dose-response curve for B the switching occurred. If it occurred at the high end of the dose-response curve for B, then use of the "standard" 1:2 ratio rather than the actual 1:10 ratio would result in the calculation of a switching dose of A that is 5 times higher than is required. At the receptor level, these differences in dose response may reflect the recently identified and characterized MOP-receptor splice variants. Thus, incomplete cross-tolerance among MOP-receptor ligands might reflect the differing selectivities of mu ligands for these MOP-receptor subtypes [47].

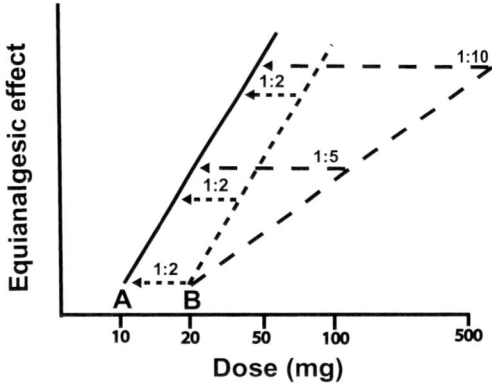

**Fig. 2.** The consequences of nonparallel analgesic dose-response curves for the estimation of the equianalgesic dose ratio as the dose is increased with the development of tolerance. The dose ratio of drug A to drug B is 1 to 2 at the low end of the curve (10 mg of A is equianalgesic to 20 mg of B). If the dose-response curves remain parallel as the dose required to produce analgesia to A is increased (presumably due to the development of tolerance), then the 1:2 equianalgesic dose conversion ratio would be correct at all doses shown (compare curve A with the dotted-line curve for B). However, if the dose-response curve for drug B (dashed line) is not parallel to that of drug A (in this case as a result of the more rapid development of tolerance to B than to A), then the initial equianalgesic dose conversion ratio of 1:2 is not correct as the dose of B is increased. In this example, the dose ratio of drug A to drug B is 1:5 in mid-range (20 mg of A is equianalgesic to 100 mg of B) and 1:10 at the higher end of the dose-response curve (compare the curve for A with the dashed curve for B). If the development of tolerance to drug B necessitated rotation to drug A, then the equianalgesic dose ratio would depend on where on the dose-response curve for B the rotation occurred. If it occurred at the high end of the dose-response curve for B, then use of the "standard" 1:2 ratio rather than the actual 1:10 ratio would result in the calculation of a rotation dose of B that is five times higher than is required.

# Mechanisms of Opioid Tolerance

The mechanisms believed to underlie opioid tolerance may be classified into two categories: within-systems and between-systems [39]. These mechanisms of tolerance are not necessarily mutually exclusive, as there is abundant evidence in support of anatomical and functional overlap of both processes [39].

## Cellular Tolerance: Within-Systems Adaptations

Within-systems processes of tolerance, often dubbed "cellular" or "homologous" tolerance, describe adaptations occurring at the level of the opioid receptors that alter the number of functional receptors or their ability to signal to downstream effectors involved in analgesia. These adaptations can include modifications of the receptor itself, such as μ-opioid-agonist-induced phosphorylation of the MOP [45,49], followed by desensitization that may include receptor internalization, endocytosis, and downregulation [5,7,27,35,52,56].

### *Receptor Desensitization, Internalization, and Recycling*

The MOP is believed to be desensitized by a mechanism that is similar to that described for the β-adrenergic receptor [26]. Fig. 3A illustrates the trafficking steps of this mechanism. Ligand activation of the MOP promotes phosphorylation of the receptor by a G-protein-coupled receptor kinase (GRK), which allows the recruitment of β-arrestin (β-arr) from the cytoplasm. This process desensitizes the receptor so that it can no longer couple to the heterotrimeric G proteins (α, β, γ), rendering it unable to signal downstream effects (cellular responses, a and b), and facilitates its endocytosis via clathrin-coated pits. Fig. 3B shows that endocytosis results in trafficking of the MOP to early endosomes, where it can be recycled back to the cell membrane or degraded. The recycling pathway has been hypothesized to be a critical step in the recovery from desensitization in which phosphatase activity is necessary for the reinsertion of receptors in the membrane [3,26].

Controversy on the role of internalization and endocytosis in the desensitization of the MOP and the development of tolerance is based in part on reports that morphine binding does not direct internalization of

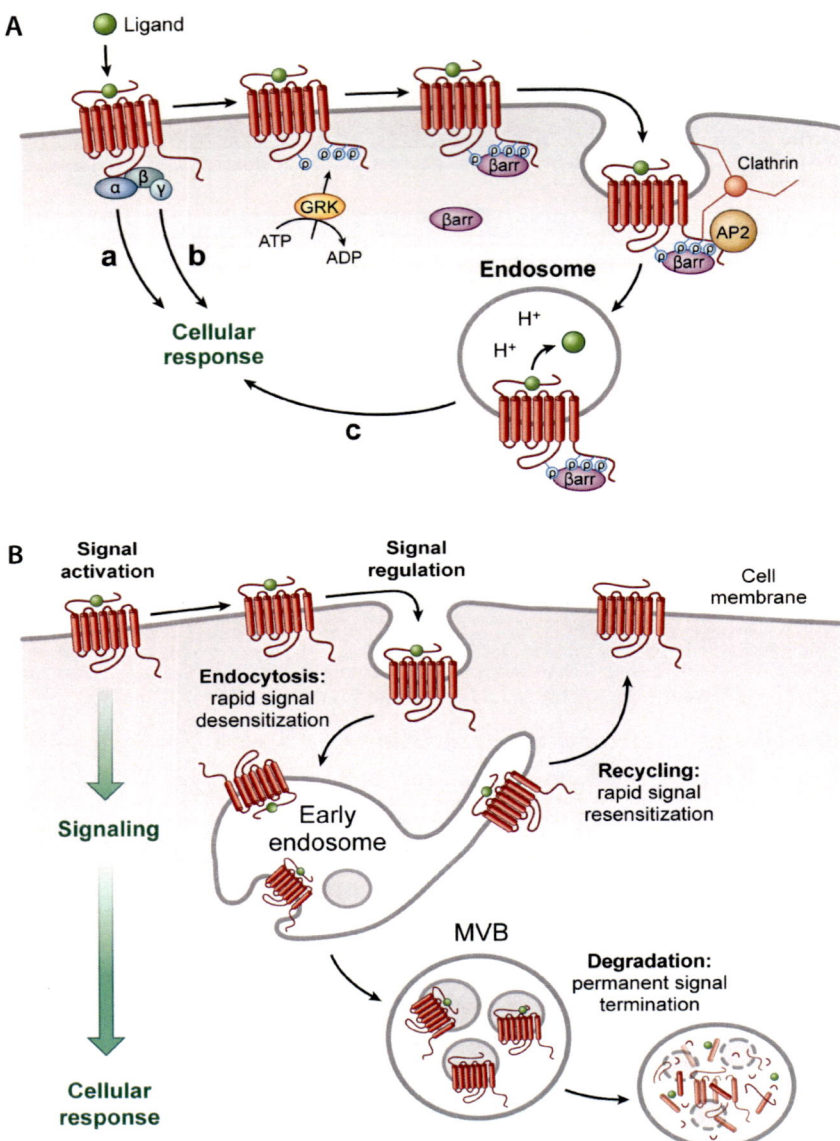

***Fig. 3.*** Receptor desensitization and internalization of G-protein-coupled receptors. (A) Ligand-bound phosphorylation of the receptor promotes the recruitment of arrestins (βarr) and receptor internalization (Endosome). ADP, adenosine diphosphate; ATP, adenosine triphosphate; GRK, G-protein-coupled receptor kinase. (B) Sorting of endocytosed receptor between divergent pathways produces recycling or degradation of the receptor. From [26] with permission from the publisher.

the MOP in some systems [20] and that MOP mutations that facilitate endocytosis actually reduce the development of cellular tolerance [20]. Using a system that allowed them to follow the internalization of the MOP into neurons under physiological conditions in real time, Arttamangkul et al. [3] studied desensitization and MOP trafficking of selected opioid agonists. Three patterns of receptor trafficking and desensitization were observed. Met-enkephalin, etorphine, and methadone produced both desensitization and receptor internalization, morphine and oxymorphone produced desensitization but not receptor internalization, and oxycodone was ineffective in both processes.

These results support the hypothesis that ligand-specific regulation of opioid receptors occurs in these brain slice neurons. However, as the authors indicate, "Given that all opioid agonists result in tolerance, it is clear that no one process can completely account for the whole animal response to opioids" [3]. In addition, they suggest that mechanisms that produce rapid desensitization of the MOP are not the only adaptations that contribute to the reduction of opioid agonist potency that manifests as opioid tolerance.

### G-Protein Signaling

Other cellular events that may contribute to tolerance include altered MOP-mediated signaling through G proteins [51]. These events include the enhanced activity of $G_s$ proteins [11,14], the release of $G_{\beta\gamma}$ subunits [11], and the modulation of G proteins by regulators of G-protein signaling proteins [23]. During chronic opioid exposure, a shift occurs in MOP-coupled signaling from predominantly $G_{i\alpha}$, an inhibitory G protein, to $G_{s\alpha}$, a stimulatory G protein, resulting in the activation of adenylyl cyclase. Gintzler and Chakrabarti [24] have reviewed these within-systems, post-receptor adaptations and proposed that this shift to $G_s$ may account for the loss of analgesic (agonist) activity and the emergence of excitatory activity during chronic opioid administration.

### Dual Receptor Targeting

The recognition that opioid receptors exist as dimers (both homodimers and heterodimers) has opened new areas of opioid pharmacophore investigation and helped to explain longstanding observations about the role of opioid receptor interactions in the modulation of tolerance [17,18].

Functional blockade of the delta-opioid receptor (DOP) by selective antagonists [1], by antisense [36], or by gene deletion [46] attenuates the development of morphine tolerance and decreases other MOP-associated
adverse effects. These observations suggested that a bivalent ligand that
would block the DOP while activating the MOP might result in a compound that would produce analgesia while limiting the development of
tolerance. Fig. 4 shows an example of a bivalent ligand that is produced by
linking oxymorphone (right; a MOP agonist) and naltrindole (left; a DOP
antagonist), which can be used to simultaneously activate the MOP and
block the DOP. A discussion of this approach is given by Dietis et al. [18].

### *Intracellular Signaling and Opioid Tolerance: Protein Kinase C*

Protein kinase C (PKC) is a family of second-messenger-dependent kinases. In vitro and in vivo (preclinical) data demonstrate that selective inhibitors of PKC isoforms α, γ, and ε can prevent or reverse the development
of morphine tolerance [4]. In vitro studies indicate that μ-opioid-mediated
stimulation leads to translocation of PKC to the plasma membrane [43] and
phosphorylation of the *N*-methyl-D-aspartate receptor (NMDAR). This
process is believed to contribute significantly to tolerance development [30]
and opioid-induced hyperalgesia (see below). Constitutively active PKC also
may phosphorylate MOP, causing its desensitization, although this effect

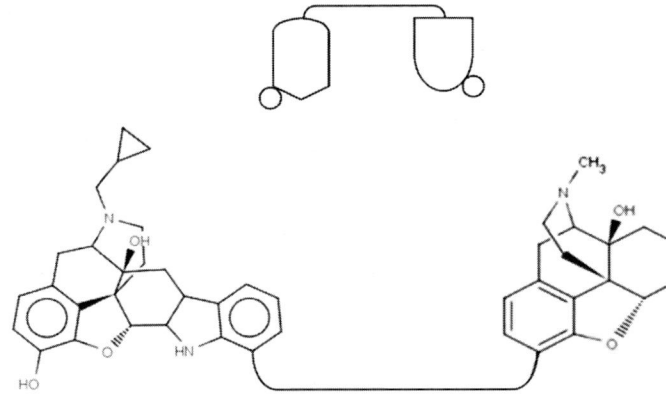

**Fig. 4.** The role of receptor heterodimers in the development of opioid tolerance. A bivalent ligand produced by linking oxymorphone (right; a μ-opioid-receptor [MOP] agonist)
and naltrindole (left; a δ-opioid-receptor [DOP] antagonist) can be used to simultaneously activate the MOP and block the DOP. From [18], with permission from the publisher.

appears to vary with cell type and μ-opioid agonist potency [4]. The intra-thecal (i.t.) administration of a PKC inhibitor [25] or an antisense oligode-oxynucleotide targeting PKC-α [29] reduced i.t. morphine tolerance in rats. Finally, intracerebroventricular (i.c.v.) coadministration of selective inhibi-tors of receptor for activated C-kinase (RACK) proteins that bind α, γ, or ε isoforms of PKC reversed systemic morphine tolerance in mice [53].

## Mechanisms of Opioid Tolerance at the Systems Level

Between-systems processes of tolerance, on the other hand, are character-ized by interactions that antagonize or compensate for the effects of an opi-oid, usually via some direct anti-opioid mechanism. These anti-opioid fac-tors may include nonopioid receptors, neurotransmitters, ion channels, and second messengers [30]. One behavioral theory that is consistent with the observation that chronic exposure to opioids is followed by a loss of analgesia and decreased pain thresholds (hyperalgesia) when opioid administration is discontinued is the opponent-process theory [38]. Applied to opioid admin-istration and pain thresholds, this theory postulates that adaptive processes are recruited to counteract the analgesic effects of the opioid and return the elevated pain threshold toward baseline values (i.e., tolerance) [10,40]. The model predicts that when opioid administration is abruptly interrupted (e.g., by an opioid antagonist), pain thresholds may transiently drop below baseline values and manifest as hyperalgesia [40]. In rodents, this pain-facil-itatory process appears to result from activation of the NMDAR [10,40] and from neuroimmune factors (described below). Furthermore, when opioid administration is stopped, a new equilibrium may develop between prono-ciceptive and endogenous antinociceptive systems [40].

### Opioid Tolerance and Opioid-Induced Hyperalgesia

Preclinical studies suggest that opioid tolerance may result from excitatory changes in the central nervous system that facilitate transmission of pain and increase pain sensitivity [2]. This condition, termed opioid-induced hyperalgesia (OIH), appears to result from the upregulation of pronoci-ceptive systems. The neuroanatomical substrates and signaling pathways involved in OIH are emerging [2].

One model is derived from the ability of NMDAR activation to mediate excitatory activity and the ability of NMDAR antagonists to attenuate or reverse opioid tolerance [16,19], OIH, and some forms of neuropathic pain. This model suggests that these phenomena share some common mechanistic components [42]. Based on studies of the effects of morphine on glutamate transporters in the spinal cord dorsal horn, some of the sequential steps in the development of morphine tolerance have emerged (Fig. 5). Morphine activates the MOP, leading to inhibition of potassium (K+) channels, one of the mechanisms responsible for the analgesic effects of morphine. With persistent morphine administration, there is a downregulation of spinal glutamate transporters (GLU). Decreased surface expression of glutamate transporters results in an increase in synaptic glutamate, which activates the NMDAR and causes an influx of calcium via the NMDAR channel into the postsynaptic cell [41]. Stimulation of the MOP also may result in the activation of PKC and other calcium-sensitive intracellular signaling cascades, producing subsequent

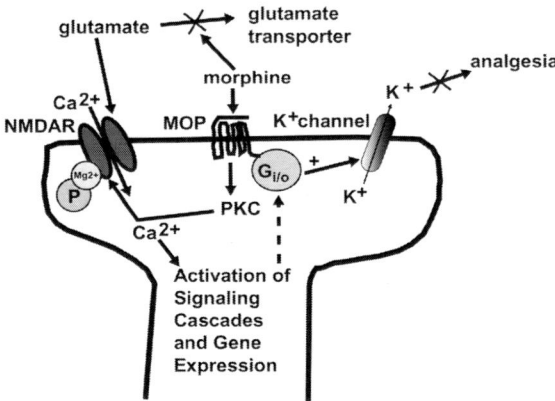

**Fig. 5.** The effects of morphine on spinal cord dorsal horn neurons may result in analgesia, hyperalgesia, and tolerance. Morphine activates the μ-opioid receptor (MOP), leading to inhibition of potassium (K+) channels, one of the mechanisms of morphine analgesia. In addition, MOP activation causes the activation of protein kinase C (PKC), and with persistent morphine administration there is a downregulation of spinal glutamate transporters (GLU). Decreased surface expression of GLU results in an increase in synaptic glutamate, which activates the N-methyl-D-aspartate receptor (NMDAR) and causes an influx of calcium via the NMDAR channel into the postsynaptic cell. [41]. Calcium-sensitive intracellular signal cascades are activated with subsequent phosphorylation of the NR1 subunit of the NMDAR. This phosphorylation removes the voltage-dependent magnesium block of the NMDAR. The resulting sustained activation of the NMDAR produces additional downstream changes in signaling cascades and gene expression that presumably result in desensitization of the MOP and tolerance.

phosphorylation of the NR1 subunit of the NMDAR, thereby removing its voltage-dependent magnesium ($Mg^{2+}$) block. The resulting sustained activation of the NMDAR produces additional downstream changes, including the activation of nitric oxide production [37]. These events ultimately lead to desensitization of the MOP. This process of sustained NMDAR activation, phosphorylation, and downstream changes in gene expression is also characteristic of central sensitization [33,58]. NMDAR-mediated central sensitization is involved in the hypersensitivity observed with inflammatory and neuropathic pain states [22].

As shown in Fig. 6, although both tolerance and OIH reduce the potency of a given dose of an opioid (X), the dose-response characteristics of a loss of opioid potency due to tolerance are different from the change in potency that is seen with OIH. Tolerance results in a shift to the right of the dose-response curve (A to C), whereas OIH results in a downward shift of the dose-response relationship (A to B) [2].

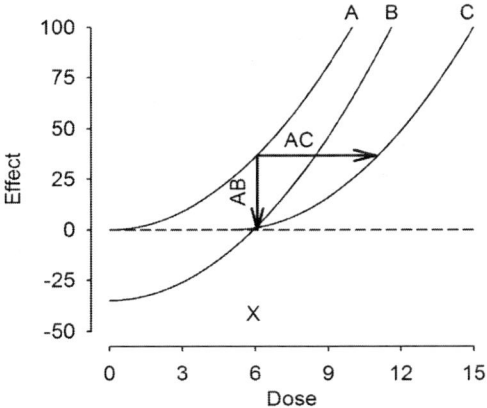

**Fig. 6.** Tolerance and opioid-induced hyperalgesia (OIH) have different effects on the analgesic dose-response relationship. However, both will increase analgesic dose requirements and therefore reduce the potency of a given dose of the opioid (X). The hypothetical dose-response curve for opioid-naive patients is shown as (A). In OIH, the dose-response curve of the chronic opioid user is shifted downward (AB), and the patient experiences increased pain in response to noxious stimuli at baseline, shown as a decreased analgesic response when the analgesic dose is zero (B). In analgesic tolerance, the slope of the dose-response curve of the chronic opioid user is shifted to the right (AC). In contrast to OIH, there is no significant change in pain sensitivity at baseline (C). This is shown as an identical analgesic response in opioid-naive subjects and chronic opioid users when the analgesic dose is zero (dashed line). From [2], with permission from the publisher.

In addition, the magnitude of the contribution of OIH to clinical opioid tolerance and the consequences for continued opioid therapy remain controversial. There is general agreement that during opioid withdrawal, OIH contributes to an exacerbation of pain [9]. Therefore, acute withdrawal should be avoided in opioid-tolerant or -dependent patients. Switching from a morphine-like opioid to a mixed agonist-antagonist (pentazocine, nalbuphine, and butorphanol) or the partial agonist buprenorphine should be avoided because these drugs can induce abrupt opioid withdrawal and cause concomitant hyperalgesia in opioid-dependent individuals [31]. In contrast, employing a combination of an opioid with a nonopioid analgesic can enhance analgesia and reduce the rate of tolerance development because tolerance does not develop to the non-opioid component of the mixture [31].

### Activation of the Immune System

The role of the immune system in maintenance of inflammatory and neuropathic pain states has been established [55]. The well-known pronociceptive actions of many cytokines have led to research on the interactions between chronic morphine administration and immune response in the presence and absence of injury states [55].

Chronic administration of morphine to rats has been shown to activate spinal glia and upregulate proinflammatory cytokines such as interleukin (IL)-1$\beta$, IL-6, and tumor necrosis factor-$\alpha$. In addition, spinal inhibition of proinflammatory cytokines restored acute morphine antinociception and significantly reversed the development of morphine tolerance and withdrawal-induced hyperalgesia and allodynia in nerve-injured or sham-operated rats [15,50,54]. These results suggest that targeting glial activation and central cytokine production may reduce the development of morphine tolerance as well as the expression of injury-induced hyperalgesic states [50].

# Summary

Establishing the mechanisms of opioid tolerance remains a continuing challenge. Some of the mechanisms described above appear to have the potential to provide new approaches for reducing or eliminating the development of opioid tolerance.

# Acknowledgments

C.E. Inturrisi is supported in part by NIDA grant DA001457 and NIDA center grant DA005130. A.M. Gregus was supported by NIDA training grant DA007274.

# References

[1]     Abdelhamid EE, Sultana M, Portoghese PS, Takemori AE. Selective blockage of delta opioid receptors prevents the development of morphine tolerance and dependence in mice. J Pharmacol Exp Ther 1991;258:299–303.

[2]     Angst MS, Clark JD. Opioid-induced hyperalgesia: a qualitative systematic review. Anesthesiology 2006;104:570–87.

[3]     Arttamangkul S, Quillinan N, Low MJ, von Zastrow M, Pintar J, Williams JT. Differential activation and trafficking of micro-opioid receptors in brain slices. Mol Pharmacol 2008;74:972–9.

[4]     Bailey CP, Smith FL, Kelly E, Dewey WL, Henderson G. How important is protein kinase C in mu-opioid receptor desensitization and morphine tolerance? Trends Pharmacol Sci 2006;27:558–65.

[5]     Bernstein MA, Welch SP. Mu-opioid receptor down-regulation and cAMP-dependent protein kinase phosphorylation in a mouse model of chronic morphine tolerance. Brain Res Mol Brain Res 1998;55:237–42.

[6]     Bespalov AY, Zvartau EE, Beardsley PM. Opioid-NMDA receptor interactions may clarify conditioned (associative) components of opioid analgesic tolerance. Neurosci Biobehav Rev 2001;25:343–53.

[7]     Bohn LM, Lefkowitz RJ, Caron MG. Differential mechanisms of morphine antinociceptive tolerance revealed in (beta)arrestin-2 knock-out mice. J Neurosci 2002;22:10494–500.

[8]     Bruera E, O'Pereira J. Neuropsychiatric toxicity of opioids. In: Jensen TS, Turner JA, Wiesenfeld-Hallin Z, editors. Proceedings of the 8th World Congress on Pain: Progress in pain research and management, Vol. 8. Seattle: IASP Press; 1997. p. 717–38.

[9]     Carroll IR, Angst MS, Clark JD. Management of perioperative pain in patients chronically consuming opioids. Reg Anesth Pain Med 2004;29:576–91.

[10]    Celerier E, Laulin J, Larcher A, Le Moal M, Simonnet G. Evidence for opiate-activated NMDA processes masking opiate analgesia in rats. Brain Res 1999;847:18–25.

[11]    Chakrabarti S, Regec A, Gintzler AR. Biochemical demonstration of mu-opioid receptor association with Gsalpha: enhancement following morphine exposure. Brain Res Mol Brain Res 2005;135:217–24.

[12]    Chou R, Fanciullo GJ, Fine PG, Adler JA, Ballantyne JC, Davies P, Donovan MI, Fishbain DA, Foley KM, Fudin J, et al. Clinical guidelines for the use of chronic opioid therapy in chronic non-cancer pain. J Pain 2009;10:113–30.

[13]    Chu LF, Clark D, Angst MS. Molecular basis and clinical implications of opioid tolerance and opioid-induced hyperalgesia. In: Sinatara A, DeLeon-Cassasola O, Viscusi E, Ginsberg B, editors. Acute pain management. New York: Cambridge University Press; 2009. p. 114–46.

[14]    Crain SM, Shen KF. GM1 ganglioside-induced modulation of opioid receptor-mediated functions. Ann NY Acad Sci 1998;845:106–25.

[15]    Cui Y, Chen Y, Zhi JL, Guo RX, Feng JQ, Chen PX. Activation of p38 mitogen-activated protein kinase in spinal microglia mediates morphine antinociceptive tolerance. Brain Res 2006;1069:235–43.

[16]    Davis AM, Inturrisi CE. Attenuation of hyperalgesia by LY235959, a competitive $N$-methyl-D-aspartate receptor antagonist. Brain Res 2001;894:150–3.

[17]    Devi LA. Heterodimerization of G-protein-coupled receptors: pharmacology, signaling and trafficking. Trends Pharmacol Sci 2001;22:532–7.

[18]    Dietis N, Guerrini R, Calo G, Salvadori S, Rowbotham DJ, Lambert DG. Simultaneous targeting of multiple opioid receptors: a strategy to improve side-effect profile. Br J Anaesth 2009;103:38–49.

[19] Elliott K, Hynansky A, Inturrisi CE. Dextromethorphan attenuates and reverses analgesic tolerance to morphine. Pain 1994;59:361–8.

[20] Finn AK, Whistler JL. Endocytosis of the mu opioid receptor reduces tolerance and a cellular hallmark of opiate withdrawal. Neuron 2001;32:829–39.

[21] Foley KM. Clinical tolerance to opioids. In: Basbaum AI, Besson JM, editors. Towards a new pharmacotherapy of pain. New York: John Wiley & Sons; 1991. p. 181–203.

[22] Garraway SM, Xu Q, Inturrisi CE. siRNA-mediated knockdown of the NR1 subunit gene of the NMDA receptor attenuates formalin-induced pain behaviors in adult rats. J Pain 2009;10:380–90.

[23] Garzon J, Rodriguez-Munoz M, de la Torre-Madrid E, Sanchez-Blazquez P. Effector antagonism by the regulators of G protein signalling (RGS) proteins causes desensitization of mu-opioid receptors in the CNS. Psychopharmacology (Berl) 2005;180:1–11.

[24] Gintzler AR, Chakrabarti S. Post-opioid receptor adaptations to chronic morphine; altered functionality and associations of signaling molecules. Life Sci 2006;79:717–22.

[25] Granados-Soto V, Kalcheva I, Hua X, Newton A, Yaksh TL. Spinal PKC activity and expression: role in tolerance produced by continuous spinal morphine infusion. Pain 2000;85:395–404.

[26] Hanyaloglu AC, von Zastrow M. Regulation of GPCRs by endocytic membrane trafficking and its potential implications. Annu Rev Pharmacol Toxicol 2008;48:537–68.

[27] He L, Fong J, von Zastrow M, Whistler JL. Regulation of opioid receptor trafficking and morphine tolerance by receptor oligomerization. Cell 2002;108:271–82.

[28] Houde RW, Wallenstein SL, Beaver WT. Evaluation of analgesics in patients with cancer pain. In: Lasagna L, editor. International encyclopedia of pharmacology and therapeutics, Vol. I. New York: Pergamon Press; 1966. p. 59–97.

[29] Hua XY, Moore A, Malkmus S, Murray SF, Dean N, Yaksh TL, Butler M. Inhibition of spinal protein kinase C alpha expression by an antisense oligonucleotide attenuates morphine infusion-induced tolerance. Neuroscience 2002;113:99–107.

[30] Inturrisi C. Preclinical evidence for a role of glutamatergic systems in opioid tolerance and dependence. Semin Neurosci 1997;9:110–9.

[31] Inturrisi CE. Clinical pharmacology of opioids for pain. Clin J Pain 2002;18:S3–S13.

[32] Inturrisi CE. Opioid rotation. In: Schmidt RF, Willis WD, editors. Encyclopedia of pain. Berlin: Springer; 2007. p. 1561–4.

[33] Ji RR, Kohno T, Moore KA, Woolf CJ. Central sensitization and LTP: do pain and memory share similar mechanisms? Trends Neurosci 2003;26:696–705.

[34] Kanner RM, Foley KM. Patterns of narcotic drug use in a cancer pain clinic. Ann NY Acad Sci 1981;362:161–72.

[35] Kelly E, Bailey CP, Henderson G. Agonist-selective mechanisms of GPCR desensitization. Br J Pharmacol 2008;153(Suppl 1):S379–88.

[36] Kest B, Lee CE, McLemore GL, Inturrisi CE. An antisense oligodeoxynucleotide to the delta opioid receptor (DOR-1) inhibits morphine tolerance and acute dependence in mice. Brain Res Bull 1996;39:185–8.

[37] Kolesnikov YA, Pan YX, Babey AM, Jain S, Wilson R, Pasternak GW. Functionally differentiating two neuronal nitric oxide synthase isoforms through antisense mapping: evidence for opposing NO actions on morphine analgesia and tolerance. Proc Natl Acad Sci USA 1997;94:8220–5.

[38] Koob GF. Drug addiction: the yin and yang of hedonic homeostasis. Neuron 1996;16:893–6.

[39] Koob GF, Bloom FE. Cellular and molecular mechanisms of drug dependence. Science 1988;242:715–23.

[40] Li H, Angst MS, Clark JD. A murine model of opioid-induced hyperalgesia. Mol Brain Res 2001;86:56–62.

[41] Mao J, Price DD, Mayer DJ. Mechanisms of hyperalgesia and morphine tolerance: a current view of their possible interactions. Pain 1995;62:259–74.

[42] Mao J, Sung B, Ji RR, Lim G. Chronic morphine induces downregulation of spinal glutamate transporters: implications in morphine tolerance and abnormal pain sensitivity. J Neurosci 2002;22:8312–23.

[43] Mayer DJ, Mao J, Price DD. The development of morphine tolerance and dependence is associated with translocation of protein kinase C. Pain 1995;61:365–74.

[44] McQuay H. Opioids in pain management. Lancet 1999;353):2229–32.

[45] Mestek A, Hurley JH, Bye LS, Campbell AD, Chen Y, Tian M, Liu J, Schulman H, Yu L. The human mu opioid receptor: modulation of functional desensitization by calcium/calmodulin-dependent protein kinase and protein kinase C. J Neurosci 1995;15:2396–406.

[46]  Nitsche JF, Schuller AG, King MA, Zengh M, Pasternak GW, Pintar JE. Genetic dissociation of opiate tolerance and physical dependence in delta-opioid receptor-1 and preproenkephalin knock-out mice. J Neurosci 2002;22:10906–13.

[47]  Pasternak GW. Incomplete cross tolerance and multiple mu opioid peptide receptors. Trends Pharmacol Sci 2001;22:67–70.

[48]  Pereira J, Lawlor P, Vigano A, Dorgan M, Bruera E. Equianalgesic dose ratios for opioids. a critical review and proposals for long-term dosing. J Pain Symptom Manage 2001;22:672–87.

[49]  Polakiewicz RD, Schieferl SM, Dorner LF, Kansra V, Comb MJ. A mitogen-activated protein kinase pathway is required for mu-opioid receptor desensitization. J Biol Chem 1998;273:12402–6.

[50]  Raghavendra V, Rutkowski MD, DeLeo JA. The role of spinal neuroimmune activation in morphine tolerance/hyperalgesia in neuropathic and sham-operated rats. J Neurosci 2002;22:9980–9.

[51]  Sharma SK, Klee WA, Nirenberg M. Dual regulation of adenylate cyclase accounts for narcotic dependence and tolerance. Proc Natl Acad Sci USA 1975;72:3092–6.

[52]  Sim-Selley LJ, Scoggins KL, Cassidy MP, Smith LA, Dewey WL, Smith FL, Selley DE. Region-dependent attenuation of mu opioid receptor-mediated G-protein activation in mouse CNS as a function of morphine tolerance. Br J Pharmacol 2007;151:1324–33.

[53]  Smith FL, Gabra BH, Smith PA, Redwood MC, Dewey WL. Determination of the role of conventional, novel and atypical PKC isoforms in the expression of morphine tolerance in mice. Pain 2007;127:129–39.

[54]  Tai YH, Wang YH, Wang JJ, Tao PL, Tung CS, Wong CS. Amitriptyline suppresses neuroinflammation and up-regulates glutamate transporters in morphine-tolerant rats. Pain 2006;124:77–86.

[55]  Watkins LR, Hutchinson MR, Johnston IN, Maier SF. Glia: novel counter-regulators of opioid analgesia. Trends Neurosci 2005;28:661–9.

[56]  Whistler JL, Chuang HH, Chu P, Jan LY, von Zastrow M. Functional dissociation of mu opioid receptor signaling and endocytosis: implications for the biology of opiate tolerance and addiction. Neuron 1999;23:737–46.

[57]  Wood JD, Galligan JJ. Function of opioids in the enteric nervous system. Neurogastroenterol Motil 2004;16(Suppl 2):17–28.

[58]  Woolf CJ, Salter MW. Neuronal plasticity: increasing the gain in pain. Science 2000;288:1765–9.

*Correspondence to:* Charles E. Inturrisi, PhD, Department of Pharmacology, Weill Cornell Medical College, 1300 York Avenue, Room LC-524, New York, NY 10065, USA. Email: ceintur@med.cornell.edu.

# Opioid Switching: A Technique for Optimizing Pain Relief and Reducing Side Effects in Cancer Pain

Kris C.P. Vissers,[a] Kees Besse,[a] Yvette M. van
der Linden,[b] Maurice Giezeman,[c] and Marieke
H.J. van den Beuken-van Everdingen[d]

[a]Department of Anesthesiology, Pain and Palliative Medicine, University Medical
Centre St. Radboud, Nijmegen, The Netherlands; [b]Radiotherapeutic Institute
Friesland, Leeuwarden, The Netherlands; [c]Department of Anesthesiology
and Pain Management, Diakonessen Hospital, Utrecht, The Netherlands;
[d]Department of Anesthesiology, Pain Management and Research Centre,
University Hospital Maastricht, Maastricht, The Netherlands

Several opioids are commercially available in various formulations for the management of severe cancer pain. Opioids are predominantly μ-opioid-receptor agonists, although the kappa and delta receptors are also potential targets of certain novel compounds. Differences in receptor affinity between opioids have been demonstrated [11]. In addition, differences in receptor activity and affinity, together with genetic factors causing differences in opioid responsiveness, support the potential utility of opioid switching in the treatment of refractory pain. Opioid switching involves changing therapy from one opioid to another with the goal of improving analgesia and reducing side effects.

## Opioids for Cancer Pain

A recent review on the prevalence of cancer pain, performed in The Netherlands, revealed that approximately 36% of patients receiving active cancer treatment experience moderate to severe cancer pain [43]. Despite the recognition that cancer pain seriously interferes with quality of life, and despite efforts to promote adequate pain management, estimates indicate that approximately 30% of cancer patients do not receive appropriate pharmacological pain treatment [35]. Several physician- and patient-related factors may contribute to the undertreatment of cancer pain. Patients may fear disease progression and be reluctant to report increasing pain. General lack of knowledge concerning opioid therapy, including overestimating the risk for addiction and side effects, may also be a contributing factor [33]. A recent survey of cancer patients suffering at least weekly pain indicated that even among those receiving prescription analgesics, 69% of patients experienced difficulties with everyday activities due to pain, and 50% believed that quality of life is not considered a priority by health care professionals [6].

Opioids are considered to be the mainstay of the pharmacological treatment of cancer-related pain. In clinical practice, opioid pharmacotherapy for cancer pain is contingent upon finding "a satisfactory balance between analgesia and side effects" [34]. In most studies, morphine is still considered the reference opioid; in oral slow-release formulation it forms the cornerstone of cancer pain management, while short-acting opioid formulations are used for breakthrough pain.

The primary goal of opioid treatment is to achieve maximum pain control. Basic analgesia is provided by means of a long-acting preparation, given by the clock. The interval between two administrations is based on the product's half-life [21]. In addition, medication for breakthrough pain should always be prescribed. For predictable incident pain, prophylactic administration is preferred. When breakthrough pain occurs at the end of dose, shortly before the next administration is planned, increasing the dose is recommended rather than shortening the interval between doses. Breakthrough pain induced by unpredictable events should be managed as needed [21].

# Limitations of Opioid Treatment

Opioid treatment is intended to reduce pain and increase quality of life. However, drug-related adverse effects often compromise the option of increasing the dose to a level required for optimal pain control. In addition, repeated exposure to an opioid may induce tolerance, causing a progressive decrease of the desired effects of the opioid. Many factors contribute to opioid tolerance [9]. Opioid receptors may be desensitized or downregulated with prolonged exposure to opioids. Chronic receptor activation induces adaptation of neuronal systems by the expression of compensating mechanisms, causing the receptor to have reduced sensitivity to the agonist. Chronic use of substances such as alcohol or barbiturates may increase the metabolization of concurrent opioids (through increased activity of cytochrome P450), resulting in a reduced opioid effect. Because of the diversity of contributing factors and the complex intracellular mechanisms involved, opioid tolerance is a difficult subject to study [42].

Mixed agonist-antagonist opioids such as pentazocine, butorphanol, and nalbuphine have a ceiling effect and are generally poor choices for patients with severe pain. Opioid cross-tolerance may develop, which is defined as tolerance to one opioid that develops as the result of the continued use of another substance with similar pharmacological actions [11]. Pain intensity can also vary, making adequate dose titration of a strong opioid difficult.

Opioid-induced hyperalgesia (OIH), a clinical entity in which patients experience worsening of pain and abnormal symptoms such as allodynia, despite increasing opioid doses, is now accepted as a clinical reality and should be differentiated from opioid tolerance [29]. OIH is thought to be caused by the simultaneous development of a pronociceptive process along with a desensitization process, although the relative contribution of each component is not yet clear [3].

# Variable Response to Opioids

The World Health Organization (WHO) introduced the stepwise use of analgesics of increasing potency by publishing recommendations for appropriate analgesic use, summarized in the WHO analgesic ladder for the management of cancer pain [45]. Morphine, an extract of the opium poppy plant, is the oldest and best studied representative of the step 3 analgesics of the WHO ladder, known as the strong opioids, and is considered the reference compound. Slow-release formulations that are released over 12 hours have made twice-daily administration possible.

Several other μ-opioid receptor agonists are available. Transdermal, intranasal, and transmucosal formulations have been developed, each with a specific time of onset and duration of action.

Clinical observation suggests that not all WHO step 3 strong opioids have a comparable pharmacological response in the same pathological condition, and there is considerable interindividual variation with regard to their effect. Intrinsic opioid receptor activity can vary significantly among the different strong opioids, perhaps due to genetic factors causing differences in opioid responsiveness [39]. Differences among strong opioids in the potential induction of tolerance and dependence have been attributed to differences in receptor affinity, potency, efficacy, bioavailability, and half-life, which define the relative activity of the particular opioid μ-receptor agonist. The majority of opioids in clinical use are μ-receptor agonist activators that induce a complex "receptor-receptor agonist" responsible for signal transduction. The quality and quantity of signaling by μ-receptor agonists is determined by a variety of properties leading to receptor activation or endocytosis and resensitization. For receptors that are recycled, such as the μ-opioid receptor, endocytosis serves as the first step toward resensitizing receptors. For receptors that are degraded, endocytosis serves as the first step in the process of receptor downregulation.

Opioid-receptor ligand activity and the degree of endocytosis are not always linear, because each opioid has a particular relative activity versus endocytosis (RAVE). The differences in RAVE are considered to be one explanation for differences in the potential for developing tolerance and dependence [23]. Opioid switching has been used empirically as a potential solution for patients who do not reach satisfactory analgesia with the opioid prescribed initially.

Clinical observations that analgesic effects and side effects differ among opioids are not yet supported by evidence from randomized controlled clinical trials. One study in rats examined the antinociceptive and adverse effects of acutely administered opioid compounds frequently used in pain management at equianalgesic doses. This study found significant differences between opioids as demonstrated by different ratios between the dose giving good analgesia and the dose inducing side effects [26].

# Factors to Be Considered when Opioid Therapy Fails

When a cancer patient has insufficient pain relief or experiences intolerable side effects from opioids, a good differential diagnosis must be considered. All potential causes of the symptoms should first be analyzed. Disease progression is an important reason for insufficient pain relief. When the patient reports symptoms related to the central nervous system, the clinician must exclude potential brain metastases, stroke, and hypercalcemia. Similar symptoms may also be caused by concomitant medications such as benzodiazepines and corticosteroids. In the case of respiratory and cardiovascular symptoms, potential hypovolemia and hyperkalemia should be assessed. Gastrointestinal symptoms may be related to chemotherapy, and constipation, a frequently occurring side effect of opioids, may also be caused by mechanical bowel obstruction.

Renal and hepatic function should be evaluated, and the implications should be assessed for the metabolism and excretion of drugs, particularly opioids. It is equally important to have a complete overview of all medication, including over-the-counter drugs the patient may be using, to be able to assess potential drug interactions [41].

## Opioid-Related Adverse Effects

Opioid-related adverse effects can reduce quality of life and, if persistent, lead to treatment discontinuation. Frequently occurring side effects such as dysphoria, nausea, and sedation may disappear in a few days when opioid treatment is continued. This phenomenon is described as the development of tolerance for side effects. Constipation, on the other hand, which is reported in up to 41% of patients receiving chronic opioid treatment, rarely disappears and is difficult to treat. Other side effects that continue during prolonged treatment are sweating, itching, and reduced libido. These side effects are often the cause of non-adherence to treatment in terms of patients reducing the dose or stopping treatment [18,25,38].

When other causes of unpleasant symptoms have been excluded, the management of opioid side effects should start with a dose reduction. It may be necessary to add a nonopioid analgesic or adjuvant drug. Cancer treatment such as chemotherapy, hormonal or radiation treatment, or surgery may be indicated to reduce tumor size and lessen pressure on the nerves and organs. When indicated, interventional pain management techniques may be used.

Symptomatic management of side effects may be appropriate. For example, laxatives should always be prescribed together with opioids to treat constipation, and antiemetics are appropriate in the case of persistent nausea and vomiting.

# Opioid Switching

After correct initiation and titration of an opioid, the drug's initial clinical efficacy may gradually wear off [19]. Patients may experience breakthrough pain despite adequate therapeutic compliance, necessitating a titration of the treatment regimen to higher doses. When higher doses provoke unwanted side effects, a different route of administration or a different opioid may be considered. Opioid switching is a therapeutic strategy in which the current opioid is stopped and replaced by a different opioid. Occasionally, opioids are switched regularly in an approach termed opioid "rotation."

Conversion from oral or transdermal administration route to parenteral administration provides adequate analgesia more rapidly [28]. Changing to the parenteral administration route provided good pain relief in 75–95% of patients [14]. Intrathecal opioid administration has been practiced since the discovery of opioid receptors in neural tissue. Administration of an appropriate opioid agonist close to the receptor site results in satisfactory analgesia at a lower dose than that required with parenteral administration. When oral administration of morphine or hydromorphone is switched to intrathecal administration, the daily dose can be substantially reduced [10]. There is little documentation concerning the reduction of side effects when switching from oral to intrathecal drug administration. An expert panel has published recommendations for the intrathecal treatment of pain, including cancer pain [2,13,40]. Intrathecal morphine may be administered using a closed implantable drug delivery system.

The success of opioid switching is thought to be due to incomplete cross-tolerance between opioid analgesics, implying distinctly different pharmacodynamics and receptor interactions between opioids. At present, there are no evidence-based guidelines for choice of opioid when switching. Changing from one opioid to another is not always easy. Some physicians may not feel at ease with this technique, because of the challenges involved in providing safe and adequate pain relief during the changeover.

## Opioid Switching: What Is the Evidence?

Opioid rotation or switching is frequently indicated in the management of cancer pain. There is only limited evidence that opioid switching results in regain of satisfactory pain control and reduced side effects. A systematic review on the management of opioid-induced side effects found no randomized controlled trials [25]. Retrospective studies suggest that opioid switching is employed in 21–44% of patients [4,7,8,12,20]. In two prospective studies, the percentages were 12% [31] and 25% [37].

There are no randomized controlled trials investigating the efficacy of opioid switching. A Cochrane review that included publications until January 2003 identified 52 publications: 14 were uncontrolled prospective trials, 15 were retrospective trials, and 23 were case reports [36]. Since then, more information has become available. The majority of published studies have been based on retrospective chart reviews, but prospective studies have also been conducted [31]. Two prospective open-label trials from 2005 and 2008 report on switching from high-dose morphine to transdermal fentanyl in 9 patients and parenteral fentanyl in 11 patients [30] and to oral oxycodone in 27 patients [32]. The reason for opioid rotation in these two cancer pain trials, the first of which was in delirious patients, was inadequate analgesia due to intolerable side effects that prevented dose increase. After switching from morphine to the alternative opioid, the dose could be increased, resulting in better pain control, without increasing the burden of intolerable side effects. A third prospective open-label trial from 2006 reports on switching to sustained-release hydromorphone. Fifty patients were switched from oral morphine, transdermal fentanyl, tramadol, oxycodone, or sublingual buprenorphine. Rotation was described as successful in 64% of patients experiencing pain and gastrointestinal and central symptoms [44].

A recent open-label study assessed the effect of switching between transdermal fentanyl and buprenorphine [1] in patients who had received a minimum of 3 months of treatment with either of the transdermal opioids. When treatment resulted in inadequate analgesia and opioid-related adverse effects, the initial opioid was switched to the alternative transdermal preparation at a dose of 50% of the calculated equianalgesic dose. Three weeks after inclusion, patients in both treatment groups reported comparable pain reduction and reduction in the incidence of nausea and vomiting. No sedation was seen in any patient 1 week after the switch in therapy.

# Opioid Switching in Practice

The major challenge during opioid switching is to ensure good pain relief during the switch. Equianalgesic tables can help physicians to estimate the optimal dose of the new opioid. Such tables only provide broad guidelines for selecting the dose. As stated above, there are large individual pharmacokinetic and even larger pharmacodynamic differences in opioid pharmacology.

Tables of equianalgesic doses often give the highest dose for comparable analgesic effects. However, these conversion tables are not based on scientific evidence [36], but often rely on the results of older single-dose clinical trials comparing the short-term efficacy of two opioids [5,16]. The treating physician should be aware of the limitations of equianalgesic tables. The key to successful conversion is continuous patient assessment.

The proposed opioid dose should be based on a theoretical dose calculation and titrated in accordance with observed clinical efficacy and the individual characteristics of the patient, such as age, renal function, side effects, and type of pain syndrome. When the current opioid dose is not adequate, it is likely that the equianalgesic dose will not provide satisfactory pain relief. Once the opioid is switched, the dose should be titrated according to the individual needs of the patient to ensure adequate pain control [5]. It is important to realize that conversion ratios may differ according to the patient population, sensitivity to opioids, and the etiology of the pain. Different pain syndromes, such as osteoarticular diseases, neuropathic pain, or oncological pain states may demonstrate a variable and highly unpredictable clinical response to opioids, thus reducing the usefulness of conversion tables [15].

In practice, the majority of patients need a dose of the new opioid that is lower than the dose calculated by using an equianalgesic table [5,22,27]. Because of incomplete cross-tolerance, it is recommended to reduce the calculated dose by approximately 33%. For safety reasons, the new opioid should be initiated at the lowest dose, which if necessary can be gradually increased to achieve adequate analgesia [5,14,17].

Reference works such as the *Textbook of Pain* [24] provide conversion tables in which parenteral morphine at a dose of 10 mg is used as the basis for calculating all other opioid doses in individual patients. A recently published evidence-based guideline for the management of cancer pain offers a conversion table based on the literature [21] (www.oncoline. nl) (see Table I). Available conversion tables generally report on opioid formulations available in the country where the study was performed. However, formulations may differ between countries, and clinicians should take this into account when using a conversion table.

As discussed above, opioid switching is performed due to (1) inadequate analgesia and (2) intolerable side effects. When switching is desirable due to adverse effects, it is recommended to start with two-thirds of

Table I
Conversion ratios for opioid rotation

| Morphine, p.o. (mg/24 h) | Morphine, s.c./i.v. (mg/24 h) | Oxycodone, p.o. (mg/24 h) | Oxycodone, s.c./i.v. (mg/24 h) | Fentanyl, t.d. (μg/h) | Hydro-morphone, p.o. (mg/24 h) |
|---|---|---|---|---|---|
| 30 | 10 | 15 | 7.5 | 12 | 4 |
| 60 | 20 | 30 | 15 | 25 | 8 |
| 120 | 40 | 60 | 30 | 50 | 16 |
| 180 | 60 | 90 | 45 | 75 | 24 |
| 240 | 80 | 120 | 60 | 100 | 32 |
| 360 | 120 | 180 | 90 | 150 | 48 |
| 480 | 120 | 240 | 120 | 200 | 64 |

*Note:* Buprenorphine was not included in the source guidelines. Mercadante [28] identified a ratio of 70:1 for oral morphine : transdermal buprenorphine and 0.6:0.8 for transdermal fentanyl : transdermal buprenorphine. i.v. = intravenous; p.o. = oral; s.c. = subcutaneous; t.d. = transdermal.

the calculated equianalgesic dose. In cases of inadequate pain control, up to 20% should be deducted from the calculated equianalgesic dose to start with. In both cases, a rescue analgesic (a short-acting opioid with a rapid onset of action) should be made available. The patient should be closely monitored with regard to analgesic effect, rescue medication requirements, and side effects. After steady state analgesia is obtained with the new opioid, the dose can be titrated either upward or downward as needed.

During the switching phase, both opioids will be present in the plasma. When a new opioid is started, the plasma half-life of the old opioid will define the time the drug is active. Excretion and hepatic and renal function should be considered, as well as potential active metabolites of the old opioid. An important consideration in relation to the "new opioid" is the time to reach maximum concentration and steady state, which will define the time to maximum analgesia and the latency time. Care should be taken that the original opioid is available in the plasma during the time it takes for the new opioid to provide maximum analgesia. Where appropriate, the dose of the original opioid is progressively tapered over the latency time of the replacement opioid.

# Future Research

Research can be divided into several categories. First is basic research that focuses on elucidating the specific mechanisms of actions of individual opioids, providing a better understanding of opioid receptor-binding properties and potential effects on other receptors, intercellular mechanisms that influence tolerance to opioids, new translational models for better pharmacological testing, and equianalgesic drug comparisons. Second is research to further clarify the mechanisms of tolerance, side effects, and efficacy in humans. Third is developing new molecules with new agonistic effects and less serious side effects, and improving knowledge of drugs and drug combinations that may reduce side effects. Finally, clinical research should be based on better documentation of the clinical effects in specific populations. Randomized controlled trials are needed to prove the equianalgesic dosages between opioids.

# Conclusions

Strong opioids play a major role in the management of cancer pain. Although morphine is still the gold standard opioid, alternative routes of administration and newer μ-receptor agonists provide the opportunity to improve the balance between pain control and side effects. It is empirically demonstrated that opioid switching is successful in approximately 70% of cancer pain patients needing this approach. With current knowledge of the mechanisms of action of individual opioids and equianalgesic doses, the selection of the appropriate opioid drug and dose will continue to be a process of "trial and error," especially in cancer patients, who often have reduced renal and hepatic function and may be taking multiple drugs concurrently.

# Acknowledgments

All authors are members of the Dutch national guideline committee for the treatment of cancer pain.

# References

[1] Aurilio C, Pace MC, Pota V, Sansone P, Barbarisi M, Grella E, Passavanti MB. Opioids switching with transdermal systems in chronic cancer pain. J Exp Clin Cancer Res 2009;28:61.

[2] Ballantyne JC, Carwood CM. Comparative efficacy of epidural, subarachnoid, and intra-cerebroventricular opioids in patients with pain due to cancer. Cochrane Database Syst Rev 2005;1:CD005178.

[3] Ballantyne JC, Shin NS. Efficacy of opioids for chronic pain: a review of the evidence. Clin J Pain 2008;24:469–78.

[4] Berger A, Hoffman DL, Goodman S, Delea TE, Seifeldin R, Oster G. Therapy switching in patients receiving long-acting opioids. Ann Pharmacother 2004;38:389–95.

[5] Brant JM. Opioid equianalgesic conversion: the right dose. Clin J Oncol Nurs 2001;5:163–5.

[6] Breivik H, Cherny N, Collett B, de Conno F, Filbet M, Foubert AJ, Cohen R, Dow L. Cancer-related pain: a pan-European survey of prevalence, treatment, and patient attitudes. Ann Oncol 2009;20:1420–33.

[7] Bruera E, Franco JJ, Maltoni M, Watanabe S, Suarez-Almazor M. Changing pattern of agitated impaired mental status in patients with advanced cancer: association with cognitive monitoring, hydration, and opioid rotation. J Pain Symptom Manage 1995;10:287–91.

[8] Cherny NJ, Chang V, Frager G, Ingham JM, Tiseo PJ, Popp B, Portenoy RK, Foley KM. Opioid pharmacotherapy in the management of cancer pain: a survey of strategies used by pain physicians for the selection of analgesic drugs and routes of administration. Cancer 1995;76:1283–93.

[9] Chu LF, Clark DJ, Angst MS. Opioid tolerance and hyperalgesia in chronic pain patients after one month of oral morphine therapy: a preliminary prospective study. J Pain 2006;7:43–8.

[10] Cohen SP, Dragovich A. Intrathecal analgesia. Med Clin North Am 2007;91:251–70.

[11] Cortazzo MH, Fishman SM. Major opioids and chronic opioid therapy. In: Benzon HT, Rathmell JP, Wu CL, Turk DC, Argoff CE. Raj's practical management of pain. Mosby: St. Louis; 2008. Chapter 32.

[12] de Stoutz ND, Bruera E, Suarez-Almazor M. Opioid rotation for toxicity reduction in terminal cancer patients. J Pain Symptom Manage 1995;10:378–84.

[13] Deer T, Krames ES, Hassenbusch SJ, Burton A, Caraway D, Dupen S, Eisenach J, Erdek M, Grigsby E, Kim P, et al. Polyanalgesic Consensus Conference 2007: Recommendations for the management of pain by intrathecal (intraspinal) drug delivery: report of an interdisciplinary expert panel. Neuromodulation 2007;10:300–28.

[14] Enting RH, van der Rijt CC, Wilms EB, Lieverse PJ, de Wit R, Smitt PA. [Treatment of pain in cancer with systemically administered opioids]. Ned Tijdschr Geneeskd 2001;145:950–4.

[15] Galer BS, Coyle N, Pasternak GW, Portenoy RK. Individual variability in the response to different opioids: report of five cases. Pain 1992;49:87–91.

[16] Gammaitoni AR, Fine P, Alvarez N, McPherson ML, Bergmark S. Clinical application of opioid equianalgesic data. Clin J Pain 2003;19:286–97.

[17] Hanks GW, Conno F, Cherny N, Hanna M, Kalso E, McQuay HJ, Mercadante S, Meynadier J, Poulain P, Ripamonti C, et al. Morphine and alternative opioids in cancer pain: the EAPC recommendations. Br J Cancer 2001;84:587–93.

[18] Harris JD. Management of expected and unexpected opioid-related side effects. Clin J Pain 2008;24(Suppl 10):S8–13.

[19] Kalso E, Allan L, Dellemijn PL, Faura CC, Ilias WK, Jensen TS, Perrot S, Plaghki LH, Zenz M. Recommendations for using opioids in chronic non-cancer pain. Eur J Pain 2003;7(5):381–6.

[20] Kloke M, Rapp M, Bosse B, Kloke O. Toxicity and/or insufficient analgesia by opioid therapy: risk factors and the impact of changing the opioid. A retrospective analysis of 273 patients observed at a single center. Support Care Cancer 2000;8:479–86.

[21] Landelijke Richtlijnwerkgroep Pijn bij Kanker. Pijn bij kanker. Available at: http://www.oncoline.nl.

[22] Lipowski A, Carr D. Re-thinking opioid equivalence. Pain: Clin Updates 2002;X(4):1–10.

[23] Martini L, Whistler JL. The role of mu opioid receptor desensitization and endocytosis in morphine tolerance and dependence. Curr Opin Neurobiol 2007;17:556–64.

[24] McMahon S, Koltzenburg M. Wall and Melzack's textbook of pain. Oxford: Elsevier; 2006.

[25] McNicol E, Horowicz-Mehler N, Fisk RA, Bennett K, Gialeli-Goudas M, Chew PW, Lau J, Carr D. Management of opioid side effects in cancer-related and chronic noncancer pain: a systematic review. J Pain 2003;4:231–56.

[26] Meert TF, Vermeirsch HA. A preclinical comparison between different opioids: antinociceptive versus adverse effects. Pharmacol Biochem Behav 2005;80:309–26.

[27] Mercadante S. Opioid rotation for cancer pain: rationale and clinical aspects. Cancer 1999;86:1856–66.

[28] Mercadante S. Opioid titration in cancer pain: a critical review. Eur J Pain 2007;11:823–30.

[29] Mitra S. Opioid-induced hyperalgesia: pathophysiology and clinical implications. J Opioid Manag 2008;4:123–30.

[30] Morita T, Takigawa C, Onishi H, Tajima T, Tani K, Matsubara T, Miyoshi I, Ikenaga M, Akechi T, Uchitomi Y. Opioid rotation from morphine to fentanyl in delirious cancer patients: an open-label trial. J Pain Symptom Manage 2005;30:96–103.

[31] Muller-Busch HC, Lindena G, Tietze K, Woskanjan S. Opioid switch in palliative care, opioid choice by clinical need and opioid availability. Eur J Pain 2005;9:571–9.

[32] Narabayashi M, Saijo Y, Takenoshita S, Chida M, Shimoyama N, Miura T, Tani K, Nishimura K, Onozawa Y, Hosokawa T, et al. Opioid rotation from oral morphine to oral oxycodone in cancer patients with intolerable adverse effects: an open-label trial. Jpn J Clin Oncol 2008;38:296–304.

[33] Pharo GH, Zhou L. Controlling cancer pain with pharmacotherapy. J Am Osteopath Assoc 2007;107(12 Suppl 7):ES22–32.

[34] Portenoy RK. Management of common opioid side effects during long-term therapy of cancer pain. Ann Acad Med Singapore 1994;23:160–70.

[35] Portenoy RK, Lesage P. Management of cancer pain. Lancet 1999;353:1695–700.

[36] Quigley C. Opioid switching to improve pain relief and drug tolerability. Cochrane Database Syst Rev 2004;3:CD004847.

[37] Riley J, Ross JR, Rutter D, Wells AU, Goller K, du Bois R, Welsh K. No pain relief from morphine? Individual variation in sensitivity to morphine and the need to switch to an alternative opioid in cancer patients. Support Care Cancer 2006;14:56–64.

[38] Shannon CN, Baranowski AP. Use of opioids in non-cancer pain. Br J Hosp Med 1997;58(9):459–63.

[39] Smith HS. Variations in opioid responsiveness. Pain Physician 2008;11:237–48.

[40] Smith TJ, Staats PS, Deer T, Stearns LJ, Rauck RL, Boortz-Marx RL, Buchser E, Catala E, Bryce DA, Coyne PJ, Pool GE. Randomized clinical trial of an implantable drug delivery system compared with comprehensive medical management for refractory cancer pain: impact on pain, drug-related toxicity, and survival. J Clin Oncol 2002;20:4040–9.

[41] Strouse TB. Pharmacokinetic drug interactions in palliative care: focus on opioids. J Palliat Med 2009;12:1043–50.

[42] Ueda H, Inoue M, Mizuno K. New approaches to study the development of morphine tolerance and dependence. Life Sci 2003;74:313–20.

[43] van den Beuken-van Everdingen MH, de Rijke JM, Kessels AG, Schouten HC, van Kleef M, Patijn J. High prevalence of pain in patients with cancer in a large population-based study in The Netherlands. Pain 2007;132:312–20.

[44] Wirz S, Wartenberg HC, Elsen C, Wittmann M, Diederichs M, Nadstawek J. Managing cancer pain and symptoms of outpatients by rotation to sustained-release hydromorphone: a prospective clinical trial. Clin J Pain 2006;22:770–5.

[45] World Health Organization. Cancer pain relief, with a guide to opioid availability, 2nd edition. Geneva: World Health Organization; 1996.

**Correspondence to:** Prof. Dr. K.C.P. Vissers, Department of Anesthesiology, Pain and Palliative Medicine, University Medical Centre St. Radboud, Huispost 550, Postbus 9101, 6500 HB Nijmegen, The Netherlands. Email: k.vissers@anes.umcn.nl.

# Drugs That Act against Opioid Tolerance

## Eija A. Kalso

*Institute of Clinical Medicine, University of Helsinki; Pain Clinic, Department of Anesthesiology, Intensive Care Medicine, Emergency Medicine and Pain Medicine, Helsinki University Central Hospital, Helsinki, Finland*

Opioids are the most important drugs in the alleviation of pain due to cancer. Development of tolerance is typical for all opioids, as discussed in Chapter 7 (Inturrisi and Gregus). In opioid tolerance, larger doses are required over time to achieve the same analgesic effect. In the clinic there are several other reasons for increased opioid requirement in order to maintain the same level of analgesia, in addition to the various pharmacological mechanisms (Table I). Larger doses of opioids usually improve analgesia when tolerance has developed. However, higher opioid doses can cause increased adverse effects. Dose escalation can also facilitate opioid tolerance by causing opioid-induced hyperalgesia.

Dose escalation of certain opioids can also be necessary for pharmacokinetic reasons (Table II). The role of drug interactions [10], and variable absorption of the opioid through the skin [33], must be considered as possible causes for decreased opioid efficacy. However, these mechanisms of opioid tolerance are not the topic of this chapter.

This chapter will discuss pharmacological strategies to reverse or prevent opioid tolerance in the management of cancer pain. Several

*Cancer Pain: From Molecules to Suffering*
edited by Judith A. Paice, Rae F. Bell, Eija A. Kalso, and Olaitan A. Soyannwo
IASP Press, Seattle, © 2010

"adjuvant" analgesics (e.g., nonsteroidal anti-inflammatory drugs, anticonvulsants, and antidepressants) can attenuate the development of opioid tolerance by decreasing the total opioid doses that are needed to control pain. Basic research has invested tremendous efforts in the study of opioid tolerance and its reversal. The literature describes many drugs that have been shown to act against opioid tolerance in rats and mice. This chapter will focus on drugs that are already used in the clinic, but usually for other indications. Evidence for the clinical effectiveness of any of these drugs used off-label against tolerance is scarce. Analgesic studies are rather challenging in cancer pain [7]. Studying interventions against opioid tolerance is particularly difficult because of the multitude of factors that may increase opioid demand. There is also some evidence to suggest a high degree of heritability of opioid tolerance [44,48]. This issue, however, has not been studied in humans.

Table I
Possible causes of clinical opioid dose
escalation to maintain analgesia

| |
| --- |
| Disease progression |
|    Tumor growth |
|    New types of pain |
|    Increased systemic inflammation |
| Pain becomes less opioid sensitive |
|    Neuropathic pain |
| Psychological reasons |
|    Anxiety |
|    Fear |
|    Depression |
| Pharmacokinetic reasons |
|    Reduced opioid absorption |
|    Drug interactions |
| Tolerance |
|    Several mechanisms (see Table II) |

# NMDA-Receptor Antagonists

N-methyl-D-aspartate (NMDA) glutamate receptors are involved in opioid-induced plasticity, including the development of both opioid tolerance and sensitization. Trujillo and Akil [61] were the first to report that a noncompetitive NMDA antagonist, MK-801 (dizocilpine), inhibited the development of

Table II
Mechanisms of opioid tolerance

---

*Pharmacodynamic Tolerance*
1) Cellular tolerance
    Changes in the number of functional receptors
    Ability of receptors to signal to downstream effectors involved in analgesia
2) Tolerance at the systems level
i) Adaptive processes: upregulation of pronociceptive systems
    Nonopioid receptors (e.g., NMDA)
    Antiopioid peptides (e.g., neuropeptide FF, cholecystokinin, dynorphin)
    Ion channels
    Second messengers
ii) Activation of the immune system
    Glial activation
    Upregulation of proinflammatory cytokines
*Pharmacokinetic Tolerance*
1) Liver metabolism
    Induction of liver enzymes (faster elimination of active drugs)
      Induction of CYP 3A4, leading to faster metabolism of methadone
    Blocking of metabolism to active metabolites (prodrugs)
      Blocking of CYP 2D6 with no metabolism of codeine to the active metabolite, morphine
2) Absorption through membranes (e.g., skin, gut, blood-brain-barrier)
    Gastrointestinal obstruction, vomiting
    Decreased absorption through the skin (e.g., transdermal fentanyl)
    Induction or inhibition of efflux and influx transporter proteins (e.g., P-glycoprotein)

---

tolerance to the antinociceptive effect of morphine without affecting acute morphine antinociception. These original findings have been confirmed by several other groups [35,38]. It has also been reported that other NMDA antagonists such as memantine and the competitive NMDA antagonist LY235959 inhibit opioid tolerance [51]. Most studies have used morphine as the opioid agonist. However, the development of tolerance to the partial opioid agonist buprenorphine and to methadone has also been inhibited by NMDA-receptor antagonists [51]. It has been suggested that the magnitude of opioid tolerance could determine the effectiveness of NMDA-receptor antagonists in attenuating opioid tolerance [1]. In addition to inhibiting opioid tolerance NDMA-receptor antagonists can also inhibit opioid-induced sensitization. Interestingly, context-dependent sensitization seems to be more resistant to NMDA-receptor blockade than context-independent sensitization [68].

Several opioids (methadone, ketobemidone, pethidine, and dextropropoxyphene) are weak noncompetitive NMDA-receptor antagonists [25,26]. However, the clinical significance of this effect has not been established. Several other clinically available drugs have shown NMDA-receptor antagonistic effects and inhibit opioid tolerance in the laboratory. These drugs include the antitussive drug dextromethorphan [2], memantine [8], and ketamine [46].

Much hope was invested in the promising results of the effects of dextromethorphan on opioid tolerance [56]. A multicenter, double-blind, randomized, placebo-controlled trial examined the efficacy and safety of 60–120 mg of dextromethorphan four times daily in morphine tolerance in 65 cancer patients [24]. Dextromethorphan and placebo groups did not differ statistically significantly in morphine consumption, and dextromethorphan caused more adverse effects (e.g., dizziness). Three multicenter, randomized, double-blind, controlled clinical trials failed to demonstrate reduction in opioid tolerance [28].

Memantine is a low-affinity, voltage-dependent noncompetitive NMDA antagonist. It is also a noncompetitive antagonist at the 5-HT$_3$ receptor [57] and at different neuronal nicotinic acetylcholine receptors [16] at potencies similar to that for the NMDA receptor. Memantine has been approved in the treatment of moderate to severe Alzheimer's disease, and it is being tested for various neuropsychiatric disorders. Memantine has not been studied in randomized and controlled trials in opioid tolerance. Case reports have been published suggesting that memantine could be effective in reversing opioid tolerance [30].

Ketamine is a truly interesting drug that was developed in the 1960s. It has been used as an anesthetic (at high doses) and as an analgesic (at low doses) in human and veterinary medicine. It produces dissociative anesthesia without respiratory depression and hypotension and is therefore used in emergency medicine. Hallucinations are the main acute adverse effect.

Ketamine is a keto-amine and a noncompetitive antagonist of the NMDA receptor, which opens in response to binding of glutamate. This effect is thought to be important in hyperalgesia and opioid tolerance. Other mechanisms of action have been suggested to be responsible for the hypnotic effect of ketamine. These include inhibition of the hyperpolarization-activated cyclic nucleotide-modulated cation channels [17].

Ketamine has been mostly used and studied in its racemic form. Its more active enantiomer, S-ketamine, is also available for medical use. It has been suggested to be 2–4 times more potent in reducing pain compared with racemic ketamine [3] and to cause less adverse effects. Ketamine is extensively metabolized in the liver by cytochrome P450 3A, 2B6, and 2C9 isoenzymes [36]. Hence, ketamine has low and variable bioavailability (17–24%) after oral administration and clinically relevant drug interactions can occur [31]. Ketamine is in the World Health Organization's Essential Drugs List, and it could be used worldwide in various indications in cancer pain management (procedural pain, neuropathic pain, opioid tolerance, and sedation). The unfortunate fact that ketamine is widely misused as a recreational drug has imposed significant restrictions on its use in many countries. Ketamine is mainly used in hospitals.

Ketamine administered systemically or spinally has been studied as an add-on drug to improve opioid analgesia in acute postoperative pain [6] and chronic pain [4]. Ketamine is widely used in cancer pain, and a large number of published case reports describe its efficacy in improving pain relief in patients receiving high doses of opioids. Unfortunately, only a few controlled studies have addressed this question [5]. A systematic review by Bell et al. [5] reported four randomized and controlled trials that were conducted in adult patients. Oral, spinal (epidural and intrathecal), and intravenous ketamine was studied in cancer patients receiving morphine without satisfactory pain relief. Different outcomes were used, and the duration of the studies ranged from 30 minutes to 30 days. Two studies qualified for the final analysis. These studies showed that intrathecal ketamine (1 mg b.i.d.) reduced intrathecal morphine requirements in cancer patients [69] and that intravenous ketamine significantly reduced pain intensity in cancer pain with a neuropathic component [52]. S-ketamine is preservative free, whereas racemic ketamine is not. However, S-ketamine has been shown to cause neuropathological changes after intrathecal administration [63]. The obvious question for clinical research would be to study how ketamine could be safely administered spinally in those patients who desperately need it. Careful patient follow-up and documentation from several centers would be one possibility to provide useful information.

The obvious research agenda is to assess the efficacy of subcutaneous administration of ketamine (or S-ketamine) in reversing opioid tolerance. The study could use a randomized crossover design where ketamine is compared with placebo infusion in several blocks lasting for a few days. Depending on the resources of the research unit, additional questions regarding the possible mechanisms and effects of different opioids and their doses could be studied.

# Pain, Stress, and Corticosteroids

The long-standing argument has been that pain has an inhibitory effect on tolerance development to some effects of opioids. Case reports have described patients on high doses of opioids who have developed respiratory depression once pain has been removed by regional anesthesia [32]. This finding could indicate that these patients have not developed tolerance to the respiratory depressant effects of opioids in a situation where pain has acted as a strong stimulator of the respiratory center. It has been reported that chronic inflammatory pain can delay the development of tolerance to morphine analgesia [39] and that this inhibitory effect of pain is mediated by the stress associated with pain and activation of the hypothalamic-pituitary-adrenal (HPA) axis [34].

Given the possible role of the HPA axis in opioid tolerance, a recent study showed that chronic administration of dexamethasone could reduce and reverse the development of tolerance in rats that received chronic injections of intraperitoneal morphine [40]. This effect was suggested to be due to the effect of dexamethasone in normalizing the balance between the levels of excitatory and inhibitory subunits of the G-proteins that couple with the opioid receptors. Dexamethasone is often given to cancer pain patients for other indications (to relieve edema or nausea and to improve appetite). The possible effect of corticosteroids on opioid tolerance has not been studied in the clinic.

# Opioid Antagonists

Opioid receptors preferentially bind the inhibitory subunits of the G-protein ($G_i$ and $G_o$) to inhibit adenyl cyclase [45], but chronic morphine exposure induces coupling of the $\mu$-opioid receptor to the stimulatory G-protein subunit ($G_s$) [15]. Very low doses of opioid antagonists have been reported to enhance opioid analgesia and reduce opioid tolerance by preventing the opioid-agonist-induced coupling switch from the inhibitory G-protein ($G_{i/o}$) to the stimulatory G-protein ($G_s$) by the μ-opioid receptor [19,20,64]. It was recently shown that naloxone binds with a 200 times higher affinity to a pentapeptide segment of the scaffolding protein filamin A compared with the μ-opioid receptor [65] to convey this effect.

Despite the promising animal studies, evidence in humans for enhanced opioid analgesia by coadministration of an ultra-low-dose opioid antagonist is scarce and conflicting. Low- or ultra-low-dose intravenous naloxone did not enhance postoperative morphine analgesia [12,13]. On the other hand, enhanced buprenorphine analgesia with the addition of ultra-low-dose naloxone has been reported in experimental pain in healthy volunteers [62], and oxycodone in combination with ultra-low-dose oral naltrexone has provided enhanced analgesia in patients suffering from osteoarthritis [18].

It seems that the dose ratio of the opioid antagonist and agonist is critical unless a $G_s$-selective antagonist is developed. Several opioid antagonist formulations have recently been introduced to prevent opioid-induced constipation. This effect should be peripheral only, whereas opioid tolerance occurs mainly in the central nervous system. Naloxone and naltrexone may, however, prevent or reverse opioid tolerance through other mechanisms, as described below in the section on glial activation.

# Adrenoceptor Antagonists

The adrenergic system has an important role in opioid withdrawal symptoms, and $\alpha_2$-adrenergic agonists (e.g., clonidine) are used to attenuate catecholamine-mediated withdrawal symptoms in the clinic. Recent studies have suggested that the adrenergic system could also be involved in the development of tolerance.

There is considerable evidence for a functional interaction between the opioid receptors and $\alpha_2$-adrenergic receptors in the spinal cord. Antinociceptive synergy has been shown between the μ-opioid and $\alpha_2$-adrenoreceptor agonists [59]. Moreover, cross-tolerance has been shown to develop between spinal opioid-mediated and $\alpha_2$-adrenoreceptor-mediated antinociception [43]. Recent studies indicate that functional μ-opioid/ $\alpha_2$-adrenoreceptor complexes can form in the spinal cord and brain [41].

Combinations of morphine and clonidine are used for spinal analgesia to manage neuropathic cancer pain [27]. It has also been suggested that adding clonidine (a nonselective $\alpha_2$-adrenoreceptor agonist) to morphine could attenuate development of tolerance to spinal opioid analgesia.

Interestingly, low doses of $\alpha_2$-adrenoreceptor antagonists have been reported to both prevent and reverse opioid tolerance [54]. All four drugs studied (atipamezole, yohimbine, mirtazapine, and idazoxan), given at doses that were clearly below those that produce spinal $\alpha_2$-adrenoreceptor blockade, significantly increased the duration of the antinociceptive effect of spinal morphine in both thermal and mechanical tests. All four drugs at similar low doses also attenuated the development of both acute and chronic morphine tolerance and reversed established tolerance. The mechanism is unclear, but one possibility is that a low dose of an $\alpha_2$-adrenoreceptor antagonist could promote a receptor state of the $\mu$-opioid/$\alpha_2$-adrenoreceptor complex in which activation of the $\mu$-opioid receptor component leads to an enhanced and sustained signaling response. Atipamezole is used in veterinary anesthesia to antagonize $\alpha_2$-adrenoreceptor-induced sedation and analgesia. It is also under research as an anti-Parkinson drug.

The role of $\beta_2$-adrenergic receptors in morphine tolerance was studied using the $\beta_2$-adrenergic antagonist butoxamine and $\beta_2$-adrenergic receptor knockout mice [49]. Systemically administered butoxamine both reversed and completely prevented acute morphine-induced tolerance. Mice that were treated only with morphine showed significantly increased mRNA expression of calcitonin gene-related peptide and substance P in the dorsal root ganglia. Mice that were given butoxamine along with morphine showed very little increase in these mRNA levels. No measurable tolerance to morphine developed in the $\beta_2$-adrenergic receptor knockout mice. Given that $\beta_2$-adrenergic receptor antagonists are widely used for their cardiovascular effects, it could be worth studying whether these drugs have any effect in clinical opioid tolerance.

## Antagonists of Antiopioid Peptides

The release of several peptides increases during chronic opioid administration. Many of these peptides have anti-opioid effects, and they are considered to be part of the homeostatic process in which the excitatory systems are activated to balance the inhibitory effects of opioids. Several peptides—cholecystokinin (CCK), neuropeptide FF (NPFF), dynorphin, nociceptin, and neuropeptide Y (NPY)—have been suggested to have anti-opioid effects.

CCK is implicated in several physiological functions, including pain and anxiety. It has a potent anti-opioid effect [14,21] and exerts a pronociceptive effect in neuropathic and anxiety-induced hyperalgesic states [50]. CCK has also been suggested to modulate negative emotional perception [29] and to play a key role in the nocebo effect [9]. In addition to being involved in opioid-induced tolerance, CCK has been suggested to mediate tolerance to the analgesic effect of transcutaneous electrical nerve stimulation (TENS) [23].

Animal studies have shown that proglumide, a nonselective antagonist of CCK types A and B, can potentiate opioid analgesia and reverse morphine tolerance [67]. The clinical evidence is very weak, however. The effect of 50 mg oral proglumide on anxiety and pain intensity was studied in cancer patients who were taking various opioids for pain relief [11]. Forty-three patients completed the randomized and placebo-controlled crossover study. The results were inconclusive.

Neuropeptide FF is another peptide that has been extensively studied in opioid analgesia and tolerance [55]. Like many other peptides, NPFF has different effects depending on whether it is administered supraspinally or at the spinal level. Intraventricular NPFF exerts anti-opioid effects, whereas intrathecal NPFF potentiates morphine antinociception.

RF9 is a potent and selective synthetic NPFF-receptor antagonist that can be administered systemically [58]. The compound itself has no effects on pain thresholds. However, its coadministration with heroin reportedly prevents the development of opioid tolerance. No clinical studies have been conducted with this compound.

# Inhibitors of Glial Activation

Inhibition of glial activation is one of the hottest areas of research in both neuropathic pain and opioid tolerance. A few laboratories have reported that opioids can activate glia, which leads to the release of proinflammatory cytokines [37,60]. It seems that opioids can activate glia through non-opioid-receptor-mediated pathways. This possibility is supported by the fact that opioid hyperalgesia can develop in triple-opioid-receptor knock-out mice [42]. One of the strongest candidates for a nonopioid gate to glial activation is toll-like receptor 4 (TLR4), an innate immune receptor expressed by glia. The prototype TLR4 agonist is the Gram-negative bacterial lipopolysaccharide.

It has been suggested that opioids activate TLR4, leading to decreased acute and chronic opioid analgesia, as well as dependence and reward [37]. Opioid antagonists (naloxone and naltrexone) block TLR4 in a nonstereoselective manner. Acute blockade of TLR4, genetic knockout of TLR4, and blockade of TLR4 downstream signaling potentiate opioid analgesia at both spinal and supraspinal sites [37].

The potential for opioid antagonists to improve opioid analgesia and prevent opioid tolerance is based on the fact that both (−) and (+)-naloxone and naltrexone antagonize TLR4 effects, whereas only the (−)-isomers bind to the opioid receptors. The (+)-isomers of naloxone and naltrexone are not easy to produce, however.

Several other drugs that are used for other indications (thalidomide, tricyclic antidepressants, minocycline, ibudilast, and propentofylline) have also been suggested to modify TLR4 signaling, with a potential for improving opioid analgesia [22,53,66]. The U.S. Food and Drug Administration (FDA) has approved ibudilast for testing its ability to increase the clinical efficacy of opioids. Ibudilast is available for oral administration and has a long history of safety in humans for the treatment of asthma and poststroke dizziness [47].

# Suggestions for Future Research

Pharmacological studies in cancer pain relief are challenging because of ethical questions, balancing patients' needs and scientific rigor, problems due to cancer as a disease with many comorbidities, and the fact that patients are usually receiving several other treatments, as discussed in Chapter 11 (Kongsgaard and Werner). When researchers address issues related to tolerance, the challenges multiply. Research on the pharmacogenetics of opioids in cancer pain has, however, engendered optimism in this field and shown that important new information can be gained even when very heterogeneous cancer pain patients are studied.

The first steps in the clinical study of opioid tolerance would be to construct an algorithm for the analysis of possible causes of this phenomenon. Fig. 1 shows a suggestion for the steps of analyzing reasons for opioid escalation. Once the putative cause of opioid escalation has been determined, a hypothesis-driven intervention can be determined. The studies could be placebo-controlled and double-blind using the "$N = 1$" principle. The more effective treatment (active treatment or placebo) could then be studied for a longer predetermined period. This study design would provide epidemiological information on causes of opioid escalation in cancer pain. It would also enable researchers to combine clinical utility with scientific rigor. Several centers would need to participate in order to provide meaningful numbers of study patients.

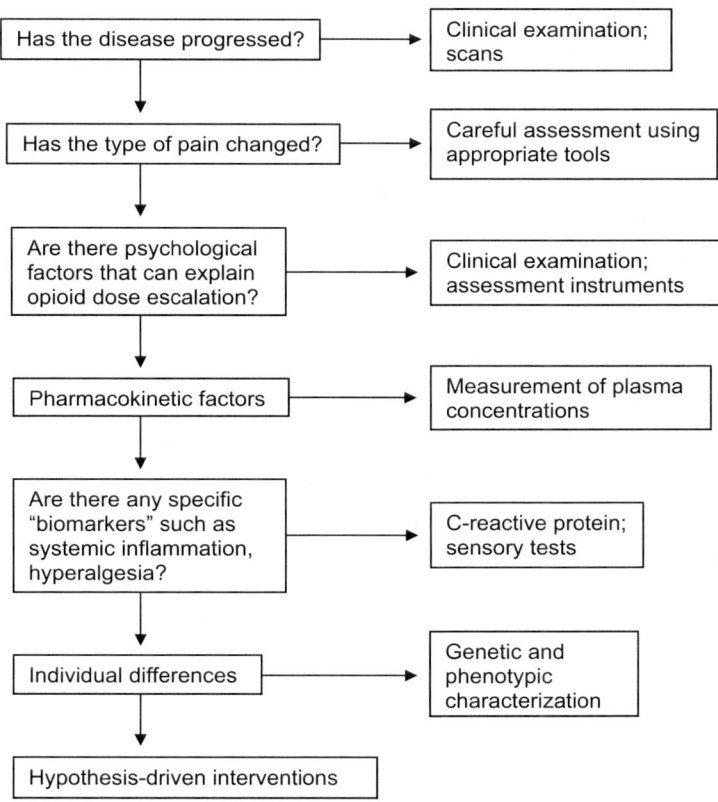

***Fig. 1.*** Procedure for assessing opioid tolerance.

# References

[1]  Allen RM, Dykstra LA. Role of morphine maintenance dose in the development of tolerance and its attenuation by an NMDA receptor antagonist. Psychopharmacology 2000;148:59–65.

[2]  Allen RM, Granger AL, Dykstra LA. Dextromethorphan potentiates the antinociceptive effects of morphine and the delta-opioid agonist SNC80 in squirrel monkeys. J Pharmacol Exp Ther 2002;300:435–41.

[3]  Arendt-Nielsen L, Nielsen J, Peterson-Felix S, Schindler TW, Zbinden AM. Effect of racemic mixture and the (S+)-isomer of ketamine on temporal summation and spatial summation of pain. Br J Anaesth 1996;77:625–31.

[4]  Bell RF. Ketamine for chronic non-cancer pain. Pain 2009;141:210–4.

[5]  Bell RF, Eccleston C, Kalso E. Ketamine as adjuvant to opioids for cancer pain. A qualitative systematic review. J Pain Symptom Manage 2003;26:867–75.

[6]  Bell RF, Dahl JB, Moore RA, Kalso E. Perioperative ketamine for acute postoperative pain, Cochrane Database Syst Rev 2006;25:CD004603.

[7]  Bell RF, Wisløff T, Eccleston C, Kalso E. Controlled clinical trials in cancer pain. How controlled should they be? A qualitative systematic review. Br J Cancer 2006;94:1559–67.

[8]  Belozertseva IV, Bespalov A. Effects of NMDA receptor channel blockers, dizocilpine and memantine, on the development of opiate analgesic tolerance induced by repeated morphine exposures or social defeats in mice. Naunyn-Schmiedebergs Arch Pharmacol 1998;358:270–4.

[9]  Benedetti F, Amanzio M, Vighetti S, Asteggiano G. The biochemical and neuroendocrine bases of the hyperalgesic nocebo effect. J Neurosci 2006;15:12014–22.

[10]  Bernard S, Bruera E. Drug interactions in palliative care. J Clin Oncol 2000;18:1780–99.

[11]  Bernstein ZP, Yucht S, Battista E, Lema M, Spaulding MB. Proglumide as a morphine adjunct in cancer pain management. J Pain Symptom Manage 1998;15:314–20.

[12]  Cepeda MS, Africano JM, Manrique AM, Fragoso W, Carr DB. The combination of low dose of naloxone and morphine in PCA does not decrease opioid requirements in the postoperative period. Pain 2002;96:73–9.

[13]  Cepeda MS, Alvarez H, Morales O, Carr DB. Addition of ultralow dose naloxone to postoperative morphine PCA: unchanged analgesia and opioid requirement but decreased incidence of opioid side effects. Pain 2004;107:41–6.

[14]  Cesselin F. Opioid and anti-opioid peptides. Fundam Clin Pharmacol 1995;9:409–33.

[15]  Chakrabarti S, Regec A, Gintzler AR. Biochemical demonstration of mu-opioid receptor association with Gs alpha: enhancement following morphine exposure. Mol Brain Res 2005;135:217–24.

[16]  Chen HS, Lipton SA. The chemical biology of clinically tolerated NMDA receptor antagonists. J Neurochem 2006;97:1611–26.

[17]  Chen X, Shu S, Bayliss DA. HCN1 channel subunits are a molecular substrate for hypnotic actions of ketamine. J Neurosci 2009;29:600–9.

[18]  Chindalore VL, Craven RA, Yu KP, Butera PG, Burns LH, Friedmann N. Adding ultralow-dose naltrexone to oxycodone enhances and prolongs analgesia: a randomized, controlled trial of Oxytrex. J Pain 2005;6:392–9.

[19]  Crain SM, Shen K-F. Ultra-low concentrations of naloxone selectively antagonize excitatory effects of morphine on sensory neurons, thereby increasing its antinociceptive potency and attenuating tolerance/dependence during chronic cotreatment. Proc Natl Acad Sci USA 1995;92:10540–4.

[20]  Crain SM, Shen K-F. Antagonists of excitatory opioid receptor functions enhance morphine's analgesic potency and attenuate opioid tolerance/dependence liability. Pain 2000;84:121–31.

[21]  Crawley JN, Corwin RI. Biological actions of cholecystokinin. Peptides 1994;15:731–55.

[22]  Cui Y, Liao X-X, Liu W, Guo R-X, Wu Z-Z, Zhao C-M, Chen P-X, Feng J-Q. A novel role of minocycline: Attenuating morphine antinociceptive tolerance by inhibition of p38 MAPK in the activated spinal glia. Brain Behav Immun 2008;22:114–23.

[23]  DeSantana JM, da Silva LFS, Sluka KA. Cholecystokinin receptors mediate tolerance to the analgesic effect of TENS in arthritic rats. Pain 2010:148:84–93.

[24]  Dudgeon DJ, Bruera E, Gagnon B, Watanabe SM, Allan SJ, Warr DG, MacDonald SM, Savage C, Tu D, Pater JL. A phase III randomized, double-blind, placebo-controlled study evaluating dextromethorphan plus slow-release morphine for chronic cancer pain relief in terminally ill patients. J Pain Symptom Manage 2007;33:365–71.

[25]  Ebert B, Andersen S, Krogsgaard-Larsen P. Ketobemidone, methadone and pethidine are non-competitive N-methyl-D-aspartate (NMDA) antagonists in the rat cortex and spinal cord. Neurosci Lett 1995;187:165–8.
[26]  Ebert B, Thorkildsen C, Andersen S, Christrup LL, Hejds H. Opioid analgesics as noncompetitive N-methyl-D-aspartate (NMDA) antagonists. Biochem Pharmacol 1998;56:553–9.
[27]  Eisenach JC, DuPen S, Dubois M, Miguel R, Allin D. Epidural clonidine analgesia for intractable cancer pain. The Epidural Clonidine Study Group. Pain 1995;61:391–9.
[28]  Galer BS, Lee DL, Ma T, Nagle B, Schlagheck TG. MorphiDex (morphine sulfate/dextromethorphan hydrobromide combination) in the treatment of chronic pain: three multicenter, randomized, double-blind, controlled clinical trials fail to demonstrate enhanced opioid analgesia or reduction in tolerance. Pain 2005;115:284–95.
[29]  Gospic K, Gunnarsson T, Fransson P, Ingvar M, Lindefors N, Petrovic P. Emotional perception modulated by an opioid and a cholecystokinin agonist. Psychopharmacology 2008;197:295–307.
[30]  Grande LA, O'Donnell BR, Fitzgibbon DR, Terman GW. Ultra-low dose ketamine and memantine treatment for pain in an opioid-tolerant oncology patient. Anesth Analg 2008;107:1380–3.
[31]  Hagelberg NM, Peltoniemi MA, Saari TI, Kurkinen KJ, Laine K, Neuvonen PJ, Olkkola KT. Claritomycin, a potent inhibitor of CYP3A4, greatly increases exposure to oral S-ketamine. Eur J Pain 2009; Epub Nov 6.
[32]  Hanks GW, Twycross TG, Lloyd JW. Unexpected complication of successful nerve block. Morphine-induced respiratory depression precipitated by removal of severe pain. Anaesthesia 1981;36:37–9.
[33]  Heiskanen T, Mätzke S, Haakana S, Gergov M, Vuori E, Kalso E. Pharmacokinetics of transdermal fentanyl in normal and cachectic patients with cancer related pain. Pain 2009;144:218–22.
[34]  Hendrie CA. ACTH: a single pre-treatment enhances the analgesic efficiency of, and prevents the development of tolerance to morphine. Physiol Behav 1988;42:41–5.
[35]  Herman BH, Vocci F, Bridge P. The effects of NMDA receptor antagonists and nitric oxide synthase inhibitors on opioid tolerance and withdrawal. Medication development issues for opiate addiction. Neuropsychopharmacology 1995;13:269–93.
[36]  Hijazi Y, Boulieu R. Contribution of CYP3A4, CYP2B6, and CYP2C9 isoforms to N-methylation of ketamine in human liver microsomes. Drug Metab Dispos 2002;30:853–8.
[37]  Hutchinson MR, Coats BD, Lewis SS, Zhang Y, Sprunger DB, Rezvani N, Baker EM, Jekich BM, Wieseler JL, Somogyi AA, et al. Proinflammatory cytokines oppose opioid-induced acute and chronic analgesia. Brain Behav Immun 2008;8:1178–89.
[38]  Inturrisi CE. Preclinical evidence for a role of glutamatergic systems in opioid tolerance and dependence. Semin Neurosci 1997;9:110–9.
[39]  Javan M, Ahmadiani A, Motamedi F, Kazemi B. Changes in G-protein gene expression in rat lumbar spinal cord support the inhibitory effect of chronic pain on the development of tolerance to morphine analgesia. Neurosci Res 2005;53:250–6.
[40]  Javan M, Kazemi B, Ahmadiani A, Motamedi F. Dexamethasone mimics the inhibitory effect of chronic pain on the development of tolerance to morphine analgesia and compensates for morphine induced changes in G proteins gene expression. Brain Res 2006;1104:73–9.
[41]  Jordan BA, Gomes I, Filipovska J, Devi LA. Functional interactions between μ opioid and $\alpha_{2A}$-adrenergic receptors. Mol Pharm 2003;64:1317–24.
[42]  Juni A, Klein G, Pintar JE, Kest B. Nociception increases during opioid infusion in opioid receptor triple knock-out mice. Neuroscience 2007;147:439–44.
[43]  Kalso EA, Sullivan AF, McQuay HJ, Dickenson AH, Roques BP. Cross-tolerance between mu-opioid and alpha2-adrenergic receptors but not between mu and delta opioid receptors in the spinal cord of the rat. J Pharmacol Exp Ther 1993;265:551–8.
[44]  Kest B, Hopkins E, Palmese CA, Adler M, Mogil JS. Genetic variation in morphine analgesic tolerance: a survey of 11 inbred mouse strains. Pharmacol Biochem Behav 2002;73:821–8.
[45]  Laugwitz KI, Offermanns S, Spicher K, Schultz G. Mu and delta opioid receptors differentially couple to G protein subtypes in membranes of human neuroblastoma SH-SY5Y cells. Neuron 1993;10:233–42.
[46]  Laulin JP, Maurette P, Corcuff JB, Rivat C, Chauvin M, Simonnet G. The role of ketamine in preventing fentanyl-induced hyperalgesia and subsequent acute morphine tolerance. Anesth Analg 2002;94:1263–9.

[47] Ledeboer A, Hutchinson MR, Watkins LR, Johnson KW. Ibudilast (AV411): a new class therapeutic candidate for neuropathic pain and opioid withdrawal syndromes. Expert Opin Investig Drugs 2007;16:935–50.

[48] Liang DY, Guo T, Liao G, Kingery WS, Peltz G, Clark JD. Chronic pain and genetic background interact and influence opioid analgesia, tolerance, and physical dependence. Pain 2006;121:232–40.

[49] Liang DY, Shi X, Li X, Li J, Clark JD. The beta2 adrenergic receptor regulates morphine tolerance and physical dependence. Behav Brain Res 2007;181:118–26.

[50] Lovic TA. Pro-nociceptive action of cholecystokinin in the periaqueductal grey: a role in neuropathic and anxiety-induced hyperalgesic states. Neurosci Biobehav Rev 2008;32:852–62.

[51] Mendez IA, Trujillo KA. NMDA receptor antagonists inhibit opiate antinociceptive tolerance and locomotor sensitization in rats. Psychopharmacology 2008;196:497–509.

[52] Mercadante S, Arcuri E, Tirelli W, Cascuccio A. Analgesic effects of intravenous ketamine in cancer patients on morphine therapy: a randomized, controlled, double-blind, crossover, double-dose study. J Pain Symptom Manage 2000;4:246–51.

[53] Mika J, Osikowicz M, Makuch W, Przewlocka B. Minocycline and pentoxifylline attenuate allodynia and hyperalgesia and potentiate the effects of morphine in rat and mouse models of neuropathic pain. Eur J Pharmacol 2007;560:142–9.

[54] Milne B, Sutak M, Cahill CM, Jhamandas K. Low doses of alpha2-adrenoreceptor antagonists augment spinal morphine analgesia and inhibit development of acute and chronic tolerance. Br J Pharmacol 2008;155:1264–78.

[55] Panula P, Kalso E, Nieminen –L, Kontinen VK, Brandt A, Pertovaara A. Neuropeptide FF and modulation of pain. Brain Res 1999;848:191–6.

[56] Popik P, Kozela E, Danysz W. Clinically available NMDA receptor antagonists memantine and dextromethorphan reverse existing tolerance to the antinociceptive effects of morphine in mice. Naunyn Schmiedebergs Arch Pharmacol 2000;361:425–32.

[57] Remmes G, Rupprecht R, Ferrari U, Ziglgänsberger W, Parsons CG. The N-methyl-D-aspartate receptor channel blockers memantine, MRZ2/579 and other amino-alkyl-cyclohexanes antagonise 5-HT$_3$ receptor currents in cultured HEK-293 and N1E-115 cell systems in a non-competitive manner. Neurosci Lett 2001;306:81–4.

[58] Simonin F, Schmitt M, Laulin J-P, Laboureyras E, Jhamandas JH, MacTavish D, Matifas A, Mollereau C, Laurent P, Parmentier M, et al. RF9, a potent and selective neuropeptide FF receptor antagonist, prevents opioid-induced tolerance associated with hyperalgesia. Proc Natl Acad Sci USA 2006;103:466–71.

[59] Sullivan AF, Kalso EA, McQuay HJ, Dickenson AH. Evidence for the involvement of the mu but not delta opioid receptor subtype in the synergistic interaction between opioid and alpha2 adrenergic anti-nociception in the rat spinal cord. Neurosci Lett 1992;139:65–8.

[60] Tawfik VL, LaCroix-Fralish ML, Nutile-McMenemy N, DeLeo JA. Transcriptional and translational regulation of glial activation by morphine in a rodent model of neuropathic pain. J Pharmacol Exp Ther 2005;313:1239–47.

[61] Trujillo KA, Akil H. Inhibition of morphine tolerance and dependence by the NMDA receptor antagonist MK-801. Science 1991;251:85–7.

[62] Vicente SF, White JM, Somogyi AA, Bochner F, Chapleo CB. Enhanced buprenorphine analgesia with the addition of ultra-low-dose naloxone in healthy subjects. Clin Pharmacol Ther 2008;83:144–52.

[63] Vranken JH, Troost D, Wegener JT, Kruis MR, van der Vegt MH. Neuropathological findings after continuous intrathecal administration of S(+)-ketamine for the management of neuropathic cancer pain. Pain 2005;117:231–5.

[64] Wang HY, Friedman E, Olmstead MC, Burns LH. Ultra-low-dose naloxone suppresses opioid tolerance, dependence and associated changes in mu opioid receptor-G protein coupling and G beta gamma signaling. Neuroscience 2005;135:247–61.

[65] Wang HY, Frankfurt M, Burns LH. High-affinity naloxone binding to filamin A prevents mu opioid receptor-Gs coupling underlying opioid tolerance and dependence. PLoS ONE 2008;3:e1554.

[66] Watkins LR, Hutchinson MR, Ricr KC, Maier SF. The "toll" of opioid-induced glial activation: improving the clinical efficacy of opioids by targeting glia. Trends Pharmacol Sci 2009;30:581–91.

[67] Watkins LR, Kinscheck IB, Mayer DJ. Potentiation of opiate analgesia and apparent reversal of morphine tolerance by proglumide. Science 1984;224:395–6.

[68] Wolf ME. The role of excitatory amino acids in behavioral sensitization to psychomotor stimulants. Prog Neurobiol 1998;54:679–720.

[69] Yang C-Y, Wong C-S, Chang J-Y. Intrathecal ketamine reduces morphine requirements in patients with terminal cancer pain. Can J Anaesth 1996;43:379–83.

***Correspondence to:*** Eija Kalso, MD, DMedSci, Pain Clinic, P.O. Box 140, 00029 HUS, Helsinki, Finland. Email: eija.kalso@hus.fi.

# Part IV

# Clinical Trial Design in Cancer Pain

# New Drugs for Cancer Pain Relief

## Andy Dray

*AstraZeneca Research & Development Montreal, Montreal, Quebec, Canada*

# The Unmet Need and Disease Complexities

Pain is the most feared symptom associated with cancer. Pain is also the most prominent symptom reported in cancer, affecting 30–40% of all patients, with increased prevalence (40–70%) during cancer treatment and even greater prevalence (70–90%) in patients in terminal supportive care [41,77] (see Chapter 8 by Vissers).

Despite the availability of a number of approaches, including the use of analgesics, anti-inflammatory agents, and tumor-shrinking paradigms such as chemotherapy and radiation, satisfactory pain management has been extremely difficult to achieve [41,45,51] (summarized in Table I; see also Chapter 8). A variety of factors, apart from the individual shortcomings of current analgesics, account for this difficulty, particularly the heterogeneity of tumor-dependent pain mechanisms [14,25,43]. For example, progressive tumor growth or secretions are algogenic, may entrap nerve fibers, and cause physical or chemical tissue injury. Tumor-driven host-defense mechanisms and powerful neuroimmune modulation [57,61,78] add

*Cancer Pain: From Molecules to Suffering*
edited by Judith A. Paice, Rae F. Bell, Eija A. Kalso, and Olaitan A. Soyannwo
IASP Press, Seattle, © 2010

Table I
Drug therapies for today's cancer pain treatment

| Drug | Mechanism | Indication | Issues |
|---|---|---|---|
| Morphine and other opioids | Mu-opioid receptors | All cancer pain; morphine is still gold standard of treatment | Many side effects; opioid switching is frequent (works in 70%); changing route of administration allows better management |
| NSAIDs and COX-2 inhibitors | COX inhibition | Moderate inflammatory pain | Drug-related side effects: GI ulcerations, renal toxicity, CV risks |
| Antidepressants (SNRIs and SSRIs) | Inhibition of NE and 5-HT reuptake | Analgesia adjuvant and mood improvement | Drug-related side effects: headache, sedation, anti-cholinergic effects, hypotension, cardiac toxicity |
| Gabapentin | Calcium channel modulation | Adjunctive therapy: neuropathic cancer pain | Drowsiness, sedation, edema, weight gain |
| Ketamine | NMDA antagonist | Adjunctive therapy: opioid resistance | Hypertension, sedation, dysphoria |
| Corticosteroids | Anti-inflammatory | Adjunctive therapy | Peptic ulceration |
| Atrasentan | ET-1 antagonist | Adjuvant in prostate cancer | Dose-limiting headache |
| Combinations | Opioids, NSAIDs, gabapentin, SNRIs | Acute and chronic pain management | Adverse effects related to individual drugs |
| Intrathecal delivery: combinations | Local anesthetics, clonidine, ziconotide, baclofen, corticosteroids | Chronic intractable pain management | Spinal toxicity |

*Abbreviations:* COX, cyclooxygenase; CV, cardiovascular; ET-1, endothelin-1; GI, gastrointestinal; 5-HT, 5-hydroxytryptamine (serotonin); NE, norepinephrine; SNRI, serotonin-norepinephrine reuptake inhibitor; SSRI, selective serotonin reuptake inhibitor.

dimensions of episodic and chronic inflammation via the secretion of other algogenic and neurotoxic chemicals such as prostanoids, chemokines, nitric oxide, and endothelins [17,74,75]. In addition, antitumor therapies such as chemotherapy may provide a high risk of additional nerve injury with associated neuropathic pain [37] (see Chapter 1 by Dougherty).

Thus, clinical presentation of cancer pain may involve a complexity of nociceptive and neuropathic pain symptoms, including tonic background pain, evoked pain, and movement-related pain, as well as episodic spontaneous and breakthrough pain. These symptoms may vary with disease progression and the extent of other therapeutic interventions. Moreover, symptoms may be compounded and exacerbated by comorbidities that include mood disorders such as depression, stress, and anxiety, as well as physical deterioration caused by nausea, vomiting, and cachexia [25,47,65] (see Chapter 5 by Fallon).

The lack of detailed understanding of the links between pain symptoms and cellular mechanisms makes individualized cancer pain management one of the most challenging of therapeutic areas. However, emerging evidence, arising from developments within animal and human pathobiology and the growth of evidence-based and translational medicine, is providing stronger rationalization for future approaches toward improved treatments. Credibility for a mechanism-based research approach is being built by systematic exploration of the relationship between symptoms, key cellular processes, and the critical molecular drivers of pain [18,33,83,84].

Major cellular mechanistic processes (summarized in Fig. 1) include peripheral and central hyperexcitability, ectopic or spontaneous generation of nerve activity, phenotypic changes in nociceptive pathways, morphological reorganizations, and neurodegenerative changes [53,83].

Mechanistic and molecular linkage in chronic pain has relied heavily on animal studies using a small number of approximated disease- or mechanism-related models. These models have emphasized key symptomatic characteristics, such as thermal or mechanical allodynia, as well as some associated specificity of neurochemical signatures [31]. More specific models of cancer-related pain are few; they include induction of bone pain via the injection of various types of tumor cells into the murine hind leg [31] (see Chapter 3 by Mantyh), induction of skin hypersensitivity via tumor cell injection into the skin [12], or the induction of spontaneous pancreatic cancer through changes in murine gene expression [40].

Usually these pain behaviors have been related to tumor progression and are accompanied by immune cell infiltration, neovascularization, proliferation of sensory and sympathetic fibers in the tumor area, and secondary changes in spinal cord cells and neurochemistry (see Chapter 3). In the case of pancreatic cancer, in which there is significant tumor and disease progression before the appearance of pain symptoms, the murine model has indicated that early pain symptoms can be precipitated by naloxone. This finding signifies the engagement of endogenous opioid pain modulation in cancer [62].

Overall, cancer pain models have reinforced a number of emerging analgesia opportunities aimed at reducing hyperexcitability in pain pathways. These potential therapies include modulators of voltage- and ligand-gated ion channels, G-protein-coupled receptors (GPCRs), and neurotrophins, which have also been identified in a variety of other studies [18,43,53].

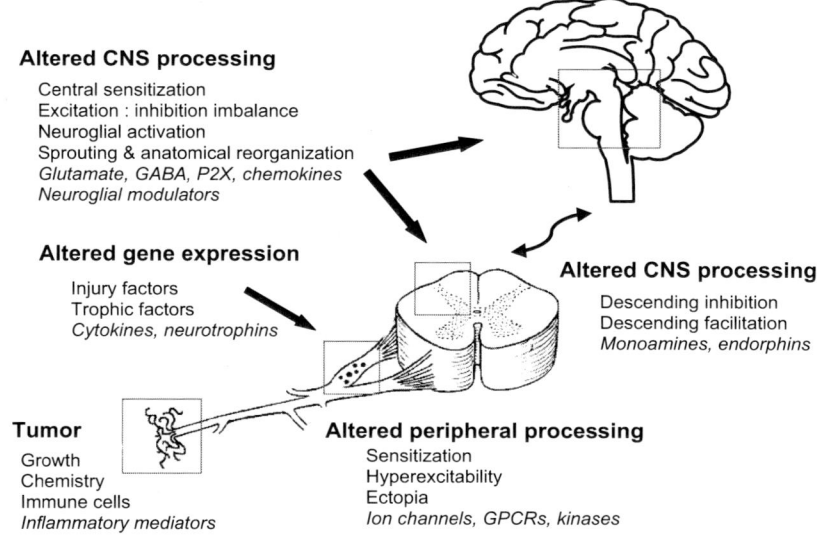

**Fig. 1.** Major cellular mechanisms operating in chronic cancer pain at different levels of pain signaling. Some analgesia targets and target families are indicated that address the variety of mechanisms. CNS = central nervous system; GABA = γ-aminobutyric acid; GPCRs = G-protein-coupled receptors.

This chapter will describe the analgesia validation of the most promising targets that have advanced to the early phases of clinical development, namely transient receptor potential vanilloid-1 (TRPV1) antagonists and anti-nerve growth factor (NGF) monoclonal antibodies. These agents have been selected from the variety of small-molecule pharmaceuticals and current biological approaches (Fig. 1).

# TRPV1 Antagonists

Targeting ion channels appears an extremely attractive option among novel analgesia approaches. Many channels are regulated by nerve and tissue injury and function to modulate the pain-related hyperexcitability of afferent and central nervous system (CNS) neurons seen across chronic inflammatory and neuropathic pain conditions [4,18,20,86]. As with other examples of targets that regulate excitable tissue, the development of analgesic efficacy, without limiting side effects (CNS or cardiovascular), has been a major challenge.

Among the most recently emerging family of channels are the ligand-gated transient receptor potential (TRP) channels. Many TRP channels are localized to sensory neurons (TRPV1, TRPV3, TRPV4, TRPA1, TRPM8) and play a major role in temperature regulation, in mechanical transduction, and particularly in pain transduction [49]. TRPV1 in particular has held center stage for many years as an important pain transducer and represents a highly valid molecular target for analgesia [69,70]. The TRPV1 receptor has been shown to be a nonselective cation channel, gated by capsaicin, noxious heat (>45°C), acids (pH < 5.3), and a variety of lipids, including anandamide [70].

The TRPV1 receptor could be considered to represent a "final" common pathway for sensitization and hyperexcitability of afferent neurons, particularly in inflammatory conditions, as it can be regulated by a variety of inflammatory agents [49]. In keeping with an important role in pain transduction, a wealth of preclinical data in a variety of animal models (nociceptive and neuropathic) support the value of TRPV1 as an analgesic target [9,21,70,81].

Although currently the major therapeutic goal for this target has been directed toward developing TRPV1 antagonists, other approaches are being exploited using TRPV1 agonists. These include capsaicin or cap-saicin-like agonists usually administered topically or locally. This approach utilizes a particular property of TRPV1 receptors in that strong or persistent activation can lead to reversible sensory nerve terminal degeneration caused by prolonged cation influx into the sensory nerve, osmotic damage and metabolic collapse [69]. This principle has been shown to be effective in the clinic. For example, topical application of high doses of capsaicin are efficacious in a number of neuropathic pain conditions, as shown in Phase III studies in patients with postherpetic neuralgia [7,81]. An injectable TRPV1-receptor agonist formulated for long-lasting pain relief is being developed [54].

Antagonist approaches can be broadly classed into those that interact with the ligand-binding sites, thus blocking the effects of capsaicin-, acid-, and heat-mediated channel activation, or those that demonstrate selectivity to capsaicin. Hitherto, there are no examples of TRPV1-selective blockers of the cation channel itself. Antagonists have been shown to be efficacious in a range of preclinical models, including a cancer pain model. In this model, TRPV1 is highly expressed in sensory fibers within the mineralized bone and bone marrow. Tumor-induced ongoing pain and movement-evoked pain behaviors could be quantified. These behaviors were attenuated by several days of treatment with the TRPV1 antagonist JNJ-17203212 [24] without notable effects on tumor growth and were absent in animals in which the TRPV1 gene had been deleted.

## Clinical Studies

A number of TRPV1 antagonist programs have advanced to early clinical development (see Table II), and there is also a highly competitive field of preclinical activities. Recent clinical studies in volunteers, using a randomized, placebo-controlled, single-blind crossover design, have shown that oral SB705498 (Glaxo-Smith-Kline) attenuated the capsaicin-evoked flare area and heat pain hyperalgesia induced by ultraviolet B irradiation [10], without notable side effects attributable to the compound. These effects were achieved at similar plasma concentrations that showed efficacy in preclinical models [52]. These studies have heralded the way for a number of Phase II clinical concept trials with TRPV1 antagonists by a number of major pharmaceutical companies. Some of these trials are

Table II
TRPV1 antagonists in clinical development

| Compound | Company | Pain Type | Phase | Status |
|---|---|---|---|---|
| AZD1386 | AstraZeneca | Dental pain | II | Active |
| ABT-102 | Abbott | Thermal sensitivity | 1 | Ongoing |
| JTS-653 | Japan Tobacco | Bladder pain | II | Ongoing |
| V-377 | PharmEste | OA | 1 | Ongoing |
| GRC 6211 | Lilly/Glenmark | Dental pain, OA | II | Suspended |
| AMG 517 | Amgen | Dental pain, OA | Ib | Terminated |
| SB-705498 | Glaxo-Smith-Kline | Migraine, IBS | II | Terminated |
| MK 2295 | Merck/Neurogen | Dental pain | II | Terminated |
| Undisclosed | Renovis/Pfizer | Not known | Not known | Not known |

*Abbreviations:* IBS, irritable bowel syndrome; OA, osteoarthritis; TRPV1, transient receptor potential vanilloid-1.

still progressing toward their intended proof of principle, but other leading compounds have been abandoned, partly because of drug-related abnormalities in body temperature regulation, including hyperthermia. For example, AM517 produced an exposure-dependent hyperthermia (maximum body temperature 39–40.2°C) in patients following third molar tooth extraction. Patients shivered and complained of being cold [23]. Although the hyperthermia could be modulated in part by acetaminophen (paracetamol), the study could not be completed to evaluate any analgesic effect of AM517.

Thus, temperature regulation has emerged as a significant challenge to developing this class of compound. Interestingly, a change in body temperature has been noted with many antagonists, but it does not appear to be a universal issue with all TRPV1 antagonists [10,39; see discussion below].

## TRPV1 and Temperature Regulation

Body temperature regulation is dynamically balanced via a number of mechanisms including vasomotor changes, thermogenesis, and shivering and sweating [22,56]. Early studies with TRPV1 knockout mice did not reveal significant thermoregulatory deficits [71]. However, responsiveness to capsaicin and pain sensitivity [13], but not heat sensitivity [82], was diminished in these animals. Interestingly, localized TRPV1 sensitization with inflammatory mediators indicated that sensory neurons can become tonically active at body temperature to transduce pain signals [50]. However, there has been little evidence that TRPV1 exists in a sensitized or activated state unless a sensitizing environment is created by pathophysiology. More recent preclinical studies, with a variety of TRPV1 antagonists, have challenged this premise. With consistent findings of hyperthermia, these newer studies suggest that TRPV1 normally exists in a tonically active state, with a significant role in maintaining normal body temperature, and that disruption of this state causes hyperthermia (for review see [22]). These data have raised questions about the physiological role of TRPV1 receptors, challenging the dogma of TRPV1 as primarily a specific pain transducer. Mechanistically, antagonists cause thermodysregulation through vasoconstriction and via increasing thermogenesis via actions outside the blood-brain barrier, possibly localized in visceral vagal afferents or within the preoptic-hypothalamic system [22,68]. Perhaps TRPV1 receptors in these areas are differentially specialized, given that several TRPV1 polymorphisms have been reported [85]. These receptors may be functionally specialized, as in, for example, the TRPV1-like salty taste transduction in mammals [42]. Additionally, there are some indications that chemical optimization of antagonists to avoid hyperthermic lability is possible [39] and that repeated administration of TRPV1 antagonists (e.g., ABT102) attenuate hyperthermia but enhance analgesic activity [30]. Thus, the prevailing view is that it still may be possible to validate the analgesic efficacy of TRPV1 antagonists without causing debilitating hyperthermia.

# Modulation of Nerve Growth Factor

Nerve growth factor (NGF) is an important member of a family of regulatory cytokines, essential for sensory nerve survival and development and for the determination of neurochemical phenotype, which is important for the regulation of excitability [67,90]. NGF is formed by cleavage of pro-NGF precursor by plasmin and has been shown, at least in the CNS, to be degraded by metalloproteinases, particularly matrix metallopeptidase

9 (MMP9) [8]. In the periphery NGF can be derived, normally and during pathological conditions, from a number of cell types, including Schwann cells, keratinocytes, and cancer cells. However, it is unclear what pathological mechanisms drive the increased expression of NGF or its receptors, although some proinflammatory cytokines have been shown to increase NGF expression [1,66].

Mature NGF signals as a homodimer, inducing dimerization of its distinct sensory neuron receptor TrkA, and activating a cascade of intracellular signaling kinases that include mitogen-activated protein kinase (MAPK), phosphoinositide 3-kinase (PI3K), and Akt [15,29,32]. These signaling protein complexes are transported to the cell body and induce further activation of gene transcription to alter the expression of a variety of membrane proteins that regulate cell excitability—including TRPV1, voltage-gated sodium channel $Na_V1.8$, acid-sensing ion channel 3 (ASIC3), and the purinoceptor $P2X_3$—and increase production of sensory neurotransmitters such as calcitonin gene-related peptide (CGRP). These membrane proteins and neurotransmitters in turn cause neural sensitization and increased excitability in pain pathways (see [29]).

NGF also interacts with p75, a ubiquitous regulatory protein that is also regulated nonspecifically by other neurotrophins such as brain-derived neurotrophic factor (BDNF). Activation of p75 by NGF has also been indicated in the regulation of sensory nerve excitability in a study showing that p75 gene deletion caused elevated thresholds to noxious stimuli [5]. However, it is less clear how p75 participates in the NGF pathway because NGF-induced hyperalgia was similar in magnitude in these animals [6]. Interestingly it has been hypothesized that pro-NGF preferentially binds a p75/sortilin complex present in peptidic sensory neurons to promote apoptosis of these cells [3,38]. It is unclear whether this mechanism affects pain transmission or how it may be integrated with other aspects of the NGF pathway.

NGF and its target receptors can be considered to have compelling preclinical as well as clinical validation with respect to pain and analgesia. For example, human gene deficits in TrkA are associated with congenital insensitivity to pain [34], and NGF loss due to Schwann cell injury in leprosy causes loss of pain sensation [2]. In addition, acute administration of NGF in human volunteers caused pain and a prolonged state of hyperalgesia [19]. Importantly, levels of NGF are elevated in various inflammatory conditions in humans such as arthritis, cystitis, prostatitis, and headache as well as in inflammation induced by ultraviolet radiation or surgical injury [26,46,59] and in neuroma tissue [28]. Targeting NGF for pain therapy is further supported by a variety of data from animal models of nociceptive and neuropathic pain [29]. For example, NGF sequestration with neutralizing antibodies or fragments attenuated inflammatory hyperalgesia [44,76,87]. Moreover, anti-TrkA neutralization reduced neuropathic pain [73,79].

With respect to cancer pain treatment, there is a compelling literature for NGF involvement in tumor growth and cancer pain. Thus, NGF and TrkA are expressed in a variety of tumor cells [16,72] and in some cases increased expression correlates strongly with perineural invasion, tumor spread, and pancreatic cancer pain [88]. Animal models of bone cancer pain have indicated a profound reduction in ongoing and evoked pain following repetitive anti-NGF treatment with tanezumab, a reduction that was equal to or better than that produced by acute doses of morphine [27,63]. In addition, NGF sequestration markedly improved cancer-associated bone fracture pain [35] and may have the potential to modify weight loss associated with cachexia [64].

## Clinical Studies

To date the major therapeutic thrust has been to develop anti-NGF monoclonal antibodies as well as inhibitors of TrkA receptors. Anti-NGF programs are clearly most advanced in the clinic (Table III). Thus, clinical efficacy has been shown using tanezumab, a humanized monoclonal anti-NGF

Table III
Anti-nerve growth factor (NGF) approaches
in clinical development

| Company | Drug | Target | Phase |
|---|---|---|---|
| Pfizer | Tanezumab | NGF | II/III |
| Amgen/Johnson & Johnson | AMG 403 | NGF | II |
| Sanofi-Aventis/Regeneron | REGN-475 | NGF | I |
| Line Genomics/Pan Genetics | PG110 | NGF | I |
| Line Genomics/Bioxell | huMNAC13 (BXL1H5) | TrkA | I |

antibody. Pfizer is leading this field and has provided validation data both in osteoarthritis (OA) and low back pain (LBP) patients for the utility of the anti-NGF approach. In a randomized, double-blind, placebo-controlled, phase II clinical trial, the safety and efficacy of tanezumab were assessed in patients with knee OA who had not fully responded to analgesic treatment [60]. After a 3-day wash-out period, 450 patients were randomized (75 in each arm of the study) to receive placebo or 1 of 5 doses of tanezumab (10, 25, 50, 100, or 200 µg/kg). Tanezumab was given by intravenous injection on days 1 and 56. Patients were followed for 16 weeks. Compared with placebo-treated patients, patients treated with tanezumab experienced significantly less knee pain on walking. The mean change in pain in the affected knee upon walking, from baseline to week 16, was a decrease of 15.5% in the placebo group and a decrease of 32.1% in the group given tanezumab at the10-µg/kg dose. Similar improvements over placebo were observed with the 25-, 50-, 100-, and 200-µg/kg doses of the drug.

Tanezumab treatment also resulted in significantly better scores on the Subject Global Assessment of therapy compared with placebo, as well as improved scores on the Western Ontario and McMaster Universities Osteoarthritis Index for pain, stiffness, and physical function. Headache, upper respiratory tract infection, and paresthesias were the three most commonly reported adverse effects associated with tanezumab, but no long-term safety issues were reported. Thus, overall tanezumab appears well tolerated and may be an effective treatment in OA knee pain. In addition, another recent multicenter study [36] in chronic LBP patients compared placebo with a single i.v. dose (200 µg) of tanezumab with twice-daily dosing of naproxen (500 mg/kg). Tanezumab showed significant, prolonged (12 weeks), and clinically meaningful pain relief that was superior to that provided by naproxen. A few patients reported some mild, transient peripheral dysesthesia with no evidence of neuropathy.

Overall, anti-NGF therapy heralds a step-change in efficacy expectations compared with current treatments for OA and low back pain. Moreover, the emerging positive clinical data signal an increased confidence in the predictability of preclinical modeling and indicate that a single peripheral drug target can provide meaningful clinical analgesic efficacy. It is hoped that these positive clinical findings will be the forerunners of other successful trials with anti-NGF treatments in cancer pain conditions, where the preclinical evidence for this approach has very high validity. Such trials are understood to be in progress.

Other drugs that are still in the preclinical phase include ALE0540 and PD90780, which inhibit NGF binding to TrkA and p75 receptors, respectively. These drugs have shown efficacy in chronic pain models [48]. In addition, HuMNAC [11], an antibody to TrkA, has also been reported to be in the preclinical phase.

To date, antibody-focused anti-NGF approaches have not highlighted major safety issues associated with physiological target disruption, such as cardiovascular changes due to alterations in the regulation of peripheral sympathetic fibers or central changes in cholinergic neuron functioning.

# Summary

Satisfactory pain treatment remains the single most important challenge to quality of life management in cancer patients. In recent years the emerging neurobiology of pain, as well as preclinical evidence drawn from animal models of pain and cancer disease mechanisms, have highlighted a multiplicity of novel analgesia opportunities. Many major pharmaceutical companies and biotechnology organizations are pursuing these avenues. This chapter has outlined two of the most advanced analgesia programs aimed at delivery of TRPV1 antagonist and anti-NGF approaches. These targets have been highly validated for analgesia by systematic preclinical studies and by early clinical readouts in support of therapeutic validation. TRPV1 antagonists show efficacy in human pain models, but further exploration appears to be challenged by target-related untoward body temperature dysregulation. On the other hand, anti-NGF treatments with the humanized monoclonal antibody tanezumab have shown high and robust efficacy in both osteoarthritis and low back pain trials, with promise of further potential in ongoing trials for cancer pain.

A potential future challenge may be the alterations in drug metabolism and drug pharmacokinetics caused by disease progression and cancer therapies [58]. Indeed, various inflammatory mediators have been shown to alter the regulation of p450 enzymes [55,89] and the structure and function of the blood-brain barrier, which may affect drug delivery and brain uptake [80].

# References

[1] Abe Y, Akeda K, An HS, Pichika R, Muehleman C, Kimura T, Masuda K. Proinflammatory cytokines stimulate the expression of nerve growth factor by human intervertebral disc cells. Spine 2007;32:635–42.

[2] Anand P. Neurotrophic factors and their receptors in human sensory neuropathies. Prog Brain Res 2004;146:477–92.

[3] Arnett MG, Ryals JM, Wright DE. Pro-NGF, sortilin, and p75NTR: potential mediators of injury-induced apoptosis in the mouse dorsal root ganglion. Brain Res 2007;1183:32–42.

[4] Bear B, Asgian J, Termin A, Zimmermann N. Small molecules targeting sodium and calcium channels for neuropathic pain. Curr Opin Drug Discov Devel 2009;12:543–61.

[5] Bergmann I, Priestley JV, McMahon SB, Bröcker EB, Toyka KV, Koltzenburg M. Analysis of cutaneous sensory neurones in transgenic mice lacking low affinity neurotrophin receptor p75. Eur J Neurosci 1997;9:18–28.

[6] Bergmann I, Reiter R, Toyka KV, Koltzenburg M. Nerve growth factor evokes hyperalgesia in mice lacking the low-affinity neurotrophin receptor p75. Neurosci Lett 1998;255:87–90.

[7] Bley KR. Recent developments in transient receptor potential vanilloid receptor 1 agonist-based therapies. Expert Opin Investig Drugs 2004;13:1445–6.

[8] Bruno MA, Cuello AC. Activity-dependent release of precursor nerve growth factor conversion to mature nerve growth factor and its degradation by a protease cascade. Proc Natl Acad Sci USA 2006;103:6730–40.

[9] Caterina MJ, Leffler A, Malmberg AB, Martin WJ, Trafton J, Petersen-Zeitz KR, Koltzenburg M, Basbaum AI, Julius D. Impaired nociception and pain sensation in mice lacking the capsaicin receptor. Science 2000;288:306–13.

[10] Chizh BA, O'Donnell MB, Napolitano A, Wang J, Brooke AC, Aylott MC, Bullman JN, Gray EJ, Lai RY, Williams PM, Appleby JM. The effects of the TRPV1 antagonist SB-705498 on TRPV1 receptor-mediated activity and inflammatory hyperalgesia in humans. Pain 2007;132:132–41.

[11] Colquhoun A, Lawrance GM, Shamovsky IL, Riopelle RJ, Ross GM. Differential activity of the nerve growth factor (NGF) antagonist PD90780 [7-benzoylamino]-4,9-dihydro-4methyl-8-oxopyrazolo-[5,1-b]-quinazoline-2-carboxylic acid] suggest altered NGF-p75NTR interactions in the presence of trkA. J Pharmacol Exp Ther 2004;310:505–11.

[12] Constantin CE, Mair N, Sailer CA, Andratsch M, Xu ZZ, Blumer MJ, Scherbakov N, Davis JB, Bluethmann H, Ji RR, Kress M. Endogenous tumor necrosis factor alpha (TNFα) requires TNF receptor type 2 to generate heat hyperalgesia in a mouse cancer model. J Neurosci 2008;28:5072–81.

[13] Davis JB, Gray J, Gunthorpe MJ, Hatcher JP, Davey PT, Overend P, Harries MH, Latcham J, Clapham C, Atkinson K, et al. Vanilloid receptor-1 is essential for inflammatory thermal hyperalgesia. Nature 2000; 405:183–7.

[14] Delaney A, Fleetwood-Walker SM, Colvin LA, Fallon M. Translational medicine: cancer pain mechanisms and management. Br J Anaesth, 2008;101:87–94.

[15] Delcroix J-D, Valletta JS, Wu C, Hunt SJ, Kowal AS, Mobley WC. NGF signaling in sensory neurons: evidence that early endosomes carry NGF retrograde signals. Neuron 2003;39:69–84.

[16] Dolle L, Yazidi-Belkoura IE, Adriaessen E, Nurcombe V, Hondermarck H. Nerve growth factor overexpression and autocrine loop in breast cancer cells. Oncogene 2003;22:5592–601.

[17] Dray A. Pharmacology of inflammatory pain. In: Merskey H, Loeser JD, Dubner R, editors. The paths of pain. Seattle: IASP Press; 2005. p. 177–90.

[18] Dray A. Neuropathic pain: emerging treatments. Br J Anaesth 2008;101:48–58.

[19] Dyck PJ, Peroutka S, Rask C, Burton E, Baker MK, Lehman KA, Gillen DA, Hokanson JL, O'Brien PC. Intradermal recombinant human nerve growth factor induces pressure allodynia and lowered heat-pain threshold in humans. Neurology 1997;48:501–5.

[20] Eglen RM, Hunter JC, Dray A. Ions in the fire: recent ion-channel research and approaches to pain therapy. Trends Pharmacol Sci 1999;8:337–42.

[21] García-Martinez C, Humet M, Planells-Cases R, Gomis A, Caprini M, Viana F, De La Pena E, Sanchez-Baeza F, Carbonell T, De Felipe C, et al. Attenuation of thermal nociception and hyperalgesia by VR1 blockers. Proc Natl Acad Sci USA 2002;99:2374–9.

[22] Gavva NR. Body-temperature maintenance as the predominant function of the vanilloid receptor TRPV1. Trends Pharmacol Sci 2008;2:550–7.

[23] Gavva NR, Treanor JJ, Garami A, Fang L, Surapaneni S, Akrami A, Alvarez F, Bak A, Darling M, Gore A, et al. Pharmacological blockade of the vanilloid receptor TRPV1 elicits marked hyperthermia in humans. Pain 2008;136:3–4.

[24] Ghilardi JR, Röhrich H, Lindsay TH, Sevcik MA, Schwei MJ, Kubota K, Halvorson KG, Poblete J, Chaplan SR, Dubin AE, et al. Selective blockade of the capsaicin receptor TRPV1 attenuates bone cancer pain. J Neurosci 2005;25:3126–31.

[25] Gutstein HB. Mechanisms underlying cancer-induced symptoms. Drugs Today (Barc) 2003;39:815–22.

[26] Halliday DA, Zettler RA, Rush R, Scicchitano R, McNeil JD. Elevated nerve growth factor level in the synovial fluid of patients with inflammatory joint disease. Neurochem Res 1998;23:919–22.

[27] Halvorson KG, Kubota K, Sevcik MA, Lindsay TH, Sotillo JE, Ghilardi JR, Rosol TJ, Boustany L, Shelton DL, Mantyh PW. A blocking antibody to nerve growth factor attenuates skeletal pain induced by prostate tumor cell growing in bone. Cancer Res 2005;65:9426–35.

[28] Harpf C, Dabernig J, Humpel C. Receptors for NGF and GDNF are highly expressed in human peripheral neuroma. Muscle Nerve 2002;25:612–5.

[29] Hefti FF, Rosenthal A, Walicke PA, Wyatt S, Vergara G, Shelton DL, Davies AM. Novel class of pain drugs based on antagonism of NGF. Trends Pharmacol Sci 2006;27:85–91.

[30] Honore P, Chandran P, Hernandez G, Gauvin DM, Mikusa JP, Zhong C, Joshi SK, Ghilardi JR, Sevcik MA, Fryer RM, et al. Repeated dosing of ABT-102, a potent and selective TRPV1 antagonist, enhances TRPV1-mediated analgesia activity in rodents, but attenuates antagonist-induced hyperthermia. Pain 2009;142:27–37.

[31] Honore P, Rogers SD, Schwei MJ, Salak-Johnson JL, Luger NM, Sabino MC, Clohisy DR, Mantyh PW. Murine models of inflammatory, neuropathic and cancer pain each generate a unique set of neurochemical changes in the spinal cord and sensory neurons. Neuroscience 2000;98:585–98.

[32] Huang EJ, Reichardt LF. Trk receptors: roles in neuronal signal transduction. Annu Rev Biochem 2003;72:609–42.

[33] Hucho T, Levine JD. Signaling pathways in sensitization: towards a nociceptor cell biology. Neuron 2007;55:365–76.

[34] Indo Y, Tsuruta M, Hayashida Y, Karim MA, Ohta K, Kawano T, Mitsubuchi H, Tonoki H, Awaya Y, Matsuda I. Mutations in the TRKA/NGF receptor gene in patients with congenital insensitivity to pain with anhydrosis. Nat Genet 1996;13:485–8.

[35] Jimenez-Andrade JM, Martin CD, Koewler NJ, Freeman KT, Sullivan LJ, Halvorson KG, Barthold CM, Peters CM, Buus RJ, Ghilardi JR, et al. Nerve growth factor sequestration therapy attenuated non-malignant skeletal pain following fracture. Pain 2007;133:183–96.

[36] Katz N, Borenstein D, Birbara C, Bramson C, Nemeth M, Smith M, Brown M. Tanezumab, an anti-nerve growth factor (NGF) antibody, for the treatment of chronic low back pain (CLBP): a randomized, controlled, double-blind, phase 2 trial. J Pain 2009;10.

[37] Lee BN, Dantzer R, Langley KE, Bennett GL, Dougherty PM, Dunn AJ, Meyers CA, Miller AH, Payne R, Reuben JM, et al. A cytokine-based neuroimmunological mechanism of cancer-related symptoms. Neuroimmunomodulation 2004;11:279–92.

[38] Lee R, Kermani P, Teng KK, Hempstead BL. Regulation of cell survival by secreted proneurotrophins. Science 2001;294:1945–8.

[39] Lehto SG, Tamir R, Deng H, Klionsky L, Kuang R, Le A, Lee D, Louis JC, Magal E, Manning BH, et al. Antihyperalgesic effects of (R,E)-N-2 hydroxy-2,3,dihydro-1H-inden-4-yl)-3-(2-(piperidin-1-yl)-4-(trifluoromethyl) phenyl)acrylamide (AMG8562), a novel transient receptor potential vanilloid type 1 modulator that does not cause hyperthermia in rats. J Pharmacol Exp Ther 2008;326:218–29.

[40] Lindsay TH, Jonas BM, Sevcik MA, Kubota K, Halvorson KG, Ghilardi JR, Kuskowski MA, Stelow EB, Mukherjee P, Gendler SJ, et al. Pancreatic cancer pain and its correlation with changes in tumor vasculature, macrophage infiltration, neuronal innervation, body weight and disease progression. Pain 2005;119:233–46.

[41] Lussier D, Huskey AG, Portenoy RK. Adjuvant analgesics in cancer pain management. Oncologist 2004;9:571–91.

[42] Lyall V, Heck GL, Vinnikova AK, Ghosh S, Phan TH, Alam RI, Russell OF, Malik SA, Bigbee JW, DeSimone JA. The mammalian amiloride-insensitive non-specific salt taste receptor is a vanilloid receptor-1 variant. J Physiol 2004;558:147–59.

[43] Mantyh PW, Clohisy, DR, Koltzenburg M, Hunt SP. Molecular mechanisms of cancer pain. Nat Rev Cancer 2002;2:201–9.

[44] McMahon SB, Bennett DL, Priestley JV, Shelton DL. The biological effect of endogenous nerve growth factor on adult sensory neurones revealed by a trkA-IgG fusion molecule. Nat Med 1995;1:774–80.
[45] Miaskowski C, editor. Principles of analgesic use in the treatment of acute pain and cancer pain, 6th edition. American Pain Society; 2008.
[46] Miller LJ, Fischer KA, Goralnick SJ, Litt M, Burleson JA, Albertsen P, Kreutzer DL. Nerve growth factor and chronic prostatitis/chronic pelvic pain syndrome. Urology 2002;59:603–8.
[47] Muscaritoli M, Bossola M, Aversa Z, Bellantone R, Fanelli FR. Prevention and treatment of cancer cachexia: new insights into an old problem. Eur J Cancer 2006;42:31–41.
[48] Owolabi JB, Rizkalla G, Tehim A, Ross GM, Riopelle RJ, Kamboj R, Ossipov M, Bian D, Wegert S, Porreca F, Lee DK. Characterization of antiallodynic actions of ALE-0540, a novel nerve growth factor receptor antagonist, in the rat. J Pharmacol Exp Ther 1999;289:1271–6.
[49] Patapoutian A, Tate S, Woolf CJ. Transient receptor potential channels: targeting pain at its source. Nature Rev Drug Disc 2009;8:55–68.
[50] Premkumar LS, Ahern GP. Induction of vanilloid receptor channel activity by protein kinase C. Nature 2000;408:985–90.
[51] Radbruch L, Elsner F. Emerging analgesia in cancer pain management. Expert Opin Emerg Drugs 2005;10:151–71.
[52] Rami HK, Thompson M, Stemp G, Fell S, Jerman JC, Stevens AJ, Smart D, Sargent B, Sanderson D, Randall AD, et al. Discovery of SB-705498: a potent, selective and orally bioavailable TRPV1 antagonist suitable for clinical development. Bioorg Med Chem Lett 2006;16:3287–91.
[53] Read SJ, Dray A. Osteoarthritic pain: a review of current, theoretical and emerging therapeutics. Expert Opin Investig Drugs 2008;17:619–40.
[54] Remadevi R, Szallisi A. Adlea (ALGRX-4975), an injectable capsaicin (TRPV1 receptor agonist) formulated for longlasting pain relief. IDrugs 2008;11:120–32.
[55] Rivory LP, Salviero KA, Clarke SJ. Hepatic cytochrome P450 3A drug metabolism is reduced in cancer patients who have an acute-phase response. Br J Cancer 2002;87:277–80.
[56] Romanovsky AA. Thermoregulation: some concepts have changed. Functional architecture of the thermoregulatory system. Am J Physiol Regul Integ Comp Physiol 2007;292:R37–R46.
[57] Rutkowski MD, DeLeo JA. The role of cytokines in the initiation and maintenance of chronic pain. Drugs News Perspect 2002;15:626–32.
[58] Sanchez RI, Mesia-Vela S, Kauffman FC. Challenges of cancer drug design: a drug metabolic perspective. Curr Cancer Drug Targets 2001;1:1–32.
[59] Sarchielli P, Alberti A, Floridi A, Gallai V. Levels of nerve growth factor in cerebrospinal fluid of chronic headache patients. Neurology 2001;57:132–4.
[60] Schnitzer TJ, Lane NE, Smith MD, Brown MT. Efficacy and safety of PF04383119 for moderate to severe pain due to osteoarthritis (OA) of the knee: a randomized trial. Abstracts: 12th World Congress on Pain. Seattle: IASP Press; 2008. PT 214.
[61] Scholz J, Woolf CJ. The neuropathic pain triad: neurons, immune cells and glia. Nat Neurosci 2007;10:1361–8.
[62] Sevcik MA, Jonas BM, Lindsay TH, Halvorson KG, Ghilardi JR, Kuskowski MA, Mukherjee P, Maggio JE, Mantyh PW. Endogenous opioids inhibit early-stage pancreatic pain in a mouse model of pancreatic cancer. Gastroenterology 2006;131:900–10.
[63] Sevcik MA, Ghilardi JR, Peters CM, Lindsay TH, Halvorson KG, Jonas BM, Kubota K, Kuskowski MA, Boustany L, Shelton DL, Mantyh PW. Anti-NGF therapy profoundly reduces bone cancer pain and the accompanying increase in markers of peripheral and central sensitization. Pain 2005;115:128–41.
[64] Shelton DL, Zeller J, Ho WH, Pons J, Rosenthal A. Nerve growth factor mediates hyperalgesia and cachexia in auto-immune arthritis. Pain 2005;116:8–16.
[65] Sindrup SH, Otto M, Finnerup NB, Jensen TS. Antidepressants in the treatment of neuropathic pain. Basic Clin Pharmacol Toxicol 2005;96:399–409.
[66] Skoff AM, Zhao C, Adler JE. Interleukin-1 alpha regulates substance P expression and release in adult sensory neurons Exp Neurol 2009;217:395–400.
[67] Sofroniew MV, Howe CL, Mobley WC. Nerve growth factor signaling, neuroprotection, and neural repair Ann Rev Neurosci 2001;24:1217–81.
[68] Steiner AA, Turek VF, Almeida MC, Burmeister JJ, Oliveira DL, Roberts JL, Bannon AW, Norman MH, Louis JC, Treanor JJ, et al. Nonthermal activation of transient receptor potential vanilloid-1 channels in abdominal visceral tonically inhibits autonomic cold-defense effectors. J Neurosci 2007;27:7459–68.

[69] Szallasi A. Blumberg PM. Vanilloid (capsaicin) receptors and mechanisms. Pharmacol Rev 1999;51:159−212.
[70] Szallasi A, Cortright DV, Blum CA Eid SR. The vanilloid receptor VR1: 10 years from channel cloning to antagonist proof-of-concept. Nat Rev Drug Discov 2007;6:357−72.
[71] Szellenyi Z, Hummel M, Szolcsanyi J, Davis JB. Daily body temperature rhythm and heat tolerance in TRPV1 knockout and capsaicin pretreated mice Eur J Neurosci 2004;19:1421−4.
[72] Tokusashi Y, Asai K, Tamakawa S, Yamamoto M, Yoshie M, Yaginuma Y, Miyokawa N, Aoki T, Kino S, Kasai S, Ogawa K. Expression of NGF in hepatocellular cells with receptors in non-tumor cell components. Int J Cancer 2005;114:39−45.
[73] Ugolini G, Marinelli S, Covaceuszach S, Cattaneo A. Pavone F. The function neutralizing anti-TrkA antibody MNAC13 reduces inflammatory and neuropathic pain. Proc Natl Acad Sci USA 2007;104:2985−990.
[74] Watkins LR, Maier S. Beyond neurons: evidence that immune and glial cells contribute to pathological pain states. Physiol Rev 2002;82:981−1011.
[75] Watkins LR, Maier SF. Glia: a novel drug discovery target for clinical pain. Nat Rev Drug Discov 2003;2:973−85.
[76] Watson JJ, Fahey MS, van den Worm E, Engels F, Nijkamp FP, Stroemer P, McMahon S, Allen SJ, Dawbarn D. TrkAd5: a novel therapeutic agent for the treatment of inflammatory pain and asthma. J Pharmacol Exp Ther 2006;316:1122−9.
[77] Weiss SC, Emanuel LL, Fairclough DL, Emanuel EJ. Understanding the experience of pain in terminally ill patients. Lancet 2001;357:1311−5.
[78] White FA, Jung H, Miller, R Chemokines and the pathophysiology of neuropathic pain. Proc Natl Acad Sci USA 2007;104:20151−8.
[79] Wild KD, Bian D, Zhu D, Davis J, Bannon AW, Zhang TJ, Louis JC. Antibodies to nerve growth factor reverse established tactile allodynia in rodent models of neuropathic pain without tolerance. J Pharm Exp Ther 2007;322:282−7.
[80] Wolka AM, Huber JD, Davis TP. Pain and the blood-brain barrier: obstacles to drug delivery. Adv Drug Deliv Rev 2003;55:987−1006.
[81] Wong GY, Gavva NR. Therapeutic potential of vanilloid receptor TRPV1 agonists and antagonists as analgesics: recent advances and setbacks Brain Res Rev 2008;60:267−77.
[82] Woodbury CJ, Zwick M, Wang S, Lawson JJ, Caterina MJ, Koltzenburg M, Albers KM, Koerber HR, Davis BM. Nociceptors lacking TRPV1 and TRPV2 have normal heat responses. J Neurosci 2004;24:6410−5.
[83] Woolf CJ, Ma Q. Nociceptors: noxious stimulus detectors. Neuron 2007;55:353−64.
[84] Woolf CJ, Salter MW. Neuronal plasticity: increasing the gain in pain. Science 2000;288:1765−9.
[85] Xu H, Tian W, Fu Y, Oyama TT, Anderson S, Cohen DM. Functional effects of non-synonymous polymorphisms in the human TRPV1 gene. Am J Physiol Renal Physiol 2007;293:F1865−76.
[86] Yaksh TL. Calcium channels as therapeutic targets in neuropathic pain. Pain 2006;7(Suppl 1): S13−S30.
[87] Zahn PK, Subieta A Park SS, Brennan TJ. Effect of blockade of nerve growth factor and tumor necrosis factor on pain behaviors after plantar incision. J Pain 2004;5:157−63.
[88] Zhu Z, Friess H, di Mola FF, Zimmermann A, Graber HU, Korc M, Büchler MW. Nerve growth factor expression correlates with perineural invasion and pain in human pancreatic cancer. J Clin Oncol 1999;17:2419−28.
[89] Zordoky BN, El-Kado AO. Role of NF-kappaB in the regulation of cytochrome p450 enzymes. Curr Drug Metab 2009;10:164−78.
[90] Zweifel LS, Kuruvilla R, Ginty DD. Functions and mechanisms of retrograde neurotrophin signaling. Nat Rev Neurosci 2005;6:615−25.

*Correspondence to:* Andy Dray, PhD, AstraZeneca Research & Development Montreal, 7171 Frederick Banting Street, Montreal, Quebec, Canada H4S 1Z9. Email: andy.dray@astrazeneca.com.

# 11

# Methodological Issues in Cancer Pain: Pharmacological Trials

## Ulf E. Kongsgaard[a,b] and Mads U. Werner[c]

[a]The Norwegian Radium Hospital, Clinic of Emergency Medicine, Oslo University Hospital, Oslo, Norway; [b]Medical Faculty, University of Oslo, Oslo, Norway; [c]Multidisciplinary Pain Center, Neuroscience Center, Rigshospitalet, Copenhagen, Denmark

Despite advances in cancer care and pain management, many patients with cancer pain obtain inadequate pain relief or experience unacceptable side effects from their treatment. Unrelieved pain impairs functional status, compromises quality of life, and may interfere with anticancer treatment. High-quality clinical studies of pharmacological treatment for cancer pain are needed to improve quality of life in these patients. The study of pain and pain management in this population has often been ignored. Pain treatment has mostly been empirical and incomplete and has often resulted in unnecessary suffering for many patients [26]. When discussing pharmacological trials for pain, why focus specifically on cancer pain? Are these patients different from other pain patients? Does the pain these patients experience differ from the pain in other painful conditions?

# Difficulties in Conducting Studies in Cancer Patients

## Cancer Patients are Heterogeneous and Have Complex Patterns of Symptoms

The efficacy of pain treatments may differ for various pain qualities. Patients with advanced cancer often present complex patterns of symptoms, of which pain is the most prevalent. Furthermore, patients regularly present with extremely heterogeneous pain profiles, particularly during unstable disease [4]. It is a challenge to describe individual patients using a common language due to this heterogeneity and complexity. Thus, clearly, a defined classification system is needed [25].

The multidimensionality of the cancer pain experience is characterized by fluctuations in pain intensity and variable responses to treatment, along with the challenge of disease progression and existential suffering. Although animal experiments are important for increased understanding of mechanisms of nociception and drug effects, extrapolation of data from animals to patients experiencing cancer pain requires caution. Furthermore, data extrapolated from healthy volunteers, from studies in acute or chronic pain, or from animal research are not proxies for clinical cancer pain (Table I). Even good pharmacological studies in cancer pain often have limitations because they are frequently based on physiologically competent subjects in an early stage of their disease and contain numerous exclusion criteria.

## Inclusion Criteria and Recruitment of Patients

Any clinical trial requires a precise definition of which patients are eligible for inclusion. Researchers must also consider how many potentially eligible patients can be included in the trial within a reasonable time frame. The achievable accrual rate of patients is often less than half of what is estimated [12,13].

Studies often include patients who are in a more stable clinical condition than those who could potentially benefit from the new treatment regimens. Ideally, strategies should be designed to include a sample population that corresponds to patients clinically most likely to benefit

Table I
Features that differentiate cancer pain
from acute pain, chronic pain, and
pain in healthy volunteers or
laboratory animals

Fever, dizziness and nausea

Fear and anxiety

Previous pain experience

Psychosocial and existential problems

Symptoms from other organs

from the intervention. This goal is not always possible with cancer patients, however [26]. Significant organ dysfunction is a major exclusion criterion in most trials of analgesics. Thus, many patients who initially qualify for inclusion may have borderline renal or hepatic dysfunction that may worsen during the study, causing them to be withdrawn from the trial. This selective withdrawal process might limit the relevance of the results obtained when applied to patients with advanced cancer. Decisions regarding the level of clinical dysfunction at which patients are still eligible for participation in clinical trials rely on the clinical judgment of researchers and represent a source of bias.

Participation in a specific drug trial excludes the patient from taking part in any other parallel investigational drug trial. In larger university centers, this limitation may restrict the potential number of patients available for a particular cancer pain study.

## Selection Bias and Confounding

Two of the major methodological challenges in observational research are selection bias and confounding, which can contribute to underestimation or overestimation of the actual efficacy of an intervention. Selection bias may be particularly problematic in observational studies of interventions or treatment when eligibility criteria limit entry into the intervention [39]. Another type of selection bias is the "healthy volunteers bias" that occurs when those who participate in research or who remain in longitudinal studies are general healthier than those who do not. Three general approaches are used to control for confounding in observation studies: the multivariate regression model, propensity scores, and instrumental variables [39]. These approaches can increase the validity of studies and the precision of estimates of treatment. The major limitations of both methods is that they can only account for what can be accurately measured—they have no direct influence on controlling the bias due to unmeasured confounders, except to the extent that those factors are highly correlated with measured characteristics. However, these methods can reduce the error associated with measured characteristics and increase the methodological rigor in observational studies [39]. In general, better methods are clearly needed to improve patient selection.

## Patient Withdrawal

Many patients entering clinical trials are likely to suffer physical or cognitive deterioration, and some may die during the trial. Loss to follow-up is a significant reason for exclusion after randomization. At times, participants lost to follow-up could still be included in the analysis if outcome information could be obtained from another source. Such opportunities, however, seldom arise. In any case, exclusions, withdrawals, and losses to follow-up should always be reported in clinical studies [33].

There are three general analytic approaches in clinical trials: analysis as randomized (referred to as intention-to-treat analysis, or ITT), compliers-only analysis (in which only those patients randomized to a treatment arm who completed the trial and complied with treatment are analyzed), and as-treated analysis (in which those who received a given treatment are counted, whether or not the patient was initially assigned to that treatment) [18]. ITT is the gold standard because it is the only analysis that preserves randomization. Withdrawals during the course of a trial can jeopardize the scientific integrity of the trial if ITT is not the primary form of analysis.

The problem of missing outcome data will always arise and needs to be specifically handled. Various methods may be used to estimate the missing responses, such as carrying forward the last observed response, or assuming that all missing responses were constant, for example by setting pain intensity to baseline. Incomplete outcome data in a randomized controlled trial (RCT) is likely to bias the final study results if the reasons for unavailability of patient data are associated with the outcome of interest [1].

## Polypharmacy: A Problem for Cancer Pain Trials

A large number of cancer pain patients, in addition to taking the trial drug, are taking other analgesics and adjuvant drugs in order to control distressing symptoms or to combat the disease itself [26]. This practice of polypharmacy may confound the interpretation of clinical trials. A study of 676 patients with advanced cancer found widespread use of adjuvant drugs for symptom control; the drugs most frequently used were major tranquilizers, sedatives, anxiolytics, antidepressants, anticonvulsants, and antiemetics [43]. The concomitant use of this heterogeneous group of drugs may affect the pharmacokinetics and pharmacodynamics of analgesics in general. The true influence of these drugs on the effects of opioids, however, may be difficult to determine. Beside drug interactions, the adverse effects of adjuvant drugs may confound the adverse effects of the trial drug, such as by causing sedation or confusion [26].

# Study Size, Duration, and Outcome

## Outcome Measures

To demonstrate the benefits of treatment, investigators must determine the appropriate endpoints for establishing both the statistical and the clinical significance level of the effects of treatment. It is important, however, to acknowledge that there is disagreement concerning which measures constitute the optimal outcome measures for clinical pain trials [16]. There is a lack of standardized and comprehensive outcome measures for pain trial that have adequate comparative information for relevant samples, that can be used across a variety of research applications, and that allow investigators to combine or compare groups with different demographic or disease characteristics [41]. Too often pain measurement tools are not appropriately used in the trial, or at least their use is not described with sufficient accuracy in the trial methods [5].

In a systematic evidence report on management of cancer pain, which included 218 relevant trials, 125 distinctly different pain outcomes were assessed [7]. A literature review on pain assessment tools in palliative care identified 80 tools that assessed pain using one or more items, of which 48 were categorized as specific pain assessments rather than general symptom or quality-of-life assessment tools [22].

Data from analgesic studies are often difficult to interpret because the clinical importance of the results is not obvious. Small and unimportant differences can achieve statistical significance in large trials and still be of no clinical importance for patients. On the other hand, in a number of analgesic studies, the percentage reduction in pain intensity, ranging from 30% to 50%, has been used to define a positive outcome [16,37]. However, setting the bar too high may result in an underestimation of efficacy. The Initiative on Methods, Measurements, and Pain Assessment in Clinical Trials (IMMPACT) has recommended that six core outcome domains should be considered when designing chronic pain clinical trials [15]. However, as pointed out by McQuay [30], these recommendations are based on opinion rather than evidence.

Tools for cancer pain assessment can be divided into two main categories: intensity scales and questionnaires intended to capture the multidimensionality of cancer pain. The most common intensity scales used are the visual analogue scales (VAS), numerical rating scales (NRS), and verbal categorical rating scales (VRS) [31]. For acute pain, NRS and VAS tools may demonstrate higher sensitivity in detecting differences in outcomes of pain intensity than VRS [3]. However, generally most of the intensity scales seem to be equally effective for pain rating [23]. Generally, pain intensity ratings (from baseline to postmedication assessment) are correlated with changes in pain relief rating, but significant differences may still exist, and therefore the use of both pain intensity and pain relief scales is recommended in analgesic trials [26]. Since we cannot rely on pain intensity or pain relief measures alone to evaluate treatment efficacy, a series of currently validated assessment instruments are available for the multidimensional evaluation of cancer pain. In some scenarios, self-reports of pain will be difficult, for instance in the cognitively impaired or in the elderly, and alternatives, such as observation of behavior or assessment of physiological variables, will need to be considered.

A global question, such as "What is your overall satisfaction with the treatment?" is an important question at the end of the study because it gives the patient an opportunity to evaluate the overall effects, both positive (analgesia, better sleep, etc), and negative (side effects), as well as the comfort and feasibility of the method employed. A patient with good analgesia but unacceptable side effects may choose to give a low score on the global assessment [40].

The increasing complexity of RCTs and the practice of obtaining a wide variety of measurements from study participants have made the consideration of multiple endpoints a critically important issue in the design, analysis, and interpretation of clinical trials [42].

## Size and Duration of Study

The sample size for a trial needs to be sufficiently large to ensure that erroneous results are not obtained by chance, and conversely, small enough to be efficient and to expose the minimum number of subjects to risk. Strict inclusion criteria are important, but they should not be so restrictive that enrollment is compromised and the findings applicable only to a small subset of the population. Large multicenter trials may be preferable and provide larger groups of study patients, although this may lead to inflation in inclusion criteria and violation of protocol adherence due to the increased number of investigators [26].

A review of 338 trials published in major journals found that 275 trials reported "negative" results, but only 16% of these "negative" trials recruited a sufficient sample size to detect a 25% relative difference between groups [32]. Underpowered studies have also been shown to overestimate treatment effect by approximately 30% [36]. Sample size calculations based on pilot results are generally more reliable than results based on results in the literature. Single small trials are unlikely to be correct. If we want to be sure of getting correct and relevant results in clinical trials, it is imperative to include a larger number of patients. Credible estimates of clinical efficacy are only likely to come from large trials or from pooling multiple trials of conventional (small) size [34].

Short, fixed periods of therapy are often satisfactory for phase II trials of short-term efficacy. However, for trials of more long-term effects, the duration of therapy may require a more complex definition that incorporates plans for dealing with side effects, dose modification, and patient withdrawal. Treatment periods should be long enough to ascertain that the patient has reached the maximal target response.

# Types of Study Design

## Randomized Controlled Trials

The RCT has become the gold standard for clinical investigations and provides the essential basic data required for evidence-based medicine. Nevertheless, a randomized placebo-controlled trial should only be used when there is genuine doubt concerning the efficacy of the treatments and when adequate precautions have been taken to secure that patients allocated to the placebo group do not experience clinically significant reduction in quality of care [26].

RCTs can mitigate the scientific, but not the ethical concerns, raised by subjecting patients to a placebo treatment. Furthermore, the rigid inclusion/exclusion criteria in the RCT design, while effective in reducing bias, severely limit the "real-world" applicability of the results. The stringent restrictions regarding concomitant medications and fixed treatment strategies bear only a modest resemblance to the ways in which patients are treated in actual practice [19]. RCTs generally include intensive medical follow-up in terms of number of medical visits, and/or type of tests, and monitoring events, which is usually not possible in routine clinical care.

The difficulties in conducting RCTs in palliative care include patient recruitment (including acceptance of the patient's participation by the relatives), gatekeeping by physicians, small sample sizes, and limited survival times.

RCTs can be impossible to conduct due to the challenges inherent in recruiting seriously ill participants, and they may not be ethically appropriate in the absence of clinical equipoise (i.e., an even balance of positive and negative clinical effects for participants) [6,39]. However, White and coworkers have shown that patients with advanced cancer are interested in participating in RCTs that focus on symptom control [44]. A directory of randomization services has been made available by Bland [2a].

## Parallel Study Designs

In a parallel study, subjects from different groups are given either the investigational drug or the comparator drug or placebo. The most commonly used design, it has the advantage of simplicity in that a single treatment or combination of treatments is given to each group with a fixed number of patients. Parallel designs are less dependent on anticipation of disease progression, and thus they are more appropriate than crossover designs when the patient's condition is expected to change over time. Parallel designs should also be favored when there is a possibility of significant carryover effects [26]. However, a large number of patients may be needed to obtain the desired statistical power. In general, parallel-group trials allow for longer follow-up with regular assessment of outcomes. Even if the duration of a parallel study is longer compared to that of a crossover study, the dropout rate may be lower [24]. In a parallel-group trial, precision may be increased when the within-subject variance is lower than that of the between-subject variance and baseline measurements are employed to provide within-subject data [26]. Table II indicates when to consider the standard parallel study design.

Table II
When to consider the standard parallel study design

| |
| --- |
| A long duration of treatment |
| A likelihood of significant carryover effects |
| A number of treatments to be compared |
| Easier patient recruitment versus the crossover design |

## Crossover Designs

In a crossover study each patient receives both drugs to be compared (usually in a random sequence). Crossover designs are used to increase the sensitivity of a study by using each patient as his or her own control [26]. This feature increases validity and reduces the sample size required compared with a parallel study design. A crossover design requires a chronic and stable condition that reverts to its original state with discontinuation of treatment. Cancer patients, however, will in most cases experience disease progression and deterioration of physical function. Therefore, crossover designs are preferred in studies of relatively short duration in order to reduce the number of withdrawals. Crossover trial designs are recommended when the therapeutic effects of the drug cease soon after it is discontinued (during the "washout" period). A difference between treatments may either be the result of a carryover effect of one treatment into the next period, or may indicate a general time effect, known as an "order" effect. During the washout period it is an obvious requirement that the design allows patients to receive adequate rescue medication [26]. Addition of other treatment sequences or a third treatment period may offer unbiased estimates of treatment effects even in the presence of various types of carryover effects. Crossover designs might be acceptable in particular circumstances, such as in the case of rare diseases, when it is difficult to recruit a sufficient number of subjects for a parallel-group study. Table III indicates when to consider the crossover study design.

Table III
When to consider a crossover trial

| |
|---|
| Carryover effects are limited. |
| Within-subject variation is restricted. |
| An extension of the treatment period does not alter the difference between the treatment effects. |
| Prolongation of the trial will result in a large number of dropouts. |
| There are difficulties in obtaining baseline measurements. |

## Enriched-Enrollment Design

Sometimes, an enriched-enrollment procedure is indicated to exclude nonresponders whose inclusion would make the study insensitive. Enriched enrollment means that only subjects who respond to the test treatment, or a similar treatment, enter the study. If the patient receives the test treatment in an open enrichment phase, the active treatment in the blinded study phase is more easily detected by the patient. Enriched enrollment into a trial, for example by including or excluding subjects who have or have not responded to a certain drug in the past, can present problems with interpretation (Table IV). Active enriched-enrollment policies are to be discouraged as they can skew the evidence base [36].

## Parallel Versus Crossover Designs

Investigators should carefully weigh the advantages and disadvantages of crossover versus parallel study designs to ensure validity without compromising effectiveness. Although certain situations will demand preferences,

Table IV
Features of the enriched enrollment study design

| |
|---|
| A variant of the crossover design |
| Useful where only a restricted number of patients respond |
| Prior exposure may jeopardize the double-blind procedures |
| May result in spurious positive results |
| Can distort the evidence base |
| Must be fully justified and transparently reported |

both designs can at times be employed, as illustrated by Deschamps et al. [10] and Parris et al. [35], who conducted trials comparing immediate-release analgesics with their sustained-release counterparts. Despite the greater numbers of subjects that must be recruited to parallel-group studies, the advantages of such a design have made it the preferred option for most investigators. Neither conventional parallel-group nor crossover designs are efficient at elucidating adverse effect frequency or drug safety, mainly due to the relatively short duration of treatment and follow-up [36]. Parallel studies are usually preferred by regulatory agencies for pivotal trials of a new drug.

## Equivalence, Superiority, and Noninferiority Studies

Ideally, a new drug is compared with a placebo, with the aim of demonstrating its superiority over the placebo [28]. A common industry-initiated study design is the equivalence or noninferiority trial. There are reasons why placebo controls are preferable to active controls, not the least of which is the ability to distinguish an effective treatment from a less effective one. However, if a new treatment is considered to be equally effective compared to an established therapy, but perhaps less expensive or invasive, or a placebo control is considered unethical, then the new treatment needs to be compared to the "gold standard" and may be considered preferable if it is just as good as, but not necessarily better than, the established therapy [19].

Underlying the interpretation of any equivalence trial is the assumption that the standard therapy is effective under the study conditions. This is not necessarily true and may confound the validity of such trials. Assay sensitivity is not proven unless a third group is added—either a placebo, two different doses of the active comparator, or two active drugs with a known difference in efficacy [40].

## Alternative Study Designs

Although some argue that any intervention can be investigated using an RCT design, such a view ignores a number of serious obstacles in the real world [2]. Difficulties in performing RCTs should not, however, preclude the use of scientific approaches. We therefore need alternative trial designs when studying drugs for cancer pain (Table V).

Well-designed observational studies can have much in common with RCTs. Important features include the use of prospective data collection, intention-to-treat analysis, contemporaneous controls, well-defined inclusion/exclusion criteria, consideration of baseline susceptibility factors, and a "zero time" for baseline measurements [20]. Properly designed observational studies permit the performance of high-quality cohort and matched case-control studies. It is of interest that observational studies incorporating the design features recommended above did not overestimate treatment effects [9]. Large-scale, well-designed observational studies demonstrated less variability and less heterogeneity when compared with RCTs studying the same conditions [9].

Table V
Alternative study designs

| |
| --- |
| Observational studies |
| Prospective open-label studies |
| Mixed-methods research (qualitative research and RCTs) |
| Fast-track research |
| Phase IV studies |
| Registry studies |

## Fast-Track Trials

Arguments against using the RCT design include the reluctance of physicians to have their patients enroll in trials in which one treatment is in opposition to their own beliefs and practice, and the ethics of denying patients treatment. One alternative that has been suggested is the fast-track trial (also known as the delayed- or deferred-intervention trial or waiting-list trial). In such trials patients are not denied access to the intervention under study, but they are randomized to either receive the intervention more quickly than they would normally have done (the fast-track group) or to receive it after a period on a waiting list (control group). Such trials have the statistical strength of the RCT but may be more acceptable to patients and physicians [17]. Although more commonly used in behavioral intervention studies, this trial design has been used to evaluate health care interventions [8].

## Phase IV Studies

Postmarketing research, postmarketing surveillance, and pharmacovigilance studies are phase IV studies. The intention is to rate the drug's effectiveness, i.e., how the product behaves in the real world, rather than their efficacy under "experimental" conditions. These studies have to some extent become misunderstood and have taken on negative connotations that have led some experts to question their validity [19]. However, these studies are definitely of importance because they can determine a new product's long-term analgesic effects and side effects, as well as patterns of physician prescribing and patient drug utilization [11,19].

# Placebo Treatment

In clinical trials, placebo effects should be balanced between groups in order to demonstrate the specific effect of the intervention. However, a placebo cannot be used if there is evidence that withholding standard treatment would be detrimental to the patient. Although it would be unethical to withhold an active analgesic for a prolonged period, administration may be delayed for a short interval, such as in postoperative pain, when the patient has immediate access to rescue medication, administered either by a nurse or via a patient-controlled device. If pain relief is not achieved, a more potent rescue treatment must be given. Thus, arguments for using a placebo in such a situation may be justified, providing the patient has given informed consent and rescue medication is available on request [26,38]. Some would argue that the use of placebo should be avoided in trials if a relevant reference drug is available. The reference drug should have a recognized evidence base for use in cancer pain, its efficacy should have been well documented, and it should be a clinically relevant comparator drug. It is a paradox, then, that controlled trials comparing morphine to placebo in cancer pain are in fact, lacking. Use of comparators with a higher analgesic efficacy than placebo will lead to fewer unintended episodes of breakthrough pain in the trial. Data from "head-to-head" active comparator-controlled trials are probably more meaningful for clinical management of pain, but unfortunately they may require very large-scale studies, unless noninferiority or equivalence trial designs are used. Using an active control is based on the assumption that the active control has been tested against placebo and found to be effective. A problem arises when the active control has not been externally validated. If this is the case, the finding that both treatments are equivalent may mean that they are equally effective, or alternatively equally ineffective. In such a situation the inclusion of a placebo control is necessary to ensure correct interpretation of the results. If the use of a placebo group is not justifiable, an alternative approach would be to use a second dose level of the standard analgesic.

The challenges associated with the use of placebo in analgesic studies have been thoroughly addressed by Max [29]. According to the World Medical Association, "The use of placebo, or no treatment, is acceptable in studies where no current proven intervention exists; or Where for compelling and scientifically sound methodological reasons the use of placebo is necessary to determine the efficacy or safety of an intervention and the patients who receive placebo or no treatment will not be subject to any risk of serious or irreversible harm. Extreme care must be taken to avoid abuse of this option." [45].

# Rescue Medication

To study the patient's perception of pain relief, the use of an additional rescue medication is a clinically appropriate and easily measured outcome. However, this approach can only be used when the study medication has a relatively fast and consistent onset and a second effective treatment is available to be used as a rescue analgesic. This option is not usually feasible except in experimental acute pain models. Instead, changes in pain scores are used as surrogate measures to assess the patient's improvement [16].

Providing patients with access to rescue analgesics makes it easier to include a placebo group in treatment efficacy studies, because patients not obtaining adequate pain relief are provided with an analgesic. However, administration of rescue treatment complicates the interpretation of differences in pain ratings between patients taking placebo or active treatment because of the reduction in pain expected to occur in patients receiving rescue treatment. The use of rescue medication is affected by both patient and provider beliefs. Patients use rescue medications to achieve varying levels of pain relief, but also for other reasons, including improving sleep or reducing anxiety, preventing increased pain resulting from physical activity, and treating pain that may be unrelated to the clinical trial [15]. Furthermore, the rescue drug (e.g., morphine) may relieve one component of the pain (e.g., nociceptive pain), but not another (e.g., neuropathic pain). Despite the complex issues involved in the interpretation of rescue medication usage in a clinical trial, patients in a placebo group are generally expected to take more rescue medication than patients taking an investigational drug. When considered together with pain intensity ratings, the consumption of rescue medication may therefore provide an important supplemental measure of the efficacy of the treatment being evaluated [15].

# Conclusion

Cancer pain remains a problem despite immense efforts aimed at improving treatment through educational campaigns, implementation of guidelines and treatment algorithms, and intense research efforts. Why have we not succeeded? Perhaps we need to consider the pertinent question: Is pain in cancer patients different from noncancer pain? There are specific pathophysiological changes in cancer patients that could explain some of the differences, such as pain due to gradual compression of nerves by tumors, chemotherapeutic agent-induced neuropathy, or release of specific cytokines from bone metastases. However, the multidimensional nature of the pain experience, including fluctuations in pain intensity and variable responses to treatment, is probably more important, along with the challenge of disease progression and existential suffering. Therefore, data extrapolated from acute pain, chronic pain, or animal research are not always representative of clinical cancer pain. Moreover, good-quality controlled trials are especially difficult to conduct in patients who are in the terminal phase of cancer [27].

Unfortunately, descriptions of cancer pain patients enrolled in clinical studies are not standardized. Homogeneous, rigorous, and sound guidelines for pain measurement, data collection, and analysis are necessary in order to improve the quality of the information provided by clinical pain trials in general [5,14]. In order to improve the quality of future pharmacological trials, in particular cancer pain trials, an international, thoroughly validated, and consensus-based classification tool is needed that has the potential to become a standard for cancer pain classification [21].

# References

[1] Akl EA, Briel M, You JJ, Lamontagne F, Gangji A, Cukierman-Yaffe T, Alshurafa M, Sun X, Nerenberg KA, Johnston BC, et al. LOST to follow-up information in trials (LOST-IT): a protocol on the potential impact. Trials 2009;10:40.

[2] Black N. Why we need observational studies to evaluate the effectiveness of health care. BMJ 1996;312:1215–8.

[2a] Bland M. Directory of randomisation software and services. Available at: http://www-users.york.ac.uk/~mb55/guide/randsery.htm.

[3] Breivik EK, Bjornsson GA, Skovlund E. A comparison of pain rating scales by sampling from clinical trial data. Clin J Pain 2000;16:22–8.

[4] Bruera E, Kim HN. Cancer pain. JAMA 2003;290:2476–9.

[5] Caraceni A, Brunelli C, Martini C, Zecca E, De Conno F. Cancer pain assessment in clinical trials. A review of the literature (1999–2002). J Pain Symptom Manage 2005;29:507–19.

[6] Carlson MD, Morrison RS. User's guide to research in palliative care: why is a new series needed? J Palliat Med 2008;11:1258–61.

[7] Carr DB, Goudas LC, Balk EM, Bloch R, Ioannidis JPA, Lau J. Evidence report on the treatment of pain in cancer patients. J Natl Cancer Inst Monogr 2004;2004:23–31.

[8] Booth S, Farquhar MC. Trial of a breathlessness intervention service for intractable breathlessness. Available at: www.clinicaltrials.gov; NCT00678405.

[9] Concato J, Shah N, Horwitz RI. Randomized, controlled trials, observational studies, and the hierarchy of research designs. N Engl J Med 2000;342:1887–92.

[10] Deschamps M, Band PR, Hislop TG, Rusthoven J, Iscoe N, Warr D. The evaluation of analgesic effects in cancer patients as exemplified by a double-blind, crossover study of immediate-release versus controlled-release morphine. J Pain Symptom Manage 1992;7:384–92.

[11] Dieppe PA, Ebrahim S, Martin RM, Jüni P. Lessons from the withdrawal of rofecoxib. BMJ 2004;329:867–8.

[12] Dugas M, Amler S, Lange M, Gerss J, Breil B, Köpcke W. Estimation of patient accrual rates in clinical trials based on routine data from hospital information systems. Methods Inf Med 2009;48:263–6.

[13] Dugas M, Lange M, Berdel WE, Müller-Tidow C. Workflow to improve patient recruitment for clinical trials within hospital information systems: a case-study. Trials 2008;9:2.

[14] Dworkin RH, Nagasako EM, Hetzel RD. Assessment of pain and pain-related quality of life in clinical trials. In: Turk D, Melzack R, editors. Handbook of pain assessment, 2nd ed. New York: Guilford Press, 2001. p 659–92.

[15] Dworkin RH, Turk DC, Farrar JT, Haythornthwaite JA, Jensen MP, Katz NP, Kerns RD, Stucki G, Allen RR, Bellamy N, et al. Core outcome measures for chronic pain clinical trials: IMMPACT recommendations. Pain 2005;113:9–19.

[16] Farrar JT, Portenoy RK, Berlin JA, Kinman JL, Strom BL. Defining the clinically important difference in pain outcome measures. Pain 2000;88:287–94.

[17] Farquhar M, Higginson IJ, Booth S. Fast-track trials in palliative care: an alternative randomized controlled trial design. J Palliat Med 2009;12:213.

[18] Glasser SP, Howard G. Clinical trial design issues: at least 10 things you should look for in clinical trials. J Clin Pharmacol 2006;46:1106–15.

[19] Glasser SP, Salas M, Delzell E. Importance and challenges of studying marketed drugs: what is a Phase IV study? Common clinical research designs, registries and self-reporting systems. J Clin Pharmacol 2007;47:1074–86.

[20] Hartrick CT. Quality assessment in clinical trials: considerations for outcomes research in interventional pain medicine. Pain Pract 2008;8:433–8.

[21] Hjermstad MJ, Gibbins J, Haugen DF, Caraceni A, Loge JH, Kaasa S; European Palliative Care Research Collaborative. Pain assessment tools in palliative care: an urgent need for consensus. Palliat Med 2008;22:895–903.

[22] Hølen JC, Hjermstad MJ, Loge JH, Fayers PM, Caraceni A, De Conno F, Forbes K, Fürst CJ, Radbruch L, Kaasa S. Pain assessment tools: is the content appropriate for use in palliative care? J Pain Symptom Manage 2006;32:567–80.

[23] Jensen MP, Chen C, Brugger AM. Postsurgical pain outcome assessment. Pain 2002;99:101–9.

[24] Kerr IG. Clinical trials to study pain in patients with advanced cancer: practical difficulties. Anticancer Drugs 1995;6(Suppl 3):18–28.

[25] Knudsen AK, Aass N, Fainsinger R, Caraceni A, Klepstad P, Jordhøy M, Hjermstad MJ, Kaasa S. Classification of pain in cancer patients: a systematic literature review. Palliat Med 2009;23:295–308.

[26] Kongsgaard UE, Werner MU. Clinical trials: cancer pain. In: Breivik H, Campell W, Nicolas MK, editors. Clinical pain management: practice and procedures, 2nd ed. London: Hodder Arnold; 2008. p. 538–51.

[27] Kongsgaard UE, Werner MU. Evidence-based medicine works best when there is evidence: challenges in palliative medicine when randomized controlled trials are not possible. J Pain Palliat Care Pharmacother 2009;23:48–50.

[28] Max MB. The design of clinical trials of pain treatment. In: Max MB, Lynn J. An interactive textbook. Available at: http://symptomresearch.nih.gov/chapter_1/index.htm.

[29] Max M. Clinical trials of pain treatment. Available at: http://symptomresearch.nih.gov/chapter_1/index/htm.

[30] McQuay H. Consensus on outcome measure for chronic pain trials. Pain 2005;113:1–2.

[31] Melzack R, Katz J: Pain assessment in adult patients. In: McMahon SB, Koltzenburg M, editors. Wall and Melzack's textbook of pain, 5th ed. Philadelphia: Elsevier Churchill Livingstone; 2006. p. 291–304.

[32] Moher D, Dulberg CS, Wells GA. Statistical power, sample size, and their reporting in randomized controlled trials. JAMA 1994; 272:122–4.

[33] Moher D, Schulz KF, Altman DG. The CONSORT statement: revised recommendations for improving the quality of reports of parallel-group randomized trials. Ann Intern Med 2001;134:657–62.

[34] Moore RA, Gavaghan D, Tramèr MR, Collins SL, McQuay HJ. Size is everything: large amounts of information are needed to overcome random effects in estimating direction and magnitude of treatment effects. Pain 1998;78:209–16.

[35] Parris WC, Johnson BW Jr, Croghan MK, Moore MR, Khojasteh A, Reder RF, Kaiko RF, Buckley BJ. The use of controlled-release oxycodone for the treatment of chronic cancer pain: a randomized, double-blind study. J Pain Symptom Manage 1998;16:205–11.

[36] Rice ASC. Clinical trials: neuropathic pain. In: Breivik H, Campell W, Nicolas MK, editors. Clinical pain management: practice and procedures, 2nd ed. London: Hodder Arnold; 2008. p. 552–65.

[37] Rowbotham MC. What is a "clinically meaningful" reduction in pain? Pain 2001;94:131–2.

[38] Stambaugh JE Jr, McAdams J. Comparison of intramuscular dezocine with butorphanol and placebo in chronic cancer pain: a method to evaluate analgesia after both single and repeated doses. Clin Pharmacol Ther 1987;42:210–9.

[39] Starks H, Diehr P, Curtis JR. The challenge of selection bias and confounding in palliative care research. J Palliat Med 2009;12:181–7.

[40] Stubhaug A, Breivik H. Clinical trials: acute and chronic pain. In: Breivik H, Campell W, Nicolas MK, editors. Clinical pain management: practice and procedures, 2nd ed. London: Hodder Arnold; 2008. p. 514–28.

[41] Turk DC, Dworkin RH, Burke LB, Gershon R, Rothman M, Scott J, Allen RR, Atkinson JH, Chandler J, Cleeland C, et al. Developing patient-reported outcome measures for pain clinical trials: IMMPACT recommendations. Pain 2006;125:208–15.

[42]  Turk DC, Dworkin RH, McDermott MP, Bellamy N, Burke LB, Chandler JM, Cleeland CS, Cow-
      an P, Dimitrova R, Farrar JT, et al. Analyzing multiple endpoints in clinical trials of pain treat-
      ment: IMMPACT recommendations. Pain 2008;139:485–93.
[43]  Walsh TD. Adjuvant analgesic therapy in cancer pain. In: Foley KM, Bonica JJ, Ventafridda V,
      editors. Second International Congress on Cancer Pain; Advances in pain research and therapy,
      Vol. 16. New York: Raven Press; 1990. p. 155–69.
[44]  White CD, Hardy JR, Gilshenan KS, Charles MA, Pinkerton CR. Randomised controlled trials of
      palliative care: a survey of the views of advanced cancer patients and their relatives. Eur J Cancer
      2008;163:341–4.
[45]  World Medical Association. Declaration of Helsinki. Ethical principles for medical research
      involving human subjects. C. Additional principles for medical research for medical research
      combined with medical care. Available at: http://www.wma.net/en/30publications/10policies/
      b3/17c.pdf.

***Correspondence to:*** Ulf E. Kongsgaard, MD, PhD, Department of Anesthesia, The Norwegian Radium Hospital, Montebello, 0310 Oslo, Norway. Email:
u.e.kongsgaard@klinmed.uio.no.

# Methodological Issues in Cancer Pain: Nonpharmacological Trials

### Michael I. Bennett

*International Observatory on End of Life Care, Lancaster University,*
*Lancaster, United Kingdom*

Nonpharmacological interventions for cancer pain are widely used in clinical practice, even though some practitioners may not recognize them as true interventions. However, establishing reliable evidence of effectiveness can be challenging when attempting to design or interpret studies of nonpharmacological interventions. This chapter will describe some of the more important and unique methodological issues for clinical trials of nonpharmacological interventions.

# Nonpharmacological Interventions in Practice

## Defining a Nonpharmacological Intervention

A fundamental aspect of researching nonpharmacological interventions is to define what this term means. An intervention is defined as "coming between" or "the act of intervening" [14]. Of course, "nonpharmacological" means anything that is not a pharmacological intervention, but it always seems harder to define (and therefore understand) something by explaining what it is not rather than by explaining what it is. These definitions tell

*Cancer Pain: From Molecules to Suffering*
edited by Judith A. Paice, Rae F. Bell, Eija A. Kalso, and Olaitan A. Soyannwo
IASP Press, Seattle, © 2010

us that we are examining some action or behavior that is not drug based and that "comes between" the pathophysiological mechanism of the cancer pain and the patient's perception of that pain.

Using this definition, nonpharmacological interventions are broad ranging and can be loosely grouped as oriented toward physical, psychological, or clinical process aspects of care; some examples are listed in Table I, which is not intended to be an exhaustive list of every type of intervention. There may also be a sociological or cultural orientation; pharmacological interventions are usually associated with physicians, whereas nonpharmacological interventions are usually associated with nursing practice and physical therapy [11]. This division seems unhelpful, especially if it results in nonpharmacological interventions being perceived as less valuable or less effective than pharmacological treatment.

Table I
Examples of nonpharmacological interventions used
in cancer pain management

| Category | Examples |
|---|---|
| Physical | Acupuncture |
| | Transcutaneous electrical nerve stimulation (TENS) |
| | Healing touch and massage |
| | Occupational therapy |
| | Music and art therapy |
| Psychological | Hypnosis |
| | Relaxation |
| | Cognitive-behavioral therapy |
| Clinical process | Pain assessment |
| | Physician's advice and communication about pain |
| | Education (for patients, professionals, family caregivers) |

## Studies of Nonpharmacological Interventions in Cancer Pain

Clinical trials of nonpharmacological interventions are easily found in the literature, but these interventions are probably overlooked as part of the management pathway for a patient with cancer pain. Health care professionals who manage cancer patients, and those in under- or postgraduate training programs, can usually describe their approaches to cancer pain as being based on the World Health Organization's analgesic ladder [20], combined with adjuvant analgesia for incident bone pain or neuropathic pain. These professionals are probably less likely to acknowledge the importance of evidence-based nonpharmacological interventions, or to consciously include them in their routine practice.

For example, from the existing literature we know that patient satisfaction with pain management is significantly associated with hearing a physician state the importance of pain management, receiving instructions for managing pain at home and dealing with side effects, and having their fears about addiction allayed [6,9]. Asking patients to self-assess their pain and their pain treatment, reviewing these data prior to consultation, discussing this information during the consultation significantly improves pain outcomes [17]. Actively using self-reported health-related quality-of-life measures has similar effects on quality of life for patients [18]. Use of specific prescribing guidelines for cancer pain results in significant benefits in pain intensity for patients compared to control groups [4,7]. However, overcoming physician barriers is important [10]; these barriers relate to technical aspects (e.g., inadequate prescription) as well as the context of the interaction with patients [15].

# Mechanisms of Action

## Pharmacological Versus Nonpharmacological Interventions

Drug-based or pharmacological interventions often have a precise and well-defined mechanism of action derived from a detailed knowledge of a particular pathophysiological mechanism involved in pain transmission, as well as an understanding of the pharmacodynamics and pharmacokinetics of the drug. The drug is designed to intervene at a specific point in the pain mechanism, perhaps by inhibiting an enzyme, or by acting as an agonist or antagonist at a specific receptor site. In clinical trials, drug-based interventions are usually given over several days or weeks, resulting in a continuous application. A useful analogy is that of a rifle continuously firing single bullets at a clear target (Fig. 1a).

In contrast, nonpharmacological interventions differ in two important respects. First, for many of these interventions, the mechanism of action is not fully understood, if at all. For example, it is not established whether acupuncture or massage affects some physiological mechanism (either in the peripheral or central nervous system) or has a psychological outcome (e.g., a reduction in anxiety or improved coping), or perhaps both. Many nonpharmacological interventions are centered on professional or patient behaviors, and so their mechanisms of action are often imprecise, multiple, and poorly defined. Second, these types of intervention are usually delivered as single or episodic applications, such as a "one-off" educational session for patients or professionals, or a series of weekly massage treatments. Therefore, the effect of the intervention is intermittent, and any benefits might be harder to identify. This effect would be analogous to a single firing of a pellet gun (Fig. 1b).

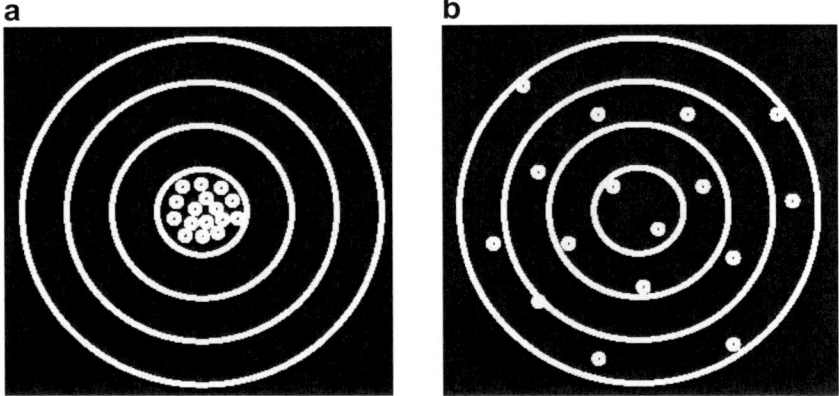

**Fig. 1.** Differences between pharmacological and nonpharmacological interventions. (a) Illustration of precise and repeated firing at a clear target from a rifle, as in a drug-based intervention. (b) Illustration of the more imprecise or dispersed firing of a single shotgun pellet, as in a nonpharmacological intervention.

## Complex Interventions

Nonpharmacological interventions are probably best regarded as complex interventions [5]. An intervention may be considered complex if it contains a combination of effects (sometimes known as bundled effects, discussed in more detail below), which act through known and unknown mechanisms. Complex interventions contain several interacting components, although the complexity may arise through several dimensions, such as the number of components within the experimental and control interventions, the number and difficulty of behaviors required by those delivering or receiving the intervention, the number of groups or organizational levels targeted by the intervention, and the number and variability of outcomes.

It is also relevant that within the context of cancer pain, complex interventions are also those that may consist of a relatively simple application within a complex biopsychosocial system. A perfect illustration of this complexity is applying an intervention to improve cancer pain in physically frail patients with advanced disease who are aware that they are facing death.

# Designing the Study

## The Intervention Arm

If we were to design a study for a drug-based intervention, we would probably already know what dose of drug was safe and in particular, the right dose and method of application to ensure that the drug would affect the pathophysiological mechanism that we want to target. In complex nonpharmacological interventions, however, it is not easy to determine the dose. For example, we might want to evaluate the effects of a massage treatment. If we can identify the mechanisms of action and understand the combined effects of these mechanisms (both physical and psychological), then we can determine whether to design the intervention arm as a single application or as multiple applications (with specified intervals). More usually, none of these aspects is really known or understood, and so the intervention (or its most important components) may be "underdosed."

Another determinant of "dose" is whether the intervention is labor intensive in its application. If an intervention is very therapist or operator dependent, then the availability or cost of such therapists may limit the number of applications or the number of patients in the intervention arm. For example, an educational intervention that requires a face-to-face hourlong session with an experienced practitioner, repeated at weekly intervals, may be financially or logistically challenging and so limit target sample size.

## The Control Arm

Establishing the appropriate dose and application of the intervention is not easy, but it is undoubtedly more challenging to do so for the control arm in these types of clinical trials. It is hard to select an appropriate control when the mechanism of action of the intervention arm is poorly understood.

This challenge is probably better understood when we consider the purpose of the control arm. When we study any intervention, the aim of the clinical trial is to distinguish the effect of the intervention (the specific effect) from the effect of other factors (the context effect). Sometimes, it is important to standardize the context effect, which is often called a placebo, rather than a comparison with usual care (a nonstandardized context effect, which is often the most poorly defined arm). The clinical trial would ideally demonstrate that while context effects may be associated with some improvement in outcomes (the placebo effect), the intervention is associated with significantly more improvement (the specific effect).

In clinical trials of nonpharmacological interventions, separation of specific effects from context effects is more difficult. For example, the effectiveness of an education program may depend on the content of the educational information (the specific effect) together with the experience and skill of the person delivering the education (the context effect) [1]. This reasoning of course assumes that the important component of this intervention is the educational information. But what if the specific effect is spending time with an experienced practitioner and the information provision is merely a context effect? Interventions of this type are then better described as "bundled effects" because it may not be possible to separate out the specific effect from the context effect. Better designed trials therefore compare usual care, a placebo control, and the intervention. They help to identify which context effects are most important in delivering the intervention, and indeed whether the context effects are just as effective, or even more effective, than the intervention itself.

Given these constraints, unless the specific effect of the intervention is understood, some control arms in trials of nonpharmacological interventions may not really standardize the context effects. For example, when simple touch (the control) was compared with massage from an experienced therapist (the intervention), significant improvements occurred in both arms of the study, with no difference over time between the two [13]. A usual care group was not included in this study, but we may conclude that the specific effects (i.e., the most important effects) of this intervention are probably simple touch combined with time and attention from a practitioner, and that there is no obvious additional benefit from specialized massage techniques (which was the presumed specific effect).

## Blinding

Blinding usually refers to keeping patients, investigators, and those collecting and analyzing clinical data unaware of the assigned treatment, so that they will not be influenced by that knowledge. Blinding is important because the expectations of both patients and investigators can influence findings—particularly in palliative care, where there is subjectivity in symptom assessment. Blinding is used to reduce this confounding.

The problem in nonpharmacological trials is that it is sometimes difficult to effectively blind the intervention and control arms. A good example is a clinical trial of transcutaneous electrical nerve stimulation (TENS), in which the control arm may consist of a device that has no electrical output [16]. It may be possible to convince the patient that the control device is active despite the absence of sensation, but the researcher still needs to distinguish between the devices. This aspect applies to a range of interventions such as educational interventions, acupuncture, and assessment procedures. In other words, a single-blind protocol (in which the patient does not know whether the treatment is active) may be possible, but double-blinding (in which neither the patient nor the researcher knows the difference) is almost impossible to achieve in nonpharmacological interventions, and this limitation may affect the validity of the design and interpretation of the findings.

## Crossover and Parallel Designs

When dealing with subjective outcomes such as pain, it is usually preferable to use a crossover design within a clinical trial so that patients can act as their own control. This design largely eliminates between-patient variation, and thus the validity and reliability of the trial are greater than for a parallel trial with the same number of patients. The corollary is that for any given level of validity, fewer patients are required in a crossover design than in a parallel design, which is attractive in a population of patients who are potentially frail, unwell, and hard to recruit.

There are problems with a crossover design, however, which can be magnified in a palliative care context. Because patients are required to cross over to a different treatment, the duration of the trial is often longer than that of a similar trial with a parallel design. Increased trial duration introduces two difficulties. First, the patient's condition or symptom may undergo natural fluctuations such that by the time of the second treatment arm, the symptoms are naturally better or worse, regardless of the arm to which the patient is currently allocated. For trials of nonpharmacological interventions, which are mostly applied intermittently (as opposed to being applied continuously, such as a drug intervention), these fluctuations can make data analysis and interpretation difficult. The second problem is that palliative care patients are, by definition, ill with advanced disease, and their health can deteriorate without warning. Patients may drop out of the trial because they are too ill to continue, or they may die unexpectedly. In trials performed in palliative care, the number of dropouts at the end of the study may be large enough to invalidate the results.

Further complications of crossover designs in nonpharmacological clinical trials include "order" or "carry-over" effects. These effects refer to the treatment effects from the first study arm on the dependent variable persisting into, and influencing, the second arm. For example, it is difficult to reverse the effect of an educational intervention if it is delivered in the first arm before the patient crosses to a control arm, and therefore a parallel design would be best for this kind of trial. Another consequence is that a crossover trial may undermine blinding, for example between active and sham TENS, in which patients quickly realize which is the active treatment when they feel a tingling sensation [2].

## Outcome Measures

Important outcomes in any pain clinical trial include pain and pain relief, and so outcome measures need to assess these intended effects [8]. However, in nonpharmacological trials, where the mechanism of action is less clearly defined, it is also important to measure additional outcomes that might help to explain the effects, and to identify other benefits. These outcomes might include coping ability, anxiety, caregiver distress, or medication adherence.

Just as critical as choosing the outcomes measures is choosing who measures the outcomes. Although blinding of the allocated intervention might be difficult (for both therapist and subject), it is possible to use a blind assessor. It is clearly biased for the person applying the treatment to also assess the outcomes in a controlled trial, but it happens [13].

An additional challenge is to determine when to measure the outcomes. Because of the intermittent or sometimes single application of the intervention, the outcomes might need to be measured immediately (e.g., for massage therapy), in the short term (e.g., for acupuncture), or in the medium to long term (e.g., for educational interventions). Clearly, the timing of assessment will be determined by the number of applications and by the expected duration of effect, provided that the mechanism is understood.

# Performing the Study

## Recruitment

Nonpharmacological interventions can be perceived as less harmful than pharmacological interventions, and so it is easy to assume that recruitment to trials of the former would be easier. There is some support for this assumption. White et al. [19] surveyed palliative care professional staff about referring patients to randomized controlled trials of various interventions. They found that the majority of staff would refer patients to nonpharmacological studies but were less willing to refer them to pharmacological trials because of possible adverse effects from the intervention.

In contrast, other authors have found that some patients view some nonpharmacological interventions with scepticism or lack of interest and so decline to take part in trials [12]. This finding highlights the importance of addressing the credibility of nonpharmacological interventions because most patients with cancer pain will usually consider drug treatment more orthodox.

## Fidelity

Treatment fidelity refers to the degree to which the trial protocol was administered as intended, and it is central to interpreting and translating research into practice. Although this issue arises in pharmacological trials—all patients must receive the right dose of drug for the same duration, and so on—it is probably more important in nonpharmacological trials because of the complex nature of the interventions.

For example, did an experienced practitioner or therapist deliver the intervention but a less skilled nurse deliver the control "treatment"? Did patients reveal to the blind assessor the fact that they experienced tingling feelings during the first application of TENS but not the second, and so reveal the allocation? Better-quality trials report aspects of fidelity such as time spent by the therapist in each arm and assessments of the success of blinding. For example, assessors may ask patients whether they think they received a placebo, and in which part of the study (in the case of crossover designs).

## Interpreting the Data

Effect sizes in nonpharmacological trials (and in many pharmacological trials) are often modest, and so large sample sizes are needed to demonstrate these effects with any reliability. If the sample size is limited by constraints (discussed under "The Intervention Arm" above), then there is a high chance that the trial may be underpowered. This is particularly likely when there are no data on which to base a power calculation before the trial is conducted.

Critics of nonpharmacological trials might think that the expectation of a positive effect is greater in nonpharmacological studies. In other words, there is a greater context effect or more placebo response. There are no data from cancer pain trials to determine this effect, but an analysis of pharmacological and nonpharmacological interventions in the treatment of major depression suggests that the placebo response is large in both types of intervention, with no significant difference between types [3].

# Some Potential Solutions

## Qualitative Interviews

Developing and testing a reliable nonpharmacological intervention for cancer pain can be improved, first by modeling the intervention (working out what to include), and second by gaining some insights into what benefits are important to measure. These improvements can be made using qualitative interviews or focus groups with patients and professionals to identify when and where it might be best to apply an educational intervention or a clinical guideline, and in what form. This process may help to identify benefits perceived by patients that are worth measuring, and it can generate hypotheses on the mechanism of action of the interventions. Feedback from patients and staff can also confirm the acceptability (or unacceptability) of any intervention.

### Feasibility Studies

Feasibility or pilot studies test trial methodology and are not designed to formally assess the effectiveness of the intervention. In trials of nonpharmacological interventions, it is crucial to understand the mechanism of action (as far as possible) before attempting a formal evaluation. Feasibility studies can help by revealing if the intervention is acceptable, whether it is possible to blind the intervention, what outcome measures are most appropriate, and whether changes occur in the intended domains; for example, does pain intensity decrease, or does coping improve and anxiety decrease instead?

## Summary

Nonpharmacological interventions are best regarded as complex interventions, and it is important to understand their mechanism of action and test the study methodology before formal evaluation. These aspects can be achieved through feasibility studies and qualitative interviews. Many of these interventions may help, particularly as supplements to pharmacological intervention, but they need rigorous evaluation.

## References

[1]  Bennett MI, Bagnall AM, Closs SJ. How effective are patient-based educational interventions in the management of cancer pain? Systematic review and meta-analysis. Pain 2009;143:192–9.
[2]  Bennett MI, Johnson MI, Brown S, Searle RD, Radford H, Brown JM. Feasibility study of transcutaneous electrical nerve stimulation (TENS) for cancer bone pain. J Pain 2009; Epub October 21.
[3]  Brunoni AR, Lopes M, Kaptchuk TJ, Fregni F. Placebo response of non-pharmacological and pharmacological trials in major depression: a systematic review and meta-analysis. PLoS One 2009;4:e4824.

[4]   Cleeland CS, Portenoy RK, Rue M, Mendoza TR, Weller E, Payne R, Kirshner J, Atkins JN, John-
      son PA, Marcus A. Does an oral analgesic protocol improve pain control for patients with can-
      cer? An intergroup study coordinated by the Eastern Cooperative Oncology Group. Ann Oncol
      2005;16:972–80.
[5]   Craig P, Dieppe P, MacIntyre S, Mitchie S, Nazareth I, Petticrew M. Developing and evaluating
      complex interventions: the new Medical Research Council guidance. BMJ 2008;337:979–83.
[6]   Dawson R, Spross JA, Jablonski ES, Hoyer DR, Sellers DE, Solomon MZ. Probing the para-
      dox of patients' satisfaction with inadequate pain management. J Pain Symptom Manage
      2002;23:211–20.
[7]   Du Pen SL, Du Pen AR, Polissar N, Hansberry J, Kraybill BM, Stillman M, Panke J, Everly R,
      Syrjala K. Implementing guidelines for cancer pain management: results of a randomized con-
      trolled clinical trial. J Clin Oncol 1999;17:361–70.
[8]   Dworkin RH, Turk DC, Farrar JT, Haythornthwaite JA, Jensen MP, Katz NP, Kerns RD, Stucki G,
      Allen RR, Bellamy N, et al. Core outcome measures for chronic pain clinical trials: IMMPACT
      recommendations. Pain 2005;113:9–19.
[9]   Gunnarsdottir S, Donovan HS, Serlin RC, Voge C, Ward S. Patient-related barriers to pain man-
      agement: the Barriers Questionnaire II (BQ-II). Pain 2002;99:385–96.
[10]  Jacobsen R, Sjøgren P, Møldrup C, Christrup L. Physician-related barriers to cancer pain man-
      agement with opioid analgesics: a systematic review. J Opioid Manag 2007;3:207–14.
[11]  Kwekkeboom KL, Bumpus M, Wanta B, Serlin RC. Oncology nurses' use of nondrug pain inter-
      ventions in practice. J Pain Symptom Manage 2008;35:83–94.
[12]  Kwekkeboom KL, Wanta B, Bumpas M. Individual difference variables and the effects of pro-
      gressive muscle relaxation and analgesic imagery interventions on cancer pain. J Pain Symptom
      Manage 2008;36:604–15.
[13]  Kutner JS, Smith MC, Corbin L, Hemphill L, Benton K, Mellis BK, Beaty B, Felton S, Yamashita
      TE, Bryant LL, Fairclough DL. Massage therapy versus simple touch to improve pain and mood
      in patients with advanced cancer: a randomized trial. Ann Intern Med 2008;149:369–79.
[14]  Oxford English Dictionary. Available at: http://www.askoxford.com.
[15]  Peretti-Watel P, Bendiane MK, Obadia Y, Favre R, Lapiana JM, Moatti JP. The South-East-
      ern France Palliative Care Group. The prescription of opioid analgesics to terminal cancer
      patients: impact of physicians' general attitudes and contextual factors. Palliat Support Care
      2003;1:345–52.
[16]  Robb KA, Newham DJ, Williams JE. Transcutaneous electrical nerve stimulation vs. transcuta-
      neous spinal electroanalgesia for chronic pain associated with breast cancer treatments. J Pain
      Symptom Manage 2007;33:410–9.
[17]  Trowbridge R, Dugan W, Jay SJ, Littrell D, Casebeer LL, Edgerton S, Anderson J, O'Toole JB.
      Determining the effectiveness of a clinical-practice intervention in improving the control of pain
      in outpatients with cancer. Acad Med 1997;72:798–800.
[18]  Velikova G, Booth L, Smith AB, Brown PM, Lynch P, Brown JM, Selby PJ. Measuring quality of
      life in routine oncology practice improves communication and patient well-being: a randomized
      controlled trial. J Clin Oncol 2004;22:714–24.
[19]  White C, Gilshenan K, Hardy J. A survey of the views of palliative care healthcare professionals
      towards referring cancer patients to participate in randomized controlled trials in palliative care.
      Support Care Cancer 2008;16:1397–1405.
[20]  World Health Organization. Cancer pain relief. Geneva: World Health Organization; 1986.

***Correspondence to:*** Michael I. Bennett, MB ChB, MD, FRCP, FFPMRCA, Professor of Palliative Medicine, International Observatory on End of Life Care, School
of Health and Medicine, Bowland Tower East, Lancaster University, Lancaster
LA1 4YT, United Kingdom. Email: m.i.bennett@lancaster.ac.uk.

# Part V

# Psychology of Cancer Pain: The Basic Research and Clinical Research Agenda

# Anxiety from an Evolutionary Perspective and the Relationship between Anxiety and Cancer Pain

## Predrag Petrovic

*Department of Clinical Neuroscience, Karolinska Institute, Stockholm, Sweden*

Both anxiety disorders and general heightened anxiety are increased in cancer patients, and this psychological stress is thought to influence the pain experience in a negative way [27]. Although this relationship is complex and bidirectional, experimental research indicates that anxiety may strongly increase pain perception [27]. Thus, in addition to providing optimal treatment for pain, it is crucial to identify and treat anxiety in cancer pain patients.

In order to understand the relationship between the stressful psychological state (i.e., anxiety) related to a cancer diagnosis and pain, we must analyze the components involved. However, anxiety is an ill-defined state, often relating to the overt context in which it is observed (such as social anxiety, obsessive-compulsive disorder, or specific phobia) and not to the experience itself or to underlying processes in the brain. It is probable that various processes involved in anxiety are fundamentally different and even suppress each other. If the different types of processes involved in anxiety are not better understood, it will be hard to fully grasp the relation between anxiety and pain in general and between anxiety and cancer pain specifically. In this chapter, I will describe the biology of anxiety by discussing the related fear

*Cancer Pain: From Molecules to Suffering*
edited by Judith A. Paice, Rae F. Bell, Eija A. Kalso, and Olaitan A. Soyannwo
IASP Press, Seattle, © 2010

states that are important from an evolutionary perspective and describe their possible relationship to the experience and processing of pain.

# The Passive Fear State

A plausible, evolutionary important fear state that may relate to anxiety is observed when an animal has detected a potential threat (e.g., a predator) in its proximity. For example, this state may be observed when an antelope has spotted a lion, or when a mouse has detected a cat. This state has been termed the "post-encounter state" and is associated with a very specific behavior pattern [8]. The animal will stop moving, and its heart rate will decrease. It will display extremely passive behavior and will focus on the source of the threat. There may be several evolutionary reasons for this behavior. Freezing will decrease the chances of being detected by a potential predator, and it will be easier for the animal to attend to external input. Importantly, this state is related to opioid-dependent analgesia, sometimes referred to as stress-induced analgesia or fear-induced analgesia.

The amygdala has been proposed to be a key region in mediating the post-encounter state [8]. Signals associated with various types of threat can activate the basolateral complex in the amygdala, and further downstream the central nucleus can activate a cascade of subcortical and brainstem regions that mediate many of the fear-related responses observed in the animal, including various autonomic responses and passive behavior (mediated by the ventrolateral periaqueductal gray [vlPAG]) [6,13]. The threat-related signals reaching the amygdala may convey fear-relevant information that can directly activate the amygdala, while more complex information about an upcoming threat is mediated via processing of the information in the cortex [6,13]. Also, the amygdala is involved in simple conditioning learning (an NMDA-mediated learning process in the basolateral nucleus), whereby previously neutral stimuli associated with a threat may induce similar activations [6,13].

The amygdala is only one of many regions belonging to a large network of cortical, subcortical, and brainstem regions that interact in mediating the post-encounter state. As mentioned above, complex analysis of external signals may require prefrontal top-down functions and the involvement of other cortical regions [15]. This analysis may relate to a better understanding of the threat and of the probability of an attack, and it also involves identifying the best possible escape route. For example, the amygdala has anatomical connections that may directly modulate the activity in the extrastriate visual pathway and thereby boost the processing of visual stimuli in order to extract as much information as possible about the impending threat [1,28]. Moreover, prefrontal regions may integrate different sources of information about the threat to select a relevant response pattern for avoiding a direct confrontation [16]. Such complex analyses take many different possible outcomes into account and may induce a large variety of responses. The theoretical drawback with this state is that the dynamic but complex processes also require a large processing capacity and are time consuming. Such processes are not optimal when a rapid response is required in order to survive.

# The Active Fear State

The most dramatic change in fear-related behavior that takes place in animals is observed when there is not merely a threat but a direct predatory attack. Under these circumstances, it is not possible to perform a complex and time-consuming analysis about the source of danger. Instead, a fast and robust response may be the only chance of survival. Behaviorally, the animal will go from an extremely passive state to an extremely active one where it tries to either escape or fight the threat, in what is known as the "fight-or-flight" reaction [8]. This state has been termed the "circa-strike state" [8]. This behavior does not require cortical input, but relies on rapid responses mediated by the brainstem, specifically the dorsolateral periaqueductal gray (dlPAG) [8]. The PAG consists of a set of vertical nuclei surrounding the aqueduct (including the vlPAG, involved in the passive fear state, and the dlPAG, involved in the active fear state) [2]. The dlPAG functions as part of a network of brainstem regions and can also communicate with prefrontal regions [2]. Different species-specific active fear responses may occur when the dlPAG is stimulated [8]. If the caudal region is stimulated, fight behavior may be induced, but if the rostral part is stimulated, flight behavior is more likely [8]. This rapid, yet complex behavior includes increased heart rate, piloerection, altered blood flow to specific muscle groups, and the fight-or-flight behavior itself [8]. Thus, no cortical input is needed in order to induce this non-dynamic but complex behavior.

One interesting feature of the circa-strike state is that it induces a powerful, non-opioid-dependent analgesic response [8]. Thus, harm to the body elicited in the attack will not induce pain and thereby slow the animal in its attempt to escape. Another interesting feature is that nociceptive signals may directly activate this state before the signals reach cortical regions [8]. In a surprise attack, these nociceptive signals may then directly induce an active fear state (which represents the animal's only chance of survival). Since early nociceptive input mediates more information about a possible threat than prolonged nociceptive input, it has been suggested that the brainstem is more involved in early versus late pain [21].

# The Relation of Fear States to Human Behavior

The fear states described above are relevant for most animals, and thus they must be relevant for humans as well [12]. But are these extreme responses relevant in situations other than life-threatening ones, and is it possible to study them experimentally? It is possible to experimentally induce low-level fear states in humans [12]. Showing standardized threatening pictures to human subjects will not only induce a feeling of unpleasantness but also cause heart-rate deceleration and an increased startle reaction, which are both indications of amygdala-dependent activation of the post-encounter phase [12]. Imaging studies in human subjects have shown that, compared with neutral pictures, threatening pictures are more likely to activate the amygdala and the extrastriate visual cortex, supporting the idea that amygdala activation enhances visual processing of the threat-related stimulus [18]. Innately threatening stimuli (such as angry and fearful faces, and even angry voices) can also activate the amygdala [28]. Interestingly, patients with bilateral sclerosis of the amygdala do not show any increased activity in the extrastriate visual cortex when fear-relevant stimuli are viewed; this further implicates the amygdala in fear-related modulation of visual processing [28]. All these studies suggest that it is possible to experimentally induce the post-encounter state in human subjects.

What about the circa-strike state? At first glance, it seems even more difficult to induce such an active state. We have previously tried to compare early nociceptive input (associated with a circa-strike phase) with later nociceptive input (associated with more chronic pain) [21]. In that study we were able to show that the brainstem (including the PAG and the pons and stretching up to the hypothalamus and thalamus) was only active in the early nociceptive phase. While the skin conductance response (an indicator of increased arousal) was more active in early rather than in late pain [21], subjects normally experience more intense pain in later phases of tonic nociceptive stimulation [22]. This result would be in line with separate systems processing nociceptive input, one based in the brainstem (and associated with the circa-strike response), and one based cortically (and associated with the pain experience).

Although that study may indicate how nociceptive information is processed in the circa-strike state, it does not tell us anything about the processes involved in active fear-related behavior. A successful model of the circa-strike state must include an active threat and the possibility of escape. We have recently constructed a model in which the subject controls a symbol that can move through a maze on the computer screen, while being chased by a virtual predator [16]. To increase the threat component, a painful shock is delivered every time the predator catches the subject. While there was no activation in cortical regions (and even a decrease of activity in the amygdala and prefrontal regions), increased activity was observed in the rostral brainstem, including the PAG, and in the cerebellum [16]. Previous studies in experimental animals have shown that circa-strike behavior is directly correlated with the distance away from the predator (the "predator imminence" effect) [8]. In our recent study we were able to show that the distance between the predator and the subject at every moment correlated positively with PAG activity and negatively with prefrontal activity [16]. Thus, the data show that it is possible to study active fear states experimentally in humans and that these states may be relevant even in situations that are not life-threatening.

## The Relation between Fear States and Anxiety

Both the animal and the human models indicate that different types of fear states vary greatly in terms of the behavior produced and the brain networks and processes involved. However, do these states have anything to do with clinical anxiety states? In a study on healthy volunteers, divided into anxiety-prone subjects and subjects with normal anxiety levels, the anxiety-prone subjects showed a greater activation of the amygdala when various threat-related stimuli were shown, including angry faces and fearful faces [25]. Interestingly, even happy faces elicited stronger amygdala activity in the anxiety-prone subjects [25]. Behaviorally, it is well known that anxiety-prone subjects are more liable to detect threat-related cues, which is in line with a stronger amygdala-induced processing of external inputs [3,25]. These findings relate the anxiety process to the passive fear state (the post-encounter state). Anxiety-prone subjects seem to have an overactive amygdala system, which may cause them to transition more easily to a post-encounter state. What about anxiety patients? A meta-analysis demonstrated that various types of anxiety patients (including those diagnosed with social phobia, post-traumatic stress disorder, and simple phobia) showed an increased activation of the amygdala and insula when they were subjected to the relevant anxiety-inducing stimulation [7]. Taken together, the evidence supports a relationship between the amygdala, the post-encounter state, and anxiety.

What about the circa-strike state? Electrical stimulation of the dorsal PAG can induce autonomic responses and a panic-like experience in humans [10]. Moreover, the activity in the PAG during the prey-predator task correlates with the degree of panic experienced [16]. In line with those findings, both structural imaging and metabolic imaging studies have implicated the brainstem, including the PAG, in panic disorder [10]. Thus, it is very likely that the PAG is crucially involved in panic attacks as well as in active fear states.

# Cancer and Pain

The fear states that we have reviewed above are not identical with the state where increased pain experience is observed in patients with cancer pain [27], because both of these fear states are associated with powerful opioid- or non-opioid-dependent analgesia. Thus, we need to expand those models in order to understand how anxiety interacts with pain. Perhaps it would be helpful to turn to human behavioral and imaging studies that focus on the relationship between emotion and pain.

While several studies have shown an augmented pain experience during experimentally induced negative emotions, other studies have shown pain-attenuating effects [23,29]. The difference may depend on how emotions interact with arousal and degree of threat [23]. The difference in how negative emotions interact with pain mirrors the difference in pain experience between the evolutionary fear states described above (associated with decreased pain) and what is observed in cancer pain (associated with increased pain). It has been proposed that the interaction between noxious input and attention determines whether pain-facilitatory or pain-inhibitory mechanisms are activated [4,27]. In hypoalgesia induced by stress or fear (as in the post-encounter state described above), pain-attenuating systems such as the endogenous opioid system are activated because the animal's attention is directed away from the pain and toward the threat. The evolutionary benefit of increased attention to the source of danger and disregard of pain is an improved chance of survival. However, if the anxiety is associated with an internal source such as fear of bodily harm, it may be of evolutionary benefit to increase the organism's attention to the painful experience. In anxiety-induced hyperalgesia (such as in cancer pain), attention is directed toward the pain, and pain-facilitatory pain systems may be activated. One example is the cholecystokinin system, which plays a key role in pain facilitation [4,14]. Systems that facilitate pain share similar networks with pain-attenuating systems [14].

Few imaging studies have been performed on the interaction between pain and emotional states. It has been shown that negative expectations of a painful event will increase both the reported pain experience and the objectively observed pain-dependent activation in the pain matrix (including the insula and the anterior cingulate cortex [ACC]) [4,11]. It has been suggested that catastrophizing is associated with increased activity in the ACC in patients with chronic pain [9]. Also, depressed patients have shown increased activity in similar regions when subjected to experimental pain [26]. Moreover, depressed patients have increased activity in the amygdala, which correlates with subjects' ratings of helplessness [26]. Interestingly, the interaction between depressive symptoms and clinical pain severity has been suggested to take place within the medial prefrontal cortex [24], a region close to the rostral ACC that is involved in cognitive regulation of pain [19,20] and anxiety [3,7].

Another clue comes from a study in healthy volunteers [17]. Subjects in this study received painful stimuli, and activity that could be attributed to general anxiety showed no interaction with pain processing.

However, pain-related brain activity was also regressed with scores on the Fear of Pain Questionnaire (FPQ), a tool that focuses on fear of bodily harm. Higher FPQ ratings correlated with stronger pain-related activity in several regions of the pain matrix. The importance of this study is that it tries to dissociate several different anxiety components, and the FPQ relates to the individual's attention to bodily pain. Thus, this finding would be in line with the suggestion that attention to internal bodily harm during anxiety increases pain processing (as opposed to an external threat, which would decrease the experience of pain) [4].

In this chapter, I have not clearly distinguished between fear and anxiety. In some of the literature, fear is defined as a situation when a threat is present, while anxiety is defined as a situation when a threat is not present [23]. However, this is clearly not the case in clinical practice. Both general anxiety (when a threat is not present) and specific anxiety (when a threat is present) are anxiety states according to international clinical classifications of anxiety. Thus, while it is important to distinguish where the threat may be in relation to the subject or patient, this parameter is not a good distinction between fear and anxiety. However, it is of interest that the dlPAG, involved in active fear states, interacts with the threatening stimulus directly, whereas in the passive fear states induced by the amygdala, the threat is more distant. Moreover, another region, called the bed nucleus of stria terminalis (BNST), seems to be important when the threat is undefined [5]. This region may also subserve fear-related processes in a similar manner to the central nucleus of the amygdala. Although the BNST and amygdala are separate structures, both the BNST and the central nucleus receive input from the basolateral nucleus, are histologically similar, and have the same output projections with the ability to induce similar fear responses [5]. It has been suggested that the BNST is involved when the source of fear is less clearly identified but more prolonged [5]. Thus, it is possible that the BNST is related with the anxiety associated with cancer and thereby is also involved in the hyperalgesic responses that occur with cancer pain.

In summary, the relationship between different anxiety states and pain is a rather complex area where little research has been performed. In this chapter, I have tried to outline some important clues to that relationship. More knowledge can help us to identify specific neuromodulatory systems (such as possibly the cholecystokinin system) that can lower the anxiety-related hyperalgesia often observed in cancer patients.

# References

[1] Amaral DG, Behniea H, Kelly JL. Topographic organization of projections from the amygdala to the visual cortex in the macaque monkey. Neuroscience 2003;118:1099–1120.

[2] Bandler R, Keay KA, Floyd N, Price J. Central circuits mediating patterned autonomic activity during active vs. passive emotional coping. Brain Res Bull 2000;53:95–104.

[3] Bishop SJ. Neurocognitive mechanisms of anxiety: an integrative account. Trends Cogn Sci 2007;11:307–16.

[4] Colloca L, Benedetti F. Nocebo hyperalgesia: how anxiety is turned into pain. Curr Opin Anaesthesiol 2007;20:435–9.

[5] Davis M. The role of the amygdala in conditioned fear. In: Aggleton JP, editor. The amygdala: neurophysiological aspects of emotion, memory, and mental dysfunction. New York: Wiley-Liss; 1992. p. 255–306.

[6] Davis M. Neurobiology of fear responses: the role of the amygdala. J Neuropsychiatry Clin Neurosci 1997;9:382–402.

[7] Etkin A, Wager TD. Functional neuroimaging of anxiety: a meta-analysis of emotional processing in PTSD, social anxiety disorder, and specific phobia. Am J Psychiatry 2007;164:1476–88.

[8] Fanselow MS. Neural organization of the defensive behavior system responsible for fear. Psychon Bull Rev 1994;1:429–38.

[9] Gracely RH, Geisser ME, Giesecke T, Grant MA, Petzke F, Williams DA, Clauw DJ. Pain catastrophizing and neural responses to pain among persons with fibromyalgia. Brain 2004;127(Pt 4):835–43.

[10] Graeff FG, Del-Ben CM. Neurobiology of panic disorder: from animal models to brain neuroimaging. Neurosci Biobehav Rev 2008;32:1326–35.

[11] Koyama T, McHaffie JG, Laurienti PJ, Coghill RC. The subjective experience of pain: where expectations become reality. Proc Natl Acad Sci USA 2005;102:12950–5.

[12] Lang PJ, Davis M, Ohman A. Fear and anxiety: animal models and human cognitive psychophysiology. J Affect Disord 2000;61:137–59.

[13] LeDoux J. The amygdala and emotion: a view through fear. In: Aggleton JP, editor. The amygdala: a functional analysis. Oxford: Oxford University Press; 2000. p. 289–310.

[14] Lovick TA. Pro-nociceptive action of cholecystokinin in the periaqueductal grey: a role in neuropathic and anxiety-induced hyperalgesic states. Neurosci Biobehav Rev 2008;32:852–62.

[15] Mesulam MM. Large-scale neurocognitive networks and distributed processing for attention, language, and memory. Ann Neurol 1990;28:597–613.

[16] Mobbs D, Petrovic P, Marchant JL, Hassabis D, Weiskopf N, Seymour B, Dolan RJ, Frith CD. When fear is near: threat imminence elicits prefrontal-periaqueductal gray shifts in humans. Science 2007;317:1079–83.

[17] Ochsner KN, Ludlow DH, Knierim K, Hanelin J, Ramachandran T, Glover GC, Mackey SC. Neural correlates of individual differences in pain-related fear and anxiety. Pain 2006;120:69–77.

[18] Petrovic P, Dietrich T, Fransson P, Andersson J, Carlsson K, Ingvar M. Placebo in emotional processing: induced expectations of anxiety relief activate a generalized modulatory network. Neuron 2005;46:957–69.

[19] Petrovic P, Ingvar M. Imaging cognitive modulation of pain processing. Pain 2002;95:1–5.

[20] Petrovic P, Kalso E, Petersson KM, Ingvar M. Placebo and opioid analgesia: imaging a shared neuronal network. Science 2002;295:1737–40.

[21] Petrovic P, Petersson KM, Ingvar M. Brainstem involvement in the initial response to pain. Neuroimage 2004;22:995–1005.

[22] Rainville P, Feine JS, Bushnell MC, Duncan GH. A psychophysical comparison of sensory and affective responses to four modalities of experimental pain. Somatosens Mot Res 1992;9:265–77.

[23] Rhudy JL, Williams AE. Gender differences in pain: do emotions play a role? Gend Med 2005;2:208–26.

[24]  Schweinhardt P, Kalk N, Wartolowska K, Chessell I, Wordsworth P, Tracey I. Investigation into the neural correlates of emotional augmentation of clinical pain. Neuroimage 2008;40:759–66.

[25]  Stein MB, Simmons AN, Feinstein JS, Paulus MP. Increased amygdala and insula activation during emotion processing in anxiety-prone subjects. Am J Psychiatry 2007;164:318–27.

[26]  Strigo IA, Simmons AN, Matthews SC, Craig AD, Paulus MP. Association of major depressive disorder with altered functional brain response during anticipation and processing of heat pain. Arch Gen Psychiatry 2008;65:1275–84.

[27]  Thielking PD. Cancer pain and anxiety. Curr Pain Headache Rep 2003;7:249–61.

[28]  Vuilleumier P, Pourtois G. Distributed and interactive brain mechanisms during emotion face perception: evidence from functional neuroimaging. Neuropsychologia 2007;45:174–94.

[29]  Wiech K, Tracey I. The influence of negative emotions on pain: behavioral effects and neural mechanisms. Neuroimage 2009;47:987–94.

*Correspondence to:* Predrag Petrovic, MD, PhD, Department of Clinical Neuroscience, Cognitive Neurophysiology MR Research Center, N-8, Karolinska Hospital, Stockholm 17176, Sweden. Email: predrag.petrovic@ki.se.

# Dealing with Cancer Pain: Coping, Pain Catastrophizing, and Related Outcomes

Tamara J. Somers, Francis J. Keefe, Sejal Kothadia,
and Agustina Pandiani

*Pain Prevention and Treatment Program and Department of Psychiatry and Behavioral
Sciences, Duke University Medical Center, Durham, North Carolina, USA*

There is growing recognition that cancer pain is a complex experience [24], along with this recognition increased interest among both clinicians and scientists in how individuals cope with cancer pain. This chapter provides an overview of the literature on coping with cancer pain. The first section describes the biopsychosocial model that serves as a conceptual foundation for studies of pain coping. The second section defines pain coping and summarizes the results of descriptive studies of pain coping in cancer patients. The third section presents research on interventions designed to enhance pain coping skills. The final section highlights important new directions for research in this area.

## The Biopsychosocial Model of Cancer Pain

Cancer pain is typically assessed and treated based on a biomedical model [11,24]. According to this model, cancer pain is caused by damage to body tissues related to disease activity (e.g., a tumor pressing on nerves) or by cancer treatments (e.g., surgery, radiation, or chemotherapy) designed to correct the underlying disease. The ideal biomedical treatment for cancer pain seeks to eliminate underlying disease activity by treating the cancer itself. However, when this approach is not sufficient, the biomedical model addresses pain either through medication management (e.g., the World Health Organization analgesic ladder) or through specialized surgical or radiation treatment approaches.

Problems with the biomedical model are widely acknowledged [11,24] and include (a) the poor correlation between underling tissue damage and level of pain, (b) variations in pain response to the same treatment protocol, and (c) the model's failure to address psychological factors (e.g., depression, anger) and social factors (e.g., social support, home/work environment) that can influence pain.

The biopsychosocial model of cancer pain is much broader than the biomedical model. Its key tenet is that biological factors (e.g., tissue damage), psychological factors (e.g., guilt, fear, and overly negative thoughts about pain), and social factors (e.g., marital satisfaction) can both influence and be influenced by pain [11,24].

To illustrate the importance of the psychological and social factors in cancer pain, consider social interactions that might occur at times of increased pain between patients with advanced cancer and their caregivers. A number of patient factors can influence pain at such times. Underlying tissue damage, for example due to cancer treatments (a biological factor), is clearly one of the factors influencing pain experienced by a patient with advanced cancer. Also important, however, are psychological factors including a patient's thoughts about the pain ("I won't be able to handle this" or "I am a burden on my partner") and related feelings (e.g., fear or guilt). Overly negative thoughts and feelings can contribute to increased pain, while more realistic thoughts can help in managing negative feelings and serve to ameliorate pain. Another key patient factor is the degree to which the patient is willing to express pain to others. Some patients hold back on expressing pain in order to buffer the impact of pain on their caregivers. For example, they may minimize the severity of pain or refuse pain medications for fear that admitting pain will upset those around them. Recent evidence suggests that holding back from disclosing pain to a partner is associated with increased pain in cancer patients.

Partner factors represent an important part of the social context of cancer pain. First, at times of increased pain, partners need to be able to decode pain expressions (i.e., interpret and understand what they mean). This task is particularly challenging if the patient is holding back on pain expression because the partner may be receiving mixed messages (e.g., the patient may verbalize that she is not having pain, whereas nonverbally it is clear that she is). Understanding pain expression is also difficult in cases where high levels of depression or anxiety influence how patients communicate their pain to others. A second important partner factor is the ability to respond appropriately to the patient's pain expression at times of increased pain. Some partners are well attuned to the patient's needs and preferences with regard to pain management. In contrast, other partners are unsure how to respond and may respond either in an unhelpful manner or in an overly solicitous fashion that increases the patient's pain and distress. A third partner factor relates to the partner's own thoughts and feelings in this situation. Partners themselves may feel helpless with regard to helping the patient control pain, and this feeling may lead them to feel anxious when confronted with an episode of increased pain [24].

Certain maladaptive thoughts and beliefs about cancer pain are common among cancer patients and those in their social context, including spouses and other caregivers [11,24,26]. First, fear of pain is a significant problem. Both patients and caregivers may believe and expect that a diagnosis of cancer means that severe pain is inevitable and unmanageable and that they are not adequately equipped to deal with it. This belief can lead to a sense of hopelessness and helplessness and lower expectations about the potential benefits of both medication and nonpharmacological pain management. Second, the recurrence of pain is often viewed as a signal of disease progression. Because pain episodes may be interpreted as a signal of impending death, patients may be acutely attuned to them. Thus, the recurrence of pain can be frightening and may lead to a variety of maladaptive responses such as heightened feelings of anxiety or avoiding a pain evaluation because of the distress it raises. Third, some patients and caregivers may view opioid medications as the only way that cancer pain can be managed. Patients and caregivers may worry about what will happen when patients develop tolerance to their pain medication and it no longer works as effectively [26]. Concerns about side effects and about managing serious adverse effects may lead to underutilization of pain medications [26]. Finally, negative attitudes and stereotypes regarding psychosocial interventions may undermine the willingness of patients and caregivers to use psychological treatments (e.g., hypnosis, imagery, and distraction techniques) that could be helpful [24].

# Pain Coping: Descriptive Studies

The biopsychosocial model of cancer pain has generated considerable interest in how patients cope with cancer pain. Coping has been defined as the cognitive and behavioral efforts that one engages in to master, reduce, or tolerate internal and external demands that are appraised as taxing or exceeding one's resources [16]. As applied to pain coping, this definition highlights two important domains: (1) coping strategies (i.e., specific efforts to manage pain) and (2) appraisals of pain coping (i.e., judgments as to the efficacy of pain coping efforts).

A number of studies have identified specific coping strategies that cancer patients use to cope with pain. Among the cognitive pain strategies used by cancer patients are ignoring pain, making coping self-statements, diverting attention from pain, having wish-fulfilling fantasies, blaming oneself, and praying or hoping [3,23]. Behavioral pain coping strategies include active coping efforts such as changing one's activity (either decreasing or increasing it), engaging in pleasant and distracting activities, communicating with others about pain or one's feelings, and seeking information or support from significant others or a health professional [3,6]. The results of studies examining the relationship between specific coping strategies and cancer pain are mixed. Some studies, for example, have reported that active behavioral coping efforts are related to less pain-related disability whereas passive coping efforts are related to higher pain-related disability [6], while other studies have not found these relationships. Taken together, these studies suggest that there is not a specific coping strategy or set of coping strategies that is associated with lower pain and better adjustment to pain in cancer patients.

Research on pain appraisals in cancer patients have focused primarily on pain catastrophizing (an overly negative appraisal of pain). Individuals who engage in pain catastrophizing tend to ruminate on how threatening a painful stimulus is and negatively evaluate their own abilities to cope with pain [13]. Pain catastrophizing has been found to relate to increased psychological distress in patients with cancer pain [27]. Why do patients with pain engage in pain catastrophizing? The communal coping theory of pain catastrophizing maintains that catastrophizing occurs because it enables patients with pain to solicit help and emotional support from others. We tested this notion in a study of pain catastrophizing in 70 patients with gastrointestinal cancer and their caregivers [14]. We found that, while patients who catastrophized reported higher levels of cancer pain, they also reported much higher levels of social support from their caregivers. Interestingly, partners of patients who were catastrophizers reported much higher caregiver stress and a lower overall quality of life. These findings suggest that while catastrophizing may enhance patients' perceptions of social support, it may inadvertently make the pain experience more aversive. The increased attention to pain that comes when significant others respond to pain catastrophizing may lead the patient to focus more on the pain experience.

## Interventions to Enhance Pain Coping

One of the most interesting outgrowths of research on pain coping in cancer has been the development of protocols designed to enhance patients' pain coping skills. Keefe et al. [15] conceptualized pain coping skills training as having three main components: (1) an educational rationale based on the gate control theory of pain that can help patients understand how their thoughts, feelings, and behaviors can influence pain and how their own efforts to manage pain can influence the pain they experience; (2) therapist-guided training in cognitive and behavioral pain coping strategies, such as progressive muscle relaxation, brief relaxation methods, goal setting, activity pacing, imagery, and cognitive restructuring (i.e., altering overly negative thoughts); and (3) training in how to apply learned coping skills to challenging pain-related situations. Pain coping skills training is typically conducted by a highly trained therapist over a series of sessions.

Syrjala conducted one of the first controlled trials of pain coping skills training in a study of patients were pain related to bone marrow transplantation [25]. In this study, 94 patients were randomized to one of four conditions: a comprehensive pain coping skills protocol that provided training in multiple pain coping skills (relaxation, imagery, cognitive restructuring, distraction, and goal setting), a simplified pain coping skills protocol that provided training in relaxation and imagery only, therapist support, or treatment as usual. Data analysis showed that patients who received either the comprehensive or simplified pain coping skills training protocols showed similar improvements in pain and that both were superior to therapist support or treatment as usual.

In another study, Dalton et al. [9] examined whether a tailored pain coping skills intervention would significantly alter pain levels in a group of patients with various types of cancer (i.e., breast, lung, lymphoma, colon, or other cancer). This approach was unique because the intervention was based on the evaluation of the patient's characteristics and needs. Following a thorough assessment, patients in the tailored intervention were matched to intervention modules that focused on their specific needs. Some examples of modules were environmental influences, loss of control, health care avoidance, past and current experience, physiological responsiveness, or thoughts of disease progression. Patients who received the tailored intervention showed improvements in pain, sleep, mobility, and relationships immediately after treatment and one month later compared to patients who received standard pain coping skills training or usual care.

Abernethy et al. [1] conducted a meta-analysis to determine the efficacy of cognitive-behavioral therapy (CBT) protocols, including pain coping skills training, for managing cancer pain. This meta-analysis included 21 trials of CBT protocols involving 2,296 participants. The efficacy of CBT was examined across three different types of intervention: imagery and hypnosis-based CBT, comprehensive CBT, and education-focused interventions. CBT protocols were effective in reducing pain in 65% of the studies, with an overall average effect size of 0.232 (95% confidence interval 0.072 to 0.392; $P = 0.004$), translating to a 7–9-point reduction in pain intensity on a 0–100 rating scale. The results from this meta-analysis suggest that systematic training in cognitive and behavioral strategies for reducing cancer pain is effective.

In recent years, there has been growing interest in the effects of cancer on both patients and their loved ones [21,19]. Patients and their partners face challenges with regards to coping with treatment effects, uncertainty of future outcomes, and in some cases, making difficult decisions pertaining to the end of life and palliative care [18]. Interestingly, spouses of cancer patients having pain often experience at least as much psychological distress as the patient. Consequently, the partner's distress can have a negative impact on the patient's outcomes [4].

Two major intervention approaches to enhancing pain coping—the partner-assisted approach and the couples-based approach—aim to address the unique circumstances faced by patients and their partners. In a partner-assisted approach, the primary focus is on the patient, and the partner acts as a coach with the goal of targeting the patient's pain coping skills. Alternatively, the couples-based approach focuses equally on both the patient and the partner. In this approach, the primary focus is to enhance interaction and communications centered around a specific topic (e.g., pain) and to emphasize ways to build the couple's relationship [10].

Keefe et al. [12] conducted the first randomized controlled trial of a partner-assisted pain coping skills training for cancer patients who were at the end of life. Participants in this study, 78 hospice-eligible cancer patients having pain and their primary caregivers, were randomly assigned to either a partner-assisted pain coping skills training protocol or usual care. The skills training was conducted in patients' homes in a series of three sessions that integrated educational information about pain with training in pain coping skills (relaxation, imagery, activity pacing, and maintenance training). During each training session, the patient's partner played a key role in assisting and guiding the patient in learning the coping skill presented. Partners were also taught how to help the patient practice these coping skills and maintain their use over time. Data analysis showed that, after completing the training, partners who received the pain coping skills training intervention reported higher self-efficacy with regard to helping the patient control pain and other symptoms, as well as lower caregiver strain. Although the pain coping skills intervention did not significantly reduce pain in patients, patients who received the intervention did report somewhat lower ratings of usual and worst pain.

Porter et al. [22] conducted another intervention adapting the partner-based approach to patients with gastrointestinal cancer and their partners. Past work had suggested that patients' inability to discuss cancer-related concerns was associated with poor coping, problems with psychological adjustment, and relationship quality. Based on these findings, Porter et al. tested the efficacy of a partner-assisted emotional disclosure protocol to promote better coping in patients with gastrointestinal cancer. Couples ($n$ = 130) were randomized to receive four sessions of either partner-assisted emotional disclosure or cancer education. The major components of the emotional disclosure intervention were to encourage patients to share their thoughts and feelings about their cancer experience (including pain) and encourage acceptance and understanding by their partner. The partner was trained to facilitate the patient's discussion of and reflection on cancer-related concerns. The education group received information on improving communication with health care providers, evaluating health information, and ways to maintain quality of life. Results suggested that the emotional disclosure intervention improved relationship quality and intimacy in couples that reported higher levels of holding back or actively inhibiting discussion of cancer-related thoughts prior to treatment. The improvements for both patients and partners in the treatment group are particularly encouraging given the relatively short nature of the treatment.

In a study of a couples-based approach to intervention, Baucom et al. [5] tested a novel relationship enhancement protocol for breast cancer patients and their partners. The intervention focused on improving the relationships by encouraging couples to approach breast cancer together with positive attitudes, improving communication skills, promoting sexual adaptation, and finding meaning in life. One of the primary goals of the intervention was to focus on the relationship between partner and patient and on ways to improve their relationship while dealing with cancer. Fourteen couples were randomized to receive either six biweekly sessions with a trained therapist or treatment as usual. Patients in the relationship enhancement group reported improvements in symptoms including pain, functional well-being, self-image, body acceptance, and relationship functioning. In partners, levels of psychological distress decreased, and post-traumatic growth (i.e., positive psychological change resulting from a challenging life circumstance) and relationship functioning improved. At a 1-year follow-up, many of these gains were maintained for both partner and patient. Applying the relationship enhancement protocol to a larger population in patients with a wider range of cancer types may be helpful in understanding the feasibility and impact of a couples-based intervention.

# New Directions

Past work has provided a strong foundation to support the importance of pain coping in cancer. As this work moves forward, it is critical to begin to examine how to more widely disseminate interventions known to be efficacious in improving coping with cancer pain symptoms. Prostate cancer, for example, is an important area where health disparities are clear. African-American men have an almost 60% higher incidence rate of prostate cancer and are more than twice as likely as Caucasians to die from the disease [2]. Further, there is literature to support that African-American men who have prostate cancer report a lower quality of life related to physical and psychological symptoms, including pain [17,20]. Investigators in our laboratory have established a program of research to begin to examine and address these disparities. In an initial intervention trial, Campbell et al. [8] explored the efficacy of a partner-assisted coping skills training to enhance coping with treatment side effects in a sample of African-American men who were prostate cancer survivors. Forty couples were randomized to receive either a telephone-based coping skills training or usual care. Partners in this protocol served as coaches for the patients with the overall goal of decreasing negative symptoms experienced by patients. Patients and their partners were given information about prostate cancer and possible long-term side effects, were taught problem-solving skills, and were trained in specific cognitive and behavioral coping skills (e.g., communication, relaxation, and activity pacing). Partners were instructed to encourage patients to incorporate these skills into their daily routines to decrease negative physical and psychological symptoms related to prostate cancer. Patients who received coping skills training demonstrated improved quality of life related to coping with the side effects (bowel, urinary, sexual, and hormonal) of prostate cancer treatment. While the focus in this intervention was on the patients, partners who received coping skills training also benefited. Partners receiving the intervention reported less caregiver strain, depression, and fatigue.

Based on the promising results from this work, Campbell and her colleagues are currently conducting two randomized controlled trials to further address ethnic disparities in recovery from prostate cancer. Both trials are testing an intervention that is designed to improve coping among African-American prostate cancer survivors. In the first trial, men are randomized either to coping skills training group intervention or to an education control group. The coping skills training in the study, along with all study material, was specifically designed to be culturally sensitive to challenges that might be unique to African-American men. For example, the interventions were tailored to address the strengths, preferences, and challenges that affect unique ways of coping for African-American males (e.g., masculine conformity and cultural context of behavior). Study materials portrayed images of African-American men and women. An important component of this trial is that interventions are co-led by men who are leaders in the African-American community. This study hypothesizes that the coping skills training will produce significant improvements in symptoms, including pain, commonly found to be problematic following prostate cancer treatment. It is also expected that patients' ability to cope with their pain and other symptoms will improve as a result of the coping skills training. The low attrition rate and clinical observations suggest that this unique coping skills training protocol is acceptable to the participants and is providing benefits in terms of symptom management and coping.

The second trial is designed to assist African-American prostate cancer survivors and their intimate partners cope more effectively with the problems and challenges experienced after radical prostatectomy for prostate cancer. In this study, couples are randomized either to partner-assisted coping skills training, cancer education, or a wait-list control. As stated above, partner-assisted coping skills training are known to benefit cancer patients and their partners [12]. Both intervention conditions (i.e., partner-assisted pain coping skills training, education) in this study consist of six sessions, delivered by telephone to the patient and partner. Partner-assisted coping skills training is expected to reduce symptom distress in the patient, decrease depressive symptoms in both the patient and partner, and reduce caregiver strain in the partner. Such training is also expected to enhance relationship functioning for both the patient and partner. Finally, increased self-efficacy for managing symptoms in both the patient and partner is expected to be associated with fewer symptoms and less caregiver strain.

This work is important because despite steadily increasing rates of minority group members in the United States, there is very limited research into providing culturally sensitive coping skills interventions for cancer and other diseases. The described interventions may provide an excellent foundation to create future coping skills interventions to apply to a wider array of individuals (including Hispanic or Asian minorities) and other disease contexts (e.g., sickle cell disease, diabetes, and HIV/AIDS). Incorporating culturally sensitive interventions into standard health care settings may assist in closing the gap in health disparities (e.g., lower rates of morbidity and mortality, better health outcomes, and higher quality of life). Culturally sensitive coping skills interventions also have the potential to lead to more confidence in the health care system among minority group members, which can lead to higher engagement in health care, including psychosocial interventions and prevention efforts.

# Summary

Evidence continues to grow suggesting that how a patient copes both cognitively and behaviorally with cancer pain can affect pain as well as adjustment to having cancer. Increasing work is also highlighting the important role of the coping strategies of the patient's partner in the patient's adjustment to cancer pain and overall disease. Approaching cancer pain and adjustment from a biopsychosocial perspective may provide the most benefit to patients and their partners who are faced with learning to cope with cancer pain. Several psychosocial intervention protocols that include patients and/or partners have been developed that are likely to improve pain coping and overall adjustment to cancer. Wider dissemination of these efficacious protocols, particularly to underserved populations, is desirable to provide both patients and their partners with coping strategies that can decrease pain and increase adjustment to having cancer.

# Acknowledgments

This work was supported by grants awarded by the National Institutes of Health: RO1 CA 122704, RO1NS053759, RO1CA107477, R01CA131148, and by the Department of Defense W81XWH-07-1-0091.

# References

[1]   Abernethy AP, Keefe FJ, McCrocy DC, Scipio C, Matchar DB. Behavioral therapies for the man-
      agement of cancer pain: a systematic review. In: Flor H, Kalso E, Dostrovsky J, editors. Proceed-
      ings of the 11th World Congress on Pain. Seattle: IASP Press; 2006. p 789–98.
[2]   American Cancer Society. Cancer facts and figures for African Americans 2009–2010. Atlanta:
      American Cancer Society; 2010.
[3]   Arraras JK, Wright SJ, Jusue G, Tejedor M, Calvo JI. Coping style, locus of control, psycho-
      logical distress and pain-related behaviours in cancer and other diseases. Psychol Health Med
      2002;7:235–41.
[4]   Badger T, Segrin C, Dorros SM, Meek P, Lopez AM. Depression and anxiety in women with
      breast cancer and their partners. Nurs Res 2007;56:44–53.
[5]   Baucom DH, Porter LS, Kirby JS, Gremore TM, Wiesenthal N, Aldrige W, Fredman S, Stanton
      SE, Scott JL, Halford KW, Keefe FJ. A couple-based intervention for female breast cancer. Psy-
      chooncology 2009;18:276–83.
[6]   Bishop SR, David W. Coping, catastrophizing and chronic pain in breast cancer. J Behav Med
      2003;26:265–81.
[7]   Campbell LC, Keefe FJ, McKee DC, Edwards CL, Herman SH, Johnson LE, Colvin OM, McBride
      CM, Donattuci CF. Prostate cancer in African Americans: relationship of patient and partner
      self-efficacy to quality of life. J Pain Symptom Manage 2004;28:433–44.
[8]   Campbell LC, Keefe FJ, Scipio C, McKee DC, Edwards CL, Herman SH, Johnson LE, Colvin
      OM, McBride CM, Donattuci CF. Facilitating research participation and improving quality of
      life for African American prostate cancer survivors and their intimate partners. A pilot study of
      telephone-based coping skills training. Cancer 2007;109(Suppl):414–24.
[9]   Dalton JA, Keefe FJ, Carlson J, Youngblood R. Tailoring cognitive-behavioral treatment for can-
      cer pain. Pain Manag Nurs 2004;5:3–18.
[10]  Epstein NB, Baucom DH. Enhanced cognitive-behavioral therapy for couples: a contextual ap-
      proach. Washington, DC: American Psychological Association; 2002.
[11]  Keefe FJ, Abernethy AP, Campbell LC. Psychological approaches to understanding
      and treating disease-related pain. Annu Rev Psychol 2005;56:601–30.
[12]  Keefe FJ, Ahles TA, Sutton L, Dalton J, Baucom D, Pope MS, Knowles V, McKinstry E, Fursten-
      berg C, Syrjala K, et al. Partner-guided cancer pain management at the end of life: a preliminary
      study. J Pain Symptom Manage 2005;29:263–72.
[13]  Keefe FJ, Lefebvre JC, Egert J, Affleck G, Sullivan MJ, Caldwell DS. The relationship of gender
      to pain, pain behavior, and disability in osteoarthritis patients: the role of catastrophizing. Pain
      2000;87:325–34.
[14]  Keefe FJ, Lipkus I, Lefebvre JC, Hurwitz H, Clipp E, Smith J, Porter L. The social context of gas-
      trointestinal cancer pain: a preliminary study examining the relation of patient pain catastroph-
      izing to patient perceptions of social support and caregiver stress and negative responses. Pain
      2003;103:151–6.
[15]  Keefe FJ, Somers TJ, Martire LM. Psychological interventions and lifestyle modifications for
      arthritis pain management. Rheum Dis Clin North Am 2008;34:351–68.
[16]  Lazarus R, Folkman S. Stress, appraisal, and coping. New York: Springer; 1984.
[17]  Lubeck DP, Grossfeld G, Ray PS, Flanders S, Penson D, Carroll PR. Health-related quality of life
      (HRQOL) and sociodemographic profiles of African American men with prostate cancer: data
      from CaPSURE. In: Program and abstracts of the American Urological Association 95th Annual
      Meeting, April 29–May 4, 2000, Atlanta, Georgia. Abstract 69.
[18]  Manne S, Badr H. Intimacy and relationship processes in couples' psychosocial adaptation to
      cancer. Cancer 2008;112(Suppl):2541–55.
[19]  Manne SL, Ostroff JS, Winkel G, Manne SL, Ostroff JS, Winkel G, Fox K, Grana G, Miller E,
      Ross S, Frazier T. Couple-focused group intervention for women with early stage breast cancer.
      J Consult Clin Psychol 2005;73:634–46.
[20]  National Cancer Institute. Prostate cancer progress report: addressing the recommendations of
      the Prostate Cancer Progress Review Group. Washington, DC: U.S. Department of Health and
      Human Services, National Institutes of Health; 2004.

[21] Northouse LL, Mood DW, Schafenacker A, Montie JE, Sandler HM, Forman JD, Hussain M, Pienta KJ, Smith DC, Kershaw T. Randomized clinical trial of a family intervention for prostate cancer patients and their spouses. Cancer 2007;110:2809–18.

[22] Porter LS, Keefe FJ, Baucom DH, Hurwitz H, Moser B, Patterson E, Kim HJ. Partner-assisted emotional disclosure for patients with cancer: results from a randomized controlled trial. Cancer 2009;115(Suppl):4326–38.

[23] Reddick BK, Nanda JP, Campbell L, Ryman DG, Gaston-Johansson F. Examining the influence of coping with pain on depression, anxiety, and fatigue among women with breast cancer. J Psychosoc Oncol 2005;23:137–57.

[24] Somers TJ, Keefe FJ, Porter LP. Understanding and enhancing patient and partner adjustment to disease-related pain: a biopsychosocial perspective. In: Moore RJ, editor. Biobehavioral approaches to pain. New York: Springer; 2009. p 95–124.

[25] Syrjala KL, Cummings C, Donaldson GW. Hypnosis or cognitive behavioral training for the reduction of pain and nausea during cancer treatment: a controlled clinical trial. Pain 1992;48:137–46.

[26] Ward SS, Donovan H, Gunnarsdottir S, Serlin R, Shapiro GR, Hughes S. A randomized trial of a representational intervention to decrease cancer pain (RIDcancerPain). Health Psychol 2008;27:59–67.

[27] Zaza C, Baine N. Cancer pain and psychosocial factors: a critical review of the literature. J Pain Symptom Manage 2002;24:526–42.

*Correspondence to:* Francis J. Keefe, PhD, Pain Prevention and Treatment Program, Duke University Medical Center, PO Box 90399, Durham, NC 27708, USA. Email: keefe003@mc.duke.edu.

# Attention Management

## Stephen Morley

*Institute of Health Sciences, University of Leeds, Leeds, United Kingdom*

Pain has a unique capacity to *interrupt;* it captures our attention and makes it difficult for us to disengage from the unwanted experience that fills our consciousness [20]. The presence of persistent pain has subtle consequences on psychological functions that depend on attention. For example, people with pain complain of difficulties in memory and concentration [31], and experimental studies confirm that these problems can be attributed to a degradation in attentional processes [16,17,29]. Despite the seemingly automatic way in which pain captures one's attention, individuals engage in effortful attempts to "push" the experience out of mind [2,6,34]. However, efforts to control mental experiences, particularly unpleasant ones, can have ironic effects and result in a rebound effect when the individual disengages from the task [27,67]. Nevertheless, the prospect of exploiting our natural predisposition to attempt to control our attention to pain to produce "psycho-analgesia" remains alluring and has been subject to considerable research at both the clinical and basic science levels.

This chapter focuses on the principles underpinning the use of psychological strategies to manipulate attention for therapeutic purposes.

*Cancer Pain: From Molecules to Suffering*
edited by Judith A. Paice, Rae F. Bell, Eija A. Kalso, and Olaitan A. Soyannwo
IASP Press, Seattle, © 2010

I have chosen to focus on pain in general rather than exclusively on pain arising as a consequence of cancer. The reason for this is twofold. The first is purely pragmatic in that there is an extensive literature on pain in general, especially with respect to experimental studies, which are essential for the development of testable models that might have clinical applications. The second is the assumption there are substantial commonalities in the experience of pain and in the psychological processes and mechanisms that underlie that experience and transcend the origin of pain. That is not to deny that different pains may invoke different processes and mechanisms to varying degrees. It is unlikely, for example, that brief controlled experimental pain or a scald received while cooking would elicit the same degree of threat as pain on movement in back pain [35] or a change in the experience of pain in a person with cancer pain [6]. However, understanding the critical parameters that relate to threat within and between pains of different origins will facilitate our ability to devise suitable clinical interventions based on sound principles.

## The Context of Interruption

Pain always occurs in the context of a larger behavioral framework, and it is convenient to consider the impact of pain at three levels: interruption, interference, and identity. Interruption refers to the capacity of pain to interrupt ongoing behavior and cognition on a moment-to-moment basis. Pain demands that attention be switched from its current focus of engagement. How pain captures attention has been the focus of an extended laboratory-based experimental research program over the last 10–15 years, and it is apparent that the characteristics of pain stimuli (bottom-up influences) are highly influential in determining the degree of interruption to ongoing behavior. Interruption is also influenced by top-down influences such a person's tendency to catastrophize. For patients with chronic pain, repeated interruption can lead to a heightened awareness of pain and hypervigilance for pain-related cues [12]. Interruption may be particularly threatening for such patients because it leads to the establishment of negative biases that may direct attention away from current tasks toward pain and the threats implied by pain, such as impending disability.

Interruption by pain such as that experienced in the laboratory or acute pain in everyday settings, although unpleasant, is not necessarily a significant problem. Pain may interrupt behavior momentarily but it may still be possible to complete a task satisfactorily. Repeated or persistent interruption by pain does, however, have an impact in that it *interferes* with a person's capacity to complete everyday tasks. The effect of interference is reflected in the frequent reports of frustration made by chronic pain patients and in the extent of disability [61]. Importantly, the degree of interference is not a direct function of the magnitude of pain sensation. There is substantial evidence that the extent of interference is related to both cognitive factors such as fear appraisals [35] and discriminative stimuli and reinforcers in the wider environment [26].

As interference persists, it affects patients' capacity to pursue their important life goals. Not only are patients unable to pursue important goals, but they may also be drawn into the futile and misdirected pursuit of the goal of eliminating pain [21]. One consequence of the unremitting pursuit of this goal is that attention to other important life goals is displaced and as a consequence these individuals' meaning in life, their very *identity*, may be deeply affected [15]. The central issue is whether repeated interference will have an impact on the self-schemata and thus on the person's identity. As Chapman and Gavrin [9] observe, "painful arthritis in the fingers would have a minor impact for most middle-aged people, but could be devastating for a professional concert musician because it affects what he or she is and *can hope to be in the future.*" It is the threat to people's sense of who they are and who they might become that generates a range of emotional responses including depression, fear, and anxiety [40,51].

This brief outline suggests several potentially key facets by which we might contextualize the experience of pain and a person's attempt to modulate their experience of it by managing attention. First, as we progress from processes related to interruption through to interference to identity, the experience of pain and associated behavior is likely to be determined by a plethora of factors not related directly to the stimulus characteristics of the pain. Second, pain generates conflict at every level: either pay attention to the pain or pursue ongoing goal-related activity (a point cogently noted by Wall [63]). Third, goal-related activity can be construed at several levels, from simple motor tasks to extended activities that are fundamental to the way in which individuals may define themselves. The interruptive impact of pain can generate emotional responses, ranging from frustration at the inability to complete a task to complex emotions related to anxiety, depression, guilt, and shame that are a function of the higher-order "identity-level" goals that are being interrupted. (See Carver and Scheier [8] for an example of an analysis of how goal interruption and conflict can color one's emotional experience.) This sequence of events provides the cognitive and affective basis for top-down influences that modulate our attention to pain and our attempts to control it.

# Attention as Limited Channel Capacity: A Brief Review and Comment on Clinical Interventions

For the most part, contemporary psychological approaches have been influenced by a view of attention derived from an essentially structural model informed by information theory. This approach, illustrated in Fig. 1, characterizes the problem of attention (how to account for why our conscious experience is restricted at any one moment to just a few of the available stimuli) as one of limited channel capacity [24,30,39]. The multiple sensory stimuli (bottom of Fig. 1) compete to enter consciousness. The limited capacity, represented by the ellipse, indicates those stimuli that are selected. Crudely speaking, willful attentional control is attained when the individual is able to redirect selection toward other stimuli, analogous to moving the ellipse right or left in the figure. Thus, with respect to pain, the aim of any intervention is to facilitate a person's ability to redirect his or her attention from painful stimuli. Two questions immediately follow: (1) What strategies are most appropriate? and (2) What are the most appropriate alternative foci for attention? The clinical approach to this problem appears to have been rather pragmatic and driven more by observations of individuals' naturally occurring strategies than by principled theoretical consideration and analysis.

In 1989 Fernandez and Turk [24] reviewed an already extensive literature. They noted the variety of strategies and terminology used and the problems that this heterogeneity posed for determining the effectiveness of strategies. They adopted an empirically derived classification developed from a sorting task given to undergraduate students. The resulting sorts were subjected to multidimensional scaling and cluster analysis from which seven classes of strategy were derived [59]. These classes are shown in Fig. 2, which also shows the results of a meta-analysis of 51 studies identified by Fernandez and Turk as reporting the effects of cognitive strategies for modifying pain. The figure shows the mean effect size ($d$) for differences between the strategy and a control and its 95% confidence interval. Inspection of these data suggests that all strategies are statistically more effective than a control, although it is not always clear what the control condition is or how well it controls for alternative plausible hypotheses. There is, however, one analysis (labeled "cognitive versus expectancy") in which a variety of strategies were tested against conditions designed to control for the effect of expectation of therapeutic gain; here the effect of treatment can still be detected. There are two other important points to note about this analysis. First, it is not clear how the outcome measures are defined; they appear to have been aggregated within the various analyses. The measures used varied widely, including estimates of pain intensity, pain affect, or overall pain severity; tolerance time; or a threshold measure. How well these measures are related to measures of clinical interest is debatable. Second, many of the studies were conducted

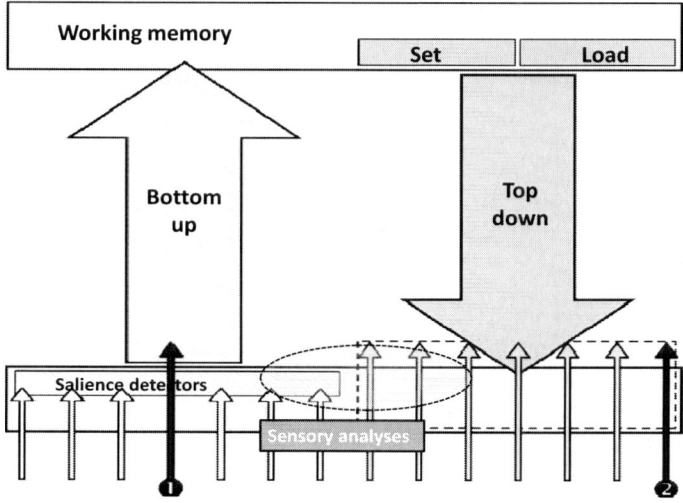

**Fig. 1.** Diagrammatic representation of the basic attentional system explained in the text. The figure is adapted with permission from Legrain et al. [36].

in nonclinical populations using a simple experimental design in which participants are exposed to a controlled pain stimulus, often the cold pressor task, and instructed to engage in an activity that directs their attention to alternative sources of stimulation. A measure of pain experience is then taken. There are obvious differences between this experimental setup and many clinical pain conditions. In experimental studies, pain is often predictable, attributable to an identifiable external source, limited in duration and intensity, escapable, and controlled—and for ethical reasons, participants are told that the stimuli are not harmful. Moreover, there is an inherent paradox in the methodology in that participants are asked to switch their attention away from pain and then make a judgment about the pain, which requires them to attend to it [18].

In another early review, also framed by the limited channel capacity model, McCaul and Malott [39] examined the evidence for four

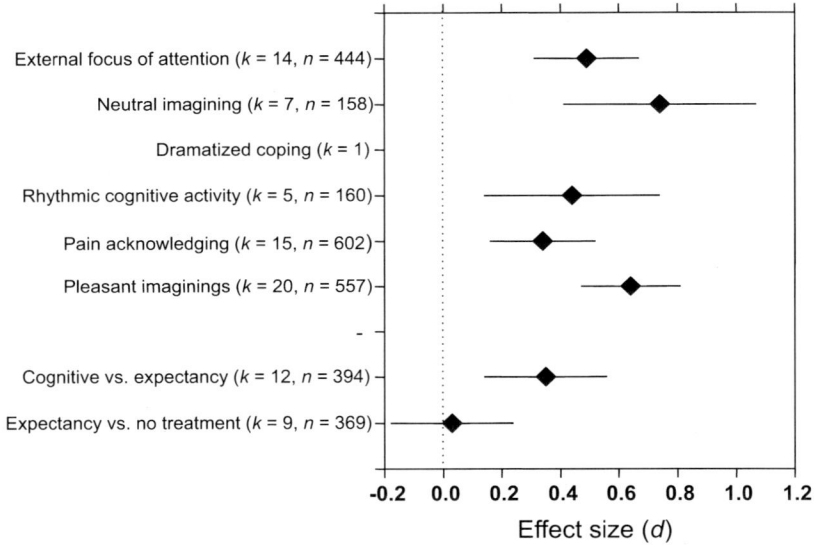

**Fig. 2.** The effectiveness of various cognitive control strategies on pain experience shown as an effect size (diamonds indicate $d$, standardized mean difference) and its 95% confidence interval (error bars). The dotted line at effect size = 0 indicates no difference between comparisons. The figure is constructed from data reported by Fernandez and Turk in Tables III to IX [24]. The number of studies ($k$) and the number of individuals ($n$) used to estimate the effect size for each class of strategy are shown. No estimate for the "dramatized coping" class is available. The lower two estimates are for comparisons of a cognitive treatment against a control for expectancy effects and for expectancy against no treatment.

principles: (1) performing an attentionally demanding task would reduce *distress* from a pain stimulus; (2) tasks that involved greater use of attentional capacity would be more effective modulators of distress; (3) distraction would be more effective for mild pain stimuli; (4) compared with re-definitional strategies (strategies that require the person to re-label the pain experience, often by focusing on nonaffective aspects of their experience), distraction would be more effective at low pain intensity, and the reverse would be true for high-intensity pain stimuli. There were data to support all of these principles, but they were not always compelling. The authors noted that "distraction is effective (within limits) for acute, and particularly for laboratory encounters with painful stimuli," but the evidence for the utility of distraction in clinical settings was less marked. With respect to the fourth principle (the interaction between attentional strategy and pain intensity), McCaul and Malott considered that the data were difficult to interpret because of marked variation between the studies. Nevertheless they expressed a degree of cautious optimism for the principle.

In a second review of this literature, Cioffi [10] addressed attention to somatic stimuli in general. She attempted to answer a different question: "Is it more adaptive to direct one's attention away from a potentially unpleasant sensation or to focus one's attention on it?" This approach indirectly picks up McCaul and Malott's issue relating to the redefinition of painful stimuli. Cioffi's attempt to provide a clear answer to this question was hampered both by methodological variability in the studies and by what she described as the failure to consistently separate the *direction* of attention from the *content* of attention. She again noted the marked differences between laboratory-based experimental studies and those in the clinical context, underlining the inherent variation in individuals' prior expectations and experiences of their somatic symptoms and their current concerns and goals. One essential element appears to be the capacity to separate the sensory experience of somatic stimuli from one's cognitive-affective response [37]. Cioffi's analysis identified several mechanisms by which sensory monitoring (paying attention to the sensory quality of bodily sensations) could produce beneficial outcomes. First, it might prevent the development of a higher-order negative affective representation of the stimulus. While this might be effective for a novel stimulus in a research setting (e.g., the cold pressor pain test), people with clinical pain have often experienced the pain repeatedly, and higher-order representations and appraisals such as catastrophizing are likely to be well established. Under these conditions, sensory monitoring might inhibit access to the affective representation of the pain and thereby reduce distress [37]. In Cioffi's words, sensory monitoring "drains the meaning out of somatic awareness." Second, sensory monitoring may allow individuals to obtain new information about the stimulus that is not otherwise available for conscious processing if they are engaged in distraction. Sensory monitoring may enable them to notice subtle fluctuations in intensity and the quality of sensation, and subsequent interpretation of this information may improve their ability to predict the event, thereby reducing the novelty and unexpectedness of the stimulus and leading to a more benign, less threatening interpretation of the event. Third, by willfully paying attention to physical sensations, individuals may gain perceived control of their mental processes, and the benefits of such control for wellbeing are well known. Finally, Cioffi raised the important question of what happens when attempts at distraction fail, as they surely must in the face of the imperative attention-demanding nature of pain [20]. The failure to exert mental control may lead to increased negative affect, an ironic increment in the experience of pain [67], and a subsequent incremental appraisal of hopelessness and despair by the sufferer. Under these conditions, an active reengagement with a sensory monitoring strategy ought to be beneficial.

## Attention Management in Clinical Practice

Despite the absence of a robust theoretical account that would direct clinical interventions, attention management has been included in many cognitive-behavioral treatment (CBT) programs. In their 1999 meta-analysis of CBT, Morley et al. [41] noted the inclusion of components of attention management in many of the CBT "packages" delivered in the trials. (An unpublished analysis showed that 16 of the 21 trials included at least one treatment arm in which some form of attention management training was given.) An example of the complex CBT intervention is given by Keefe and his colleagues [33,66], who describe a manualized protocol that has been used in several high-quality randomized controlled trials and can be implemented in routine treatment [43]. The overall program comprises four behavioral components (activity pacing, pleasant event scheduling, social reinforcement, and time-contingent medication) and four cognitive components (cognitive restructuring, problem solving, distraction, and relapse prevention). Distraction—the attention management strategy—has three components. The first component is training in progressive muscle relaxation in which patients are encouraged to engage in mini-practice trials throughout the day. The second is the use of visual imagery, including (a) learning to generate pleasant imagery and emphasizing the inclusion of imagined material from all senses; (b) training in focal point distraction, i.e., willfully directing one's attention to a feature in the immediate environment; and (c) a counting task that involves counting backwards from a given number. This task can be enhanced by asking the individual to generate a visual image of the numbers on a screen. The third component is active homework in which patients are encouraged to practice the strategies for brief period (a minute or so) up to 20 times a day. While these strategies have obvious face validity, estimating the effectiveness of this component of treatment is impossible because it is embedded in a range of other intervention strategies, and there does not appear to be a systematic series of studies investigating the impact of the various treatment components.

The attention management strategies reported by Keefe and his colleagues represent a small sample of those available [24], but until recently there was no treatment manual that provided an integrated approach to the various components. Morley and colleagues [42] described a demonstration project to develop a treatment manual that incorporated many of the attention management strategies reported in the literature. Following an extensive literature search, including obtaining unpublished treatment manuals, they developed a manual that was reviewed by a small panel of expert clinicians who critically evaluated the material and its sequencing. Revisions were undertaken to incorporate relevant feedback. An outline of the manual's structure is given in Table I. There has only been one attempt to evaluate this package of techniques using a simple uncontrolled design comparing performance on range of pre- and post-treatment measures [23]. Although statistical change was observed, it is impossible to make any strong inferences about the clinical utility of the treatment.

Table I
Outline of a treatment manual for attention management

*Module 1: Engaging the Patient and Basic Attention Management Skills*
Aims: To assess the patients' current use of attention management strategies; to assess the patient's attitude towards using and developing these strategies; to collaboratively reformulate patients' experience of pain to include its modulation by psychological factors; to outline the idea of attention management and the course; to demonstrate (experientially) the basic features of attention; to provide an opportunity to rehearse basic skills of attention management.
Sample procedures:
1.      Group sharing of current strategies of pain management
2.      Demonstrations of attention (a) directed listening; (b) paradoxical instructions: "Don't think of pink elephants"
3.      Mini-relaxation

*Module 2: Attention Diversion Strategies*
Aims: To make links between patients' current practice of attention strategies and their use as effective skills; to improve concentration, through the use of "mindfulness"; to broaden the concept of attention-diversion to include focal points; to consider the ways in which attention diversion may be used appropriately; to instill the need to practice manipulating attention as a skill to be developed; to discuss pain vigilance and consider how attention management may help patients broaden their identity beyond their pain.
Sample procedures:
1.      Increasing mindfulness: describing a candle in detail
2.      Focal points, e.g., switching attention within the body: breathing

*Module 3: Imagery and Imagination*
Aims: To assess patients' own use of imagery when coping with pain; to involve patients in elaborating images, making particular use of the sensory modalities; to re-conceptualize the use of imagery and imagination as useful tools in coping with pain; to collaboratively explore the potential of pain transformation techniques; to give support and advice on how to use imagery and imagination strategies.
Sample procedures:
1.      Guided imagery, e.g., cutting a lemon
2.      Transforming an image; exploring metaphors for pain

*Module 4: Intense Pain and Flare-ups*
Aims: To identify negative thoughts and images that patients experience when in severe pain, and to explore whether patients have means of coping with intense pain; to establish the ways in which negative thoughts and images contribute to patients' experience of pain; to establish a basic principle in dealing with severe pain—a non-confrontational approach; to guide patients through the use of specific coping skills—the "signal breath" and coping self-statements; to encourage patients to use the coping techniques through structured advice and homework.
Sample procedures:
1.      Assessing catastrophizing—identifying vicious cycles
2.      Signal breath technique—defusing catastrophic thoughts
3.      Developing coping statements

*Source:* Morley et al. [42]; reproduced by permission of Taylor and Francis. The complete manual and supplementary documentation are available in pdf format at: http://www.leeds.ac.uk/lihs/psychiatry/staff/morley.htm.

# Hypnosis as Attention Management

As is apparent in guides to its clinical implementation, hypnosis would appear to be a procedure, *par excellence,* that seeks to alter the focus of a person's attention [3,52]. Price and Barrell's phenomenological analysis [4,46] identified five common features of hypnotic experience, including "an absorbed and sustained focus of attention." (The other four characteristics were a feeling of wellbeing; a absence of censorious, judgmental monitoring of experience; reduced orientation toward time, place, and self; and finally, the experience of automaticity of one's actions.)

Several recent narrative reviews have summarized the evidence for the effectiveness of hypnosis. These related reviews provide qualitative comparisons of hypnosis with various controls but have not combined the various studies to produce quantitative estimates (effect sizes) of its impact.

Patterson and Jensen [44] reviewed the available data from randomized controlled trials for procedural pain such as burn care wound dressing and bone marrow aspiration, and also for chronic pain (headache, fibromyalgia, and cancer-related breast pain). The review was confined to adults and concluded that hypnosis directed at producing analgesia was superior to no treatment, to standard or routine care, and to control treatments that had attempted to control for nonspecific factors such as the degree of therapeutic attention given to participants. However, there was no evidence that hypnosis was superior to other active nonhypnotic treatments, namely autogenic training and progressive muscular relaxation. The same authors recently updated their review [50] and reached similar conclusions. Hypnosis has also been used to manage procedure-related pain in children, and in a review of controlled trials, Accardi and Milling [1] came to a conclusion that was highly congruent with the data from studies on adults: hypnosis is more effective than standard medical care in reducing pain and discomfort and is equivalent to distraction-based techniques.

Stoelb et al. [50] noted the equivalence of hypnosis to "treatments that contain hypnotic elements." Why relaxation and imagery should be regarded as specific to hypnosis is debatable, but this comment does underscore problems in evaluating the mechanisms of complex multicomponent treatments such as hypnotic and nonhypnotic approaches to control attention. The traditional strategy in psychotherapy research is to use dismantling designs [32] to conduct a component analysis. As with so much of research on the effects of psychological treatments for pain, there is evidence for superiority when judged against a set of controls that arguably cannot truly match the treatment for a variety of known nonspecific effects such as expectation and the structure and experience of treatment. As a consequence, it is difficult to conclude if the observed treatment effects are due to specific components that are unique to hypnosis or other methods of attention management or whether nonspecific effects account for the observed differences between treatments [22,41,64,65].

We need to turn to experimental analyses of the procedure to gain some insight into possible mechanisms. A series of experiments by Rainville and Price and their collaborators are illuminating in this respect [49]. The framework for these studies is an account of pain that distinguishes between the sensory intensity component and the affective component of pain [45,60]. Briefly, in addition to generating sensory experience, nociceptive input is associated with an immediate appraisal of intrusion and threat, accompanied by autonomic and somatic arousal. The immediate experience of pain unpleasantness is one of momentary emotional states of distress, annoyance, and fear linked to the intensity of the stimulation. This immediate component of pain affect is distinguished from the more extended, or secondary, affective component, which is the consequence of appraising the longer-term implications of pain and results in frustration, misery, anger, and anxiety. The distinction between sensory-intensity and affective components is reflected in neuroimaging studies [49,53].

Hypnosis has been used as a tool to explore the phenomenological distinctions made in the model. These studies indicate that *specific* hypnotic instructions directed at the sensory and affective components have relatively specific effects. Suggestions to decrease or increase the sensory component were accompanied by corresponding changes in ratings of both sensory-intensity *and* unpleasantness, whereas suggestions to modulate the affective component produced corresponding changes in unpleasantness only [48]. Further studies demonstrated that hypnotic induction of negative emotions consistently increased ratings of pain unpleasantness, as did a hypnotic suggestion aimed to increase a person's desire for pain relief [47]. These, and other studies, demonstrate a degree of specificity between the hypnotic instruction and particular outcomes. They also indicate the critical role of affect in modulating pain experience. Such refined distinctions are often lost in clinical studies that tend to use measures that essentially aggregate experience and use many facets of hypnotic procedures in an attempt to affect pain experience.

# A Functional Account of Pain and Attention

In the mid-1990s, Eccleston and Crombez and their colleagues began a research program guided by a different conceptualization of attention [20]. While they still acknowledged many aspects of the general limited channel capacity model, their approach was essentially functional. They asked the question: "What is the function of attention?" Attention is construed as a process that allows the organism to select an appropriate behavior for action. In essence, the function of attention is to manage the efficient engagement of resources necessary to fulfil the requirements of an ongoing task, but also to retain an awareness of the demands of higher-priority tasks. This approach is inherently a goal-action perspective in which individuals regulate their behavior to achieve multiple goals. It recognizes the importance of both top-down influences (cognitive and affective representations of goal elements) and bottom-up influences (e.g., stimulus characteristics) in determining the immediate focus of attention. The functional perspective had been elaborated with respect to attention in other sensory modalities and by other pain researchers [62,63], but Eccleston and Crombez employed a systematic experimental approach to answer the question "How and why does pain first capture attention?" [20], arguing that answers to this question will help us to understand how pain may be displaced from focal awareness. A simple but radically different experimental model was required to answer the question. Rather than induce pain and impose a distraction, the investigators require participants to engage in a task while pain stimuli are presented. The attentional properties of the pain can be assessed by examining the extent to which task performance is changed (usually degraded). This *primary task paradigm* is diagrammed in Fig. 3. The paradigm allows systematic examination of three components: the stimulus characteristics,

the competitive nature of the primary task, and variations in the participant's characteristics. Whereas the latter are mainly assessed by correla-
tional methods, both the stimulus and task characteristics are capable of
experimental analysis.

It is clear that pain stimuli that are intense, novel, and threatening
and have the capacity to capture attention with a degree of automaticity.
Moreover, there is evidence that characteristics such as heightened fear
of pain and the tendency to make catastrophizing appraisals enhance the
disruptive effects of pain stimuli [13,14,28]. It is also apparent that once
pain has captured attention from the ongoing task, it is difficult to disengage from the pain, and this too is enhanced by characteristics such as
catastrophizing [54–56]. Applying the primary task paradigm to clinical
pain is problematic because experimental control of the pain stimulus
is not possible. It is, however, possible to vary the demands of the primary task and correlate the interruptive effect of naturally varying pain
levels. For example, Eccleston [19] showed that chronic pain patients

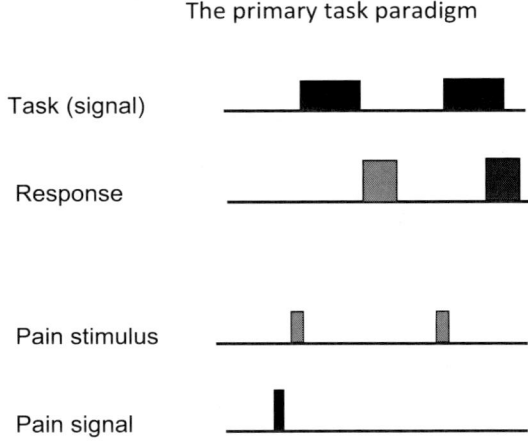

**Fig. 3.** This figure presents the basic experimental operations in the primary task paradigm as four traces. The primary task is defined in the upper two traces, in which a brief
signal is presented to which the participant must make a response. The reaction time to
the task signal is recorded. The third trace represents the experimental pain stimulus (frequently electric shock). The timing of the pain stimulus relative to the task signal may
be systematically varied and its effect on the response observed. Typically pain occurring
in the early part of the task signal is more interruptive than pain in the latter part. The
fourth trace represents the addition of a nonpainful stimulus signaling the future occurrence of pain. The interruptive effect of this stimulus may also be quantified.

with high-intensity pain showed significantly impaired performance on an attentionally demanding task when compared with pain patients with low levels of reported pain and control participants without pain. Differences between the groups were not observed when the primary task was less attentionally demanding.

More recently, Goubert et al. [27] examined the impact of distraction (a relatively simple button-pressing task in response to randomly presented tones) when chronic pain patients performed a bag-lifting task. The bag-lifting procedure may be threatening to a proportion of patients, and it generally results in a temporary increase in pain. Although there was no difference between the distraction and non-distraction conditions in the increase in pain during bag lifting, further analyses revealed that participants' tendency to catastrophize about their pain was related to greater attention to pain and less engagement with the distracting task, as evidenced by reaction times to the signal tone. Finally, Goubert et al. observed the paradoxical effect of *increased* pain levels after patients had made the effort to engage in the distracting task. This phenomenon—the reemergence of mental content after effortful attempts to suppress it—is known as ironic control [67,68] and has been observed in for a range of unwanted experiences. It has been observed in laboratory models of pain [11], but it does not appear to have been systematically documented or explored in the clinical setting, yet it clearly has major implications for clinical interventions of attentional control.

Despite the theoretical advantages of the functional approach to attention, experimental investigation using the primary task paradigm has been constrained by the difficulties in developing primary tasks that might plausibly match even mild experimental pain with respect to their affective-motivational characteristics. Anecdotally, it would appear that attention to pain stimuli is effectively "trumped" only under conditions when the competing goal is very demanding, when there is a motivational state that is more threatening than pain (e.g., imminent death [5]) or where a high level of behavioral activity is demanded and the goal is highly focused, as in competitive sports [63]. Unfortunately, neither of these conditions suggests a plausible candidate for a clinical intervention, and they are either difficult to replicate in the laboratory or it would be ethically dubious to do so.

Reframing the problem as one of goal conflict may be beneficial. Pain stimuli elicit a threat to bodily integrity and the urge to escape and avoid: an avoidance goal. The theory suggests that primary tasks that have greater priority for the individual will be less likely to be interrupted by pain stimuli. Competitor tasks may vary on many features, such as affective valence, cognitive complexity, and behavioral response requirements, as is evident by the range of strategies observed in clinical studies of distraction and documented by Fernandez and Turk [24]. At best, laboratory tasks have been mildly affectively positive in tone and probably not significantly meaningful to elicit a significant motivational state. In a simple two-goal situation, such as "avoid harm versus pursue social engagement," maintaining attention to the social task will be governed by the interplay of the bottom-up and top-down influences of both the pain and social engagement task. If we assume constancy in pain stimulus characteristics, then reducing the threat value of the pain stimuli will facilitate attention to the social engagement task. As noted above, focusing on the sensory characteristics of the pain may facilitate this reduction in threat value. Exposure to stimuli is established as an effective method for reducing threat, with successful application in pain [25,35]. Increasing the stimulus demands of the distraction strategies (e.g., with elaborated imagery [24]) and the affective-motivational characteristics of the competing goal [57] should facilitate the study participants' ability to switch their attention away from pain. This somewhat brief analysis does not take into account two other potentially important elements. First, the motivational valence of the nonpain task is likely to be influential. Tasks with an avoidance motive (to *avoid* social disapproval) may be less suitable distracters as they are thought to be underpinned by the same neurobiological functions responsible for aversion and punishment as well as pain, which may detract from their effectiveness. Second, at a practical level, failure to achieve success in the distracting task is likely to elicit negative affect that may make switching attention from pain more problematic. As a consequence, the introduction of attention management protocols calls for careful analysis of both the pain and the competing tasks and requires the development of strategies that are sensitive to the dynamic fluctuation of affect. Many skillful and sensitive clinicians and clinical researchers have provided excellent accounts of how to work in this area [52,66].

The functional model put forward by Eccleston and Crombez [20] suggests that under most circumstances, it is implausible to *prevent* pain from capturing attention; pain simply has motivational priority in most circumstances. The problem of attention management is therefore one of developing strategies that enable the individual to disengage from the motivational urge to escape pain on a moment by moment basis.

# Conclusions

Trying to distract oneself from ongoing pain is a natural response to an unwanted mental experience. It seems that the development of most clinical strategies has been driven by implementing these naturally occurring strategies and adding a general psychological model to provide a rationale for any effects observed. The evidence that the treatments, whether they be various distraction effects or hypnotic procedures, are effective in clinical practice is modest, and if they do work, the mechanisms by which any effects are obtained are debatable. In contrast to laboratory studies, methods used in clinical settings are often complex and contain multiple components. These components may affect any one of a number of psychological processes, thus presenting us with considerable methodological challenges.

This model of attention to painful stimuli is predicated on an analysis of attention that is independent of any specific pathology. It is essentially a normative account that can be applied to any pain arising from any pathology. However, it is likely that features associated with particular diagnostic classes will present specific challenges to the therapeutic application of the model. There are two features of cancer-related pain that may present therapeutic problems. The first example illustrates a potential influence on the threat value of pain that may be difficult to modify. Some patients with cancer-related pain report using pain to monitor the progress of their disease. Subtle shifts in the spatial-temporal and sensory characteristics of pain may be particularly threatening if they are interpreted as indicative of disease progression [6,35]. This presents challenges to clinical interventions that might be aimed at understanding and modifying individuals' common-sense model of their illness or attempts at threat reduction through the use of exposure-based methods

[25]. The second example concerns the salience and availability of competitive alternative goals with significant, positive, affective-motivational characteristics to which attention may be diverted. This problem may be especially prominent at the end of life when a person's cognitive and behavioral functioning is severely limited.

Undoubtedly, clinicians will continue to use attention management methods. The inherent plausibility and apparent absence of harmful effects of these methods will ensure their continued attractiveness as psychological management strategies. Attention management may hold greater promise as our scientific understanding of attention develops [36,58] and is translated into clinical practice. Construing the problem as a process in which individuals learn to disengage from the imperative of pain stimuli on a moment to moment basis will have implications for the design of clinical outcome studies. For example, the use of pre- or post-treatment designs is probably inappropriate because they cannot capture the momentary impact of applying a treatment strategy, and post-treatment retrospective ratings are likely to be biased. Studies that can capture the dynamics of treatment will need to be developed. The application of daily process methodology [38] to understanding the dynamic relationship between the pain experience and the pursuit of goal-related activity and its capacity to moderate pain is promising. Such methods allow us to investigate important general processes in the context of individual variation, which is so evident in clinical research.

# Acknowledgments

My thanks go to Geert Crombez, Chris Eccleston, Johan Vlaeyen, and Stefaan van Damme for collegial discussions and friendship over the years. Many of the ideas in this chapter come from their insights and would be better expressed by them.

# References

[1]   Accardi MC, Milling LS. The effectiveness of hypnosis for reducing procedure-related pain in children and adolescents: a comprehensive methodological review. J Behav Med 2009;32:328–39.
[2]   Affleck G, Urrows S, Tennen H, Higgins P, Abeles M. Sequential daily relations of sleep, pain intensity, and attention to pain among women with fibromyalgia. Pain 1996;68:363–8.

[3]    Barber J. Hypnosis and suggestion in the treatment of pain: a clinical guide. New York: Norton; 1996.
[4]    Barber J. Hypnotic analgesia: mechanisms of action and clinical implications. In: Price DD, Bushnell MC, editors. Psychological methods of pain control: basic science and clinical perspectives. Seattle: IASP Press; 2004. p. 269–300.
[5]    Beecher HK. The measurement of subjective responses. Oxford: Oxford University Press; 1959.
[6]    Buck R, Morley S. A daily process design study of attentional pain control strategies in the self-management of cancer pain. Eur J Pain 2006;10:385–98.
[7]    Carver CS. Self-regulation of action and affect. In: Baumeister RF, Vohs KD, editors. Handbook of self-regulation: research and applications, New York: Guilford Press; 2004. p. 13–39.
[8]    Carver CS, Scheier MF. On the self-regulation of behavior. Cambridge: Cambridge University Press; 1998.
[9]    Chapman CR, Gavrin J. Suffering: the contributions of persistent pain. Lancet 1999;353:2233–7.
[10]   Cioffi D. Beyond attentional strategies: a cognitive-perceptual model of somatic interpretation. Psychol Bull 1991;109:25–41.
[11]   Cioffi D, Holloway J. Delayed costs of suppressed pain. J Pers Soc Psychol 1993;64:274–82.
[12]   Crombez G. Hypervigilance and attention to pain: experimental and clinical evidence. In: Flor H, Kalso E, Dostrovsky JO, editors. Proceedings of the 11th World Congress on Pain. Seattle: IASP Press; 2006. p. 515–28.
[13]   Crombez G, Eccleston C, Baeyens F, Eelen P. When somatic information threatens, catastrophic thinking enhances attentional interference. Pain 1998;75:187–98.
[14]   Crombez G, Eccleston C, Baeyens F, Van Houdenhove B, Van Den Broeck A. Attention to chronic pain is dependent upon pain-related fear. J Psychosom Res 1999;47:403–10.
[15]   Crombez G, Morley S, McCracken L, Sensky T, Pincus T. Self, identity, and acceptance in chronic pain. In: Dostrovsky JO, Carr DB, Koltzenburg M, editors. Proceedings of the 10th World Congress on Pain: Progress in pain research and management, Vol. 24. Seattle: IASP Press; 2003. p. 651–9.
[16]   Dick BD, Rashiq S. Disruption of attention and working memory traces in individuals with chronic pain. Anesth Analg 2007;104:1223–9.
[17]   Dick BD, Verrier MJ, Harker KT, Rashiq S. Disruption of cognitive function in fibromyalgia syndrome. Pain 2008;139:610–6.
[18]   Eccleston C. The attentional control of pain: methodological and theoretical concerns. Pain 1995;63:3–10.
[19]   Eccleston C. Chronic pain and distraction: an experimental investigation into the role of sustained and shifting attention in the processing of chronic persistent pain. Behav Res Ther 1995;33:391–405.
[20]   Eccleston C, Crombez G. Pain demands attention: a cognitive-affective model of the interruptive function of pain. Psychol Bull 1999;125:356–66.
[21]   Eccleston C, Crombez G. Worry and chronic pain: a misdirected problem solving model. Pain 2007;132:233–6.
[22]   Eccleston C, Williams AC de C, Morley S. Psychological therapies for the management of chronic pain (excluding headache) in adults. Psychological therapies for the management of chronic pain (excluding headache) in adults. Cochrane Database Syst Rev 2009(2).
[23]   Elomaa MM, Williams AC de C, Kalso EA. Attention management as a treatment for chronic pain. Eur J Pain 2009;13:1062–7.
[24]   Fernandez E, Turk DC. The utility of cognitive coping strategies for altering pain perception: a meta-analysis. Pain 1989;38:123–35.
[25]   Flink IK, Nicholas MK, Boersma K, Linton SJ. Reducing the threat value of chronic pain: a preliminary replicated single-case study of interoceptive exposure versus distraction in six individuals with chronic back pain. Behav Res Ther 2009;47:721–8.
[26]   Fordyce WE. Behavioral methods for chronic pain and illness. St Louis: Mosby; 1976.
[27]   Goubert L, Crombez G, Eccleston C, Devulder J. Distraction from chronic pain during a pain-inducing activity is associated with greater post-activity pain. Pain 2004;110:220–7.
[28]   Goubert L, Crombez G, Van Damme S. The role of neuroticism, pain catastrophizing and pain-related fear in vigilance to pain: a structural equations approach. Pain 2004;107:234–41.
[29]   Grisart JM, Plaghki LH. Impaired selective attention in chronic pain patients. Eur J Pain 1999;3:325–33.
[30]   Hanson RW, Gerber KE. Coping with chronic pain. New York: Guilford Press; 1990.

[31] Jamison RN, Sbrocco T, Parris WC. The influence of problems with concentration and memory on emotional distress and daily activities in chronic pain patients. Int J Psychiatry Med 1988;18:183–91.

[32] Kazdin AE. Research design in clinical psychology, 3rd ed. Boston: Allyn & Bacon; 1998. p. 524.

[33] Keefe FJ, Beaupré PM, Gil KM, Rumble ME, Aspnes AK. Group therapy with patients with chronic pain. In: Turk DC, Gatchel RJ, editors. Psychological approaches to pain management: a practitioner's handbook. New York: Guilford Press; 2002. p. 234–55.

[34] Keefe FJ, Kashikar-Zuck S, Robinson E, Salley A, Beaupré P, Caldwell D, Baucom D, Haythornthwaite J. Pain coping strategies that predict patients' and spouses' ratings of patients' self-efficacy. Pain 1997;73:191–9.

[35] Leeuw M, Goossens MEJB, Linton SJ, Crombez G, Boersma K, Vlaeyen JWS. The fear-avoidance model of musculoskeletal pain: current state of scientific evidence. J Behav Med 2007;30:77–94.

[36] Legrain V, Damme SV, Eccleston C, Davis KD, Seminowicz DA, Crombez G. A neurocognitive model of attention to pain: behavioral and neuroimaging evidence. Pain 2009;144:230–2.

[37] Leventhal H, Everhart D. Emotion, pain and physical illness. In: Izard CE, editor. Emotions in personality and psychopathology. New York: Plenum Press; 1979. pp. 263–99.

[38] Litt MD, Shafer DM, Ibanez CR, Kreutzer DL, Tawfik-Yonkers Z. Momentary pain and coping in temporomandibular disorder pain: exploring mechanisms of cognitive behavioral treatment for chronic pain. Pain 2009;145:160–8.

[39] McCaul KD, Malott JM. Distraction and coping with pain. Psychol Bull 1984;95:516–33.

[40] Morley S, Eccleston C. The object of fear in pain. In: Asmundson GJ, Vlaeyen J, Crombez G, editors. Understanding and treating fear of pain. Oxford: Oxford University Press; 2004. p. 163–88.

[41] Morley S, Eccleston C, Williams A. Systematic review and meta-analysis of randomized controlled trials of cognitive behaviour therapy and behaviour therapy for chronic pain in adults, excluding headache. Pain 1999;80:1–13.

[42] Morley S, Shapiro DA, Biggs J. Developing a treatment manual for attention management in chronic pain. Cogn Behav Ther 2004;33:1–11.

[43] Naylor MR, Keefe FJ, Brigidi B, Naud S, Helzer JE. Therapeutic Interactive Voice Response for chronic pain reduction and relapse prevention. Pain 2008;134:335–45.

[44] Patterson DR, Jensen MP. Hypnosis and clinical pain. Psychol Bull 2003;129:495–521.

[45] Price DD. Psychological mechanisms of pain and analgesia. Seattle: IASP Press; 1999.

[46] Price DD, Barrell JJ. The structure of the hypnotic state: a self directed experiential study. In: Barrell JJ, editor. The experiential method: exploring the human experience. Acton, MA: Copely; 1990. p. 85–97.

[47] Rainville P, Bao QVH, Chretien P. Pain-related emotions modulate experimental pain perception and autonomic responses. Pain 2005;118:306–18.

[48] Rainville P, Carrier B, Hofbauer RK, Bushnell MC, Duncan GH. Dissociation of sensory and affective dimensions of pain using hypnotic modulation. Pain 1999;82:159–71.

[49] Rainville P, Price DD. The neurophenomenology of hypnosis and hypnotic analgesia. In: Price DD, Bushnell MC, editors. Psychological methods of pain control: basic science and clinical applications. Seattle: IASP Press; 2004. p. 235–67.

[50] Stoelb BL, Molton IR, Jensen MP, Patterson DR. The efficacy of hypnotic analgesia in adults: a review of the literature. Contemp Hypn 2009;26:24–39.

[51] Sutherland R, Morley S. Self-pain enmeshment: future possible selves, sociotropy, autonomy and adjustment to chronic pain. Pain 2008;137:366–77.

[52] Syrjala KL, Abrams JR. Hypnosis and imagery in the treatment of pain. In: Turk DC, Gatchel RJ, editors. Psychological approaches to pain management: a practitioner's handbook. New York: Guilford Press; 2002. p. 187–209.

[53] Tracey I. Imaging pain. Br J Anaesth 2008;101:32–9.

[54] Van Damme S, Crombez G, Eccleston C. Retarded disengagement from pain cues: the effects of pain catastrophizing and pain expectancy. Pain 2002;100:111–8.

[55] Van Damme S, Crombez G, Eccleston C. Disengagement from pain: the role of catastrophic thinking about pain. Pain 2004;107:70–6.

[56] Van Damme S, Crombez G, Eccleston C, Goubert L. Impaired disengagement from threatening cues of impending pain in a crossmodal cueing paradigm. Eur J Pain 2004;8:227–36.

[57] Verhoeven K, Crombez G, Van Damme S, Eccleston C, Van Ryckegem D, Morley S. Motivated distraction works for those who catastrophize about pain: an experimental analysis. Pain; in press.

[58]   Villemure C, Bushnell M. Cognitive modulation of pain: how do attention and emotion influence pain processing? Pain 2002;95:195–9.

[59]   Wack JT, Turk DC. Latent structure of strategies used to cope with nociceptive stimulation. Health Psychol 1984;3:27–43.

[60]   Wade JB, Dougherty LM, Archer CR, Price DD. Assessing the stages of pain processing: a multivariate analytical approach. Pain 1996;68:157–67.

[61]   Wade JB, Price DD, Hamer RM, Schwartz SM, Hart RP. An emotional component analysis of chronic pain. Pain 1990;40:303–10.

[62]   Wall PD. Introduction to the edition after this one. In: Wall PD, Melzack R, editors. The textbook of pain. Edinburgh: Churchill Livingston; 1994. p. 1–7.

[63]   Wall PD. Pain: the science of suffering. London: Weidenfeld & Nicholson; 1999.

[64]   Wampold BE. The great psychotherapy debate: models, methods, and findings. Mahwah, NJ: Lawrence Erlbaum Associates; 2001.

[65]   Wampold BE, Mondin GW, Moody M, Stich F, Benson K, Ahn HN. A meta-analysis of outcome studies comparing bona fide psychotherapies: empirically, "all must have prizes." Psychol Bull 1997;122:203–15.

[66]   Waters SJ, Campbell LC, Keefe FJ, Carson JW. The essence of cognitive-behavioral pain management. In: Dworkin RH, Breitbart W, editors. Psychosocial aspects of pain: a handbook for health care providers. Seattle: IASP Press; 2004. p. 261–83.

[67]   Wegner DM. Ironic processes of mental control. Psychol Rev 1994;101:34–52.

[68]   Wenzlaff RM, Wegner DM. Thought suppression. Ann Rev Psychol 2000;51:59–91.

**Correspondence to:** Stephen Morley, MPhil, PhD, Institute of Health Sciences, University of Leeds, Charles Thackrah Building, 101 Clarendon Road, Leeds, LS2 9LT, United Kingdom. Email: s.j.morley@leeds.ac.uk.

# Part VI

# Interaction, Education, Resources: How to Make a Difference

# Empathy in Cancer Pain

## Amanda C. de C. Williams[a] and Sue Gessler[b,c]

[a]Research Department of Clinical, Health and Educational Psychology,
[b]Gynaecological Cancer Centre, and [c]Elizabeth Garrett Anderson Institute for
Women's Health, University College London, London, United Kingdom

"The pain grew steadily worse and I grew more and more furious because nobody had ever talked about the physical pain."
Audre Lorde [34]: diary entry several days after her mastectomy

Pain is the greatest fear of the newly diagnosed cancer patient; it remains a serious concern at all stages of treatment, regardless of severity of illness [20]. Near the end of life, pain control is among the highest priorities for terminally ill patients and for those close to them [14]. However, it is also a common source of dissatisfaction and frustration throughout the course of cancer care. Coyle [11] provides eloquent descriptions from terminal cancer patients concerning opioids, "both a blessing and a burden," symbolizing disease progression, deterioration, and the end of hope for survival, but at the same time offering relief from pain that can make patients wish to die. These concerns may be difficult for patients to express or for health care professionals to intuit, concerned as they are with treatment or palliation by all means possible.

There are many reasons why cancer pain might not be talked about. Some in the medical establishment wish it away with generous doses of opioids; both patients and those treating them may prioritize cancer treatment and its adverse effects over pain; those around the patient may find it easier to empathize with more abstract existential dilemmas than with the reality of cancer pain. Empathy involves sharing, at least in part, the experience of the other, emotions as well as perspective, and that may be very hard to do within clinical settings. Surprisingly, pain is little mentioned in the literature on empathy in medical settings, a disproportionate amount of which concerns consultations in cancer, particularly around diagnosis ("breaking bad news"), treatment decisions, and the transition from treatment to palliative care.

The concept of empathy originated in aesthetics, referring to an active process of engaging with a work of art. It is now commonly used in psychology to refer to the capacity to *allow* one's own feelings to be engaged with the other, as well as an active and deliberate process of engagement.

## Empathy and Clinicians' Communication

Empathy is best understood, by reference to evolutionary theory, as a probable extension of parental care [60]. At its most elaborated, it refers to sharing the other's emotional state, understanding the reasons for this state, and adopting the other's perspective: many nonhuman species show emotional sharing, which underpins evolutionarily advantageous altruistic behaviors widespread in social animals [60]. Communication skills teaching, almost universal in medical and nursing curricula, embraces not only perspective-taking and emotional sharing but conveying empathy through behavior.

Empathic skills can be improved in medical students, at least in the short term, by training specific behavioral skills such as eye contact, active listening, and open questioning [55]: these practices emphasize perspective-taking more than emotional sharing [22]. Despite their plausibility, narrative and similar means are less effective in inducing empathic feelings and changing behavior. Unfortunately, these skills may show little change with training [3,37,47,49], or they may decline over time and with seniority, despite the evident benefits for patient and clinician of increased disclosure, adherence to advice, and patient and clinician satisfaction

[36,47]. One intensive training scheme [18] showed improvement over time in several skills, such as responsiveness to patient cues, but verbal expressions of empathy decreased (although subsequent reviews of the lower-scoring doctors' videos showed that they may have translated some empathic communication into nonverbal signs and gestures that were not scored). There is some evidence that prompting the patient to list his or her concerns, as on a quality of life or distress questionnaire, results in improvement to the medical content of the consultation [59], but only when the content is then jointly addressed.

The "communication in cancer" debate in the literature has been dominated by the issue of "telling the truth" [17], an area of considerable conflict and of cultural change in cancer medicine over the last 50 years [57]. The often-quoted figure is that most doctors will have 200,000 consultations in their lifetime, 20,000 of which will involve "breaking bad news": diagnosis, progression, or recurrence of disease, or the move from active to palliative treatment [32]. The emphasis on skills in the training literature, particularly when aiming to develop standardized training in medical schools [5], or in an entire country's oncology service (www.connected.nhs.uk/ in the United Kingdom), requires the specification and measurement of transferable skills. In practice, many communications skills courses include large elements of redirecting clinicians' attention from their own needs to the patient's agenda, and they tend to focus on what can be measured, such as information giving. The U.K. Department of Health has recently launched an "Information Prescription" for all adult oncology patients (www.informationprescription.info) with the laudable aim of better meeting patients' need for information, but it does not address empathy, and thus it risks promoting a more comprehensive but less responsive mode of delivering information, at the cost of listening to the patient.

The emotional skills of empathy may be much more difficult to specify and to teach or learn than more easily defined communication skills. Razavi [50] showed that even after training, clinicians' heart rates still peaked just before delivering bad news, interpreting this finding as a demonstration that clinicians retain an empathic response to the patient, in addition to executing newly-learned skills. This is a key area of interest for current communications skills research: How can these skills be learned and practiced without sacrificing emotional engagement? Arguably, empathy is expressed in the way in which effective clinicians conduct their consultations, rather than as a minimum quantity of particular components. Baider [4] asserts that empathy cannot be taught, but it can, regrettably, be extinguished, so that the aim of training health care workers should be to prevent this. She suggests that many young physicians are overwhelmed by compassion for the patient and that their attempts to manage this problem can lead to less effective relationships with patients. Her oncology internist training, "Partnership of Care," aims to enable the physician to retain and express empathy while managing the considerable medical demands and responsibilities, both cognitive and emotional. By extension, Baider is promoting the physician's development of emotional resilience, a key element in a profession known to be of high risk to the mental wellbeing of its members [48,58].

Empathic behavior is more evident where clinician and patient are more alike (for example, in age), but there is very little research on how ethnic and cultural differences may affect patient care [27]. It is not clear that training addresses the extra demands made by extremes of disparity, nor the ways in which disclosure risks widening an uncomfortable power gap [41]. However, compassion for the patient can adversely affect the factual content of consultations. Prognoses given by doctors are often seriously inaccurate [35,39,43], 90% of them in an unduly optimistic direction [16], and the better the doctor knows the patient, the more likely he or she is to overestimate the chances of survival [10].

The starting point, however, is not necessarily that patients express their emotions in a way that is easy to read. Patients may make considerable effort not to do so, or they may offer the clinician "empathic opportunities," which, if the clinician does not respond empathically or at least with curiosity, are not necessarily repeated [15,38]. The list of reasons for which patients may withhold disclosure to the clinician include several that are important in cancer: the belief that nothing can be done, the desire not to seem ungrateful, the wish not to be pitied, the worry that their worst fears may be confirmed, and a reluctance to burden the doctor [36]. When these patient factors are combined with clinicians' tendency to prioritize medical information-giving and not to enquire after patients' emotional state [19], their wish not to distress the patient, the concern that they have neither the time nor the means to deal with what is disclosed, and self-protection needs, it is clear that much goes unsaid in cancer consultations. A qualitative study of consultations between male physicians and patients with prostate cancer—men being less communicative, both as patients and as clinicians—provides a telling in-depth account of difficulties in understanding [41] in an area with a plethora of conflicting sources of information about best treatment.

## Empathy from Patients' Perspectives

It is noticeable how much research on empathy in cancer takes the perspective of medical staff and neglects patients' viewpoints [42,62]. Patients' accounts of empathic and unempathic behavior of clinical staff take a broader perspective than communication skills, integrating a wide range of nonverbal behaviors into global judgments. If a patient feels able to trust a doctor (perhaps entirely on the basis of nonverbal behaviors), or feels cared for or recognized as an individual, then he or she may show more initiative in communicating emotional needs, and some clumsiness on the part of the doctor may well be tolerated (Wright et al. [62] quote a patient who trusted her doctor and excused him for a poor bedside manner as "not really a cold person").

   When patients were asked about a recent consultation in which they received bad news about their cancer, they rated as most important that the clinician was familiar with current research evidence on the particular cancer, described the treatment options, gave full attention, and answered questions honestly. The lowest-rated behaviors were touching the arm or hand while breaking the news (possibly a learned communication skill), and discussing how the patient should tell others [42]. Another study of patients' preferences after a consultation provided a similar emphasis on technical expertise and honest answers to questions, and few patients mentioned discussion of emotion [62]. Acts of kindness or signs of respect or recognition of individuality were highly valued; by contrast, if trust was lost by apparent lack of honesty (in the patient's judgment), then the therapeutic relationship foundered. In a study of transitions in cancer, patients reported that their sense of vulnerability and uncertainty was reduced by clinicians eliciting concerns and expressing empathy, providing realistic information as well as plans for what could be done to help, however limited [15]. However, the fact that the great majority of patients expected and desired information from clinicians did not imply that patients felt able to make decisions where they believed doctors were far more competent.

Patients with anxiety and depression at clinical levels of severity may prefer to receive psychological care within the broader oncology or palliative care team rather than by referral to a separate psychology or psychiatry service [25,56]; it is not uncommon, however, for patients to be offered neither option [2]. In a Scottish study of predominantly female cancer patients, nearly three-quarters wanted only talk therapy (counseling, psychology, or psychotherapy) for depression, whereas over half of their primary care physicians would prescribe antidepressants alone or in addition [25]. Physicians made this choice despite evidence that psychological interventions may help to prevent unnecessary anxiety about recurrence after successful cancer treatment [52]. Various risk factors are associated with higher scores on measures of depression; in a large mixed sample, these factors included active disease (but not seriousness of diagnosis), female gender, and being under 65 years old [56], and in a review of ovarian cancer studies they included younger age, more advanced disease, more symptoms, and more recent diagnosis [2]. Personal variables, such as ethnicity, may also affect levels of distress (although they can also be associated with differences in prognosis). For example, an Australian study of palliative care showed poorer understanding of diagnosis (in advanced malignant disease) among non-English speakers, with less control of non-pain symptoms, higher levels of distress, and less adequate palliative care [8]. Pain and fear of pain are not routinely sampled in studies of predictors of distress in cancer patients, although treatment is an important cause of distress, and intervention around surgery can help not only mood but pain [1].

## Social Support and Mutual Support

The early reports of longer survival attributable to psychotherapy have not withstood the test of randomized trials, although the methodological problems in this field are considerable [12,44]. However, social support may have some impact on the progression of breast cancer, in which this factor has been most studied [40]; social support is measured in terms of structural qualities, such as the size of the support network or the number of confidants, rather than by functional qualities. There are many problems with designing studies: When and how should social support be measured? Does its impact vary according to the baseline level of support (that is, is there mainly a benefit for people with inadequate support at the outset of the study)? How can researchers quantify support from the clinical team as cancer progresses? In the populations studied, lay support has occurred alongside medical care, but in other countries with poor medical resources, it may be the only help available. Difficulties arise in conducting studies and interpreting findings because of the many possible routes by which such support could work: through behavior related to health and treatment requirements; through a direct impact on sympathetic mechanisms and on the immune system; through psychological health and its ramifications for physical wellbeing [12,40]. Again, pain rarely appears as a variable in these studies.

Researchers are increasingly focusing on social support through patient groups, through informal opportunities (such as cancer day centers for those undergoing outpatient treatments), and through volunteer survivor mentors (such as Imerman Angels in the United States: www.imermanangels.com; Hope and Cope in Canada www.hopecope.jgh.ca; and Women helping Women: www.nlcn.nhs.uk/whwhome). Coyne et al. [12], in their systematic review of psychological therapy for people with cancer, comment on the wide variance in effects, including negative consequences such as increasing preoccupation with cancer. Volunteers may be more helpful than partners [45], and the extent of psychological distress in partners should not be underestimated [26]. Where treatment is a significant source of difficulty or there are related issues such as coping with loss of function or changes in appearance, volunteers may be more able to share the patient's experience, normalizing the distress and possibly offering strategies for managing the problems. However, discussing shared experience is not necessarily supportive, and self-disclosure by the volunteer may not be helpful unless it occurs within a framework of empathic communication [46].

# Pain in Cancer

Many cancer-free people with severe pain or pain that persists unaccountably will fear that cancer is the cause of pain. Many health systems have moved away from exhaustive investigations to exclude cancer as the cause of a new episode of pain, particularly in the musculoskeletal system (both for reasons of economy and to avoid unnecessary medicalization for problems that are best managed by rehabilitation and judicious use of analgesics). This development can mean that patients' anxieties about cancer continue unresolved, and that rare cases of cancer may be diagnosed late, with serious consequences for the patient.

Both clinicians and people with a cancer diagnosis perceive pain as a high priority, and it is perhaps due to a dualistic heritage that pain is mainly discussed in terms of analgesic technology, with the psychological focus on the impact of cancer on quality of life and on facing death. After diagnosis, pain and other symptoms that occurred before diagnosis but were not acted upon by patient or physician may be seen as missed opportunities for earlier diagnosis and, perhaps, a better prognosis.

Once the diagnosis has been established, pain is a predominant cause of fear: it may be assumed to signal disease progression and dissemination, and patients may worry that it will increase to unbearable levels. Yet surveys have repeatedly found a lack of routine enquiry about pain by clinical staff, even with inpatients, and these findings have contributed to the campaign to make pain "the fifth vital sign." Where treatment is successful, and during rehabilitation, the patient may feel that a complaint of pain is anathema to health care staff: patients may be admonished to be more grateful for their survival, even though recognition and treatment of pain at this stage is most likely to improve wellbeing and active recovery. Pain retains its sinister meaning for many cancer survivors: Audre Lorde [34] wrote that "I do not forget cancer for very long, ever. That keeps me armed and on my toes, but also with a slight background noise of fear." Fears about recurrence, which may be exacerbated by persistent pain following surgery, radiotherapy, or chemotherapy, may prompt unproductive repeated visits to health care providers for reassurance.

# Experiencing Another's Pain

Humans have the ability to read pain in others' faces [61], with automatic activation of both sensory and affective pathways in processing facial expressions of pain [51] or of other pain cues [28]. These responses, which can be shown by functional magnetic resonance imaging, are proportional to empathy scores in the observer [51]. Better temporal resolution using event-related brain potential analysis suggests that empathy for another's pain may be a two-stage process [23], with an early emotional response that differentiates pain from non-pain, and a later more cognitive response that is more sensitive to context. In one study, pictures of needles piercing the skin were rated as much less painful by acupuncturists (who believed acupuncture to be painless) than by controls, although empathy scores were comparable [9], and this way of processing observed pain was associated with activity in areas associated with emotion regulation, but again only in acupuncturists. It may be that replication with other clinicians would not produce similar results if they expected to observe pain in the patient, but findings suggest that familiarity with particular procedures, and/or focus on clinical tasks, may be associated with suppression of emotional and perhaps even cognitive empathic responses [9]. This suppression, in turn, could be required in order to exercise clinical skills effectively (a popular lay model of the dispassionate clinician), or it may have a self-protective function. After all, seeing another in pain can sensitize the observer, as shown in a study finding that pain sensitivity in mice could be modulated by observation of a littermate experiencing pain [33].

While patients may communicate their pain through many channels, leaving the observer with little need to interpret, health care workers cannot afford to share the patient's full emotional experience. Skepticism about the extent of patients' pain has been repeatedly demonstrated in clinical settings [30], although it is not universal. Lower estimations of another's pain can be cued by relying on facial expression without verbal report of pain, and by the suggestion that pain may be simulated [31]. In that study, although doctors' and nurses' mean estimate was that 25% of patients exaggerate their pain (and higher exaggeration estimates were associated with lower pain estimates), oncology staff gave lower exaggeration estimates than did staff in emergency rooms. Whether this difference is related to their work experience or to the fact that they differ in other ways is unknown.

Clinicians are gatekeepers for society's limited health resources, their own time and skills, costly treatments, and some resources that are subject to further restrictions, such as opioids. Skepticism about patients' pain or insufficient allocation of these resources will probably result in undertreatment of patients with genuine pain. Unquestioning acceptance of patients' reports of pain raises fears of exploitation, loss of professional status in the eyes of peers, and in extreme cases, restriction of prescribing and other rights. It is not uncommon for clinicians to express doubts about the authenticity of patients' pain-related behaviors, particularly when these behaviors appear inconsistent with the clinician's belief about an "appropriate" level of pain and ways to express it [13]. However, the assumption that responsivity of behavior to social context indicates simulation or exaggeration is poorly supported; it is equally or more likely that it indicates release of suppression in the presence of carers or potential carers [61].

Social pressure to judge "deservingness" in allocating resources; the need to control emotional response to distressed patients; possible metacognitive processes overriding emotional responding; the anomaly of pain as a symptom in a health system focused on diagnosis and treatment of underlying disease: all contribute to difficulty empathizing with a patient's pain. It is not evident that training in communication skills, and lowering of formal barriers between clinicians and patients, will necessarily improve empathy.

## Research Issues

Research bearing on empathy for pain appears to fall into several categories with little permeability between them, and the lack of theory or of application of available theories makes for difficulty in integrating research findings. Pain is noticeably absent from the literature on communication between clinician and patient, but whether that is because the data have not been collected, or because patients do not speak about it, pain remains an important concern for patients that should be included. Conversely, some of the detailed methods for studying consultation behaviors could usefully be exported into the broader field of pain research. There seems to be a relative neglect of the use of cognate areas of research, particularly that of reassurance, and the persistence of anxiety and distress despite the delivery of what the clinician believes to be reassurance is now well recognized.

A search of the empathy literature discovered 59 different measures, less than 10 of which had any supporting data on their quality as measures, least of all predictive validity in medical settings, and many of which did not make explicit links to any operationalized construct or theory of empathy [24]. Although empathy is often assumed to be a trait, self-ratings of empathy have fairly low stability across time, and the evolutionarily based theories of empathy (such as de Waal [60]) propose a much more contextual experience than do personality theories. Hemmerdinger and colleagues [24] also question whether empathy is a continuous variable, as modeled by all rating scales, when it might operate by a threshold effect. These are fundamental concerns for effective investigation of empathy.

The equation of empathy with communication skills is a medical institutional view that favors cognitive engagement over emotional engagement [22] and does not serve the field well [7]. The diversity of constructs within communication skills, from global ratings of consultations to microanalyses of particular behaviors, while a strength of the research canon, makes integration and application of findings a challenging task, the more so as agreement between studies is not high. Bower and Mead [7] are also critical of researching all aspects of care using a drug metaphor in which increased dose produces a greater outcome, without attention to need at baseline. For instance, social support might only make a difference to patients who lack it, with no measurable benefit to those who already have adequate quantity and quality of support. More use of patients rather than research staff as raters of recorded communication, more use of actual rather than simulated consultations, and a move away from detailed counts of particular clinician communication events toward a recognition of the place of patients' global judgments and how these affect the impact of consultation skills: all would contribute to greater understanding of patients' experience and how it could be improved.

Patients themselves are not a homogeneous group, and there is surprisingly little research on differences attributable to gender or culture [27].

Most cancer research concerns Caucasian males, but undermedication of ethnic minority patients has repeatedly been shown in the pain field [21], with lower fluency in English correlating with poorer palliative care [8]. Interestingly, Surbone's [57] review of different cultural responses to truth-telling in cancer offers a model for physicians responding to their patients in a patient-led, culturally aware way that might be tested in the area of cancer pain.

Crossover between biomedically focused studies and psychosocially informed studies would significantly enrich the field, given the lack of understanding, and even of coherent theory in some areas, of mechanisms affecting patients' wellbeing [2]. Interactions of psychological and biological variables emerging in the field of pain are surprising and fascinating [6]. Few psychosocial studies include biological markers; few biological ones sample psychosocial variables.

# Issues for Clinicians

Direct regular questioning about pain, observation of patients' faces and behavior, and challenging beliefs about how pain should or should not be felt or expressed are the basis for good care of pain. Asking about pain should not only be a request to rate it on a simple scale: patients can be asked about their concerns about pain or apprehensions about its meaning or course. Patients may hold vivid images or narratives about pain being unbearable, uncontrollable, and robbing them of dignity, control, and humanity. They may assume that increased pain always implies progress of cancer and brings death nearer. Sontag [54] describes at length the common use of cancer as an analogy for "whatever seemed ruthless, implacable, predatory."

Fears about pain are rarely volunteered, but they can be disclosed to an empathic clinician who is in a crucial position to offer realistic reassurance. Some protocols may be particularly useful in breaking unwelcome news [15,29], or in trying to check that the patient has understood such information. For instance, in response to patients who try to induce the clinician to provide an unrealistically optimistic prognosis, Evans et al. [15] suggest the formulation of "hoping for the best, preparing for the worst." Even when little can be done to relieve patients' physical state, something can almost always be done to help meet their psychological and social needs.

## Conclusion

Some of the material reviewed above questions how realistic it is to assume that more empathy is always better for both patient and clinician. The expectation that the clinician is fully engaged both cognitively and emotionally with the patient is an ideal that takes little account of the clinician's own feelings, fears, and reluctance to cause or exacerbate distress. The trajectory of the physician's or surgeon's anxiety may be very different from that of the patient, decreasing markedly with a diagnosis and treatment plan, whereas for the patient such an outcome may be the end of hopes that cancer was not the cause of the symptoms and may precipitate anxiety about pain. Emotions help us make quick decisions according to priorities, rather than carefully calculated algorithms of pros and cons: if the clinician's priority is, for instance, to avoid causing distress or exposing him or herself to more distress from patients, or to be liked, then the result is likely to be overoptimistic predictions to the patient or withholding or minimization of unwelcome information. Unfortunately, we know less about this propensity in relation to pain than in relation to other causes of distress for the cancer patient. The skills of balancing emotional engagement with the patient with calculation or communication of clinical data are hard to specify and quantify and, no doubt, to learn. The emphasis on empathy needs to be tempered by the context in which it is used, and by the way patients formulate and value it in the context of the clinical consultation.

## References

[1]    Andersen BL, Simonelli LE. Cancer: general. In: Ayers S, Baum A, McManus C, Newman S, Wallston K, Weinman J, West R, editors. Cambridge handbook of psychology, health & medicine, 2nd edition. Cambridge: Cambridge University Press; 2007. p 584–91.

[2]    Arden-Close E, Gidron Y, Moss-Morris R. Psychological distress and its correlates in ovarian cancer: a systematic review. Psycho-Oncology 2008;17:1061–72.

[3]    Back AL, Arnold RM, Baile WF, Fryer-Edwards KA, Alexander SC, Barley GE, Gooley TA, Tulsky JA. Efficacy of communication skills training for giving bad news and discussing transitions to palliative care. Arch Intern Med 2007;167:453–60.

[4]    Baider L. Physicians' hidden distress: confrontation with their own emotions. Psycho-Oncology 2009;18:S5–6.

[5]   Baile WF, Aaron J. Patient-physician communication in oncology: past, present, and future. Curr Opin Oncol 2005;17:331–5.
[6]   Benedetti F, Lanotte M, Lopiano L, Colloca L. When words are painful: unraveling the mechanisms of the nocebo effect. Neuroscience 2007;147:260–1.
[7]   Bower P, Mead N. Patient-centred healthcare. In: Ayers S, Baum A, McManus C, Newman S, Wallston K, Weinman J, West R, editors. Cambridge handbook of psychology, health and medicine, 2nd edition. Cambridge: Cambridge University Press; 2007. p 468–72.
[8]   Chan A, Woodruff RK. Comparison of palliative care needs of English and non-English-speaking patients. J Palliat Care 1999;15:26–30.
[9]   Cheng Y, Lin CP, Liu HL, Hsu YY, Lim KE, Hung D, Decety J. Expertise modulates the perception of pain in others. Curr Biol 2007;17:1708–13.
[10]  Christakis NA, Lamont EB. Extent and determinants of error in doctors' prognoses in terminally ill patients: prospective cohort study. BMJ 2000;320:369–72.
[11]  Coyle N. In their own words: seven advanced cancer patients describe their experience with pain and the use of opioid drugs. J Pain Symptom Manage 2004;27:300–9.
[12]  Coyne JC, Stefanek M, Palmer SC. Psychotherapy and survival in cancer: the conflict between hope and evidence. Psychol Bull 2007;133:367–94.
[13]  Craig KD, Badali MA. Introduction to the special series on pain, deception and malingering. Clin J Pain 2004;20:377–82.
[14]  Downey L, Engelberg RA, Curtis JR, Lafferty WE, Patrick DL. Shared priorities for the end-of-life period. J Pain Symptom Manage 2009;37:175–88.
[15]  Evans WG, Tulsky JA, Back AL, Arnold RM. Communications at times of transitions: how to help patients cope with loss and re-define hope. Cancer J 2006;12:417–24.
[16]  Fallowfield L, Jenkins V. Communicating sad, bad and difficult news in medicine. Lancet 2004;363:312–9.
[17]  Fallowfield L, Jenkins V, Beveridge HA. Truth may hurt, but deceit hurts more. Palliat Med 2002;16;296–303.
[18]  Fallowfield L, Jenkins V, Farewell V, Solis-Trapata I. Enduring impact of communication skills training: results of a 12-month follow-up. Br J Cancer 2003;89:1445–9.
[19]  Ford S, Fallowfield L, Lewis S. Doctor-patient interactions in oncology. Soc Sci Med 1996;42:1511–9.
[20]  Graves KD, Arnold SM, Love CL, Kirsh KL, Moore PG, Passik SD. Distress screening in a multidisciplinary lung cancer clinic: prevalence and predictors of clinically significant distress. Lung Cancer 2007;55:215–24.
[21]  Green CR, Anderson KO, Baker TA, Campbell LC, Decker S, Fillingim RB, Kaloukalani DA, Lasch KE, Myers C, Tait RC, Todd KH, Vallerand AH. The unequal burden of pain: confronting racial and ethnic disparities in pain. Pain Med 2003;4:277–94.
[22]  Halpern J. What is clinical empathy? J Gen Intern Med 2003;18:670–4.
[23]  Han S, Fan Y, Mao L. Gender difference in empathy for pain: an electrophysiological investigation. Brain Res 2008;1196:85–93.
[24]  Hemmerdinger JM, Stoddart SDR, Lilford RJ. A systematic review of tests of empathy in medicine. BMC Med Educ 2007;7:24–31.
[25]  Hodges L, Butcher I, Kleiboer A, McHugh G, Murray G, Walker J, Wilson R, Sharpe M. Patient and general practitioner preferences for the treatment of depression in patients with cancer: how, who, and where? J Psychosom Res 2009;67:399–402.
[26]  Hodges LJ, Humphris GM, Macfarlane G. A meta-analytic investigation of the relationship between the psychological distress of cancer patients and their carers. Soc Sci Med 2005;60:1–12.
[27]  Im E-O, Chee W. A feminist critique of research on cancer pain. West J Nurs Res 2001;23:726–52.
[28]  Jackson PL, Meltzoff AN, Decety J. How do we perceive the pain of others? A window into the neural processes involved in empathy. Neuroimage 2005;24:771–9.
[29]  Joekes K. Breaking bad news. In: Ayers S, Baum A, McManus C, Newman S, Wallston K, Weinman J, West R, editors. Cambridge handbook of psychology, health & medicine, 2nd edition. Cambridge: Cambridge University Press; 2007. p 423–6.
[30]  Kappesser J, Williams ACdeC. Pain estimation: asking the right questions. Pain 2010;148:184–7.
[31]  Kappesser J, Williams ACdeC, Prkachin KM. Testing two accounts of pain underestimation. Pain 2006;124:109–16.

[32] Kurtz S, Silverman J, Draper J. Teaching and learning communication skills in medicine. Oxford: Radcliffe Medical Press; 1998.

[33] Langford DJ, Crager SE, Shehzad Z, Smith SB, Sotocinal SG, Levenstadt JS, Chanda ML, Levitin DJ, Mogil JS. Social modulation of pain as evidence of empathy in mice. Science 2006;312:1967–70.

[34] Lorde A. The cancer journals. San Francisco: Sheba Feminist Publishers; 1980.

[35] Mackillop WJ, Quirt CF. Measuring the accuracy of prognostic judgments in oncology. J Clin Epidemiol 1997;50:21–9.

[36] Maguire P, Pitceathly C. Key communication skills and how to acquire them. BMJ 2002;325:697–700.

[37] Merckaert A, Libert Y, Delvaux N, Marchal S, Boniver J, Etienne A-M, Klastersky J, Reynaert C, Scalliet P, Slachmuylder J-L, Razavi D. Factors that influence physicians' detection of distress in patients with cancer. Cancer 2005;104:411–21.

[38] Morse DS, Edwardsen EA, Gordon HS. Missed opportunities for interval empathy in lung cancer communication. Arch Intern Med 2008;168:1853–8.

[39] Muers MF, Shevlin P, Brown J. Prognosis in lung cancer: physicians' opinions compared with outcome and a predictive model. Thorax 1996;51:894–902.

[40] Nausheen B, Gidron Y, Peveler R, Moss-Morris R. Social support and cancer progression: a systematic review. J Psychosom Res 2009;67:403–15.

[41] Oliffe J, Thorne S. Men, masculinities, and prostate cancer: Australian and Canadian patient perspectives of communication with male physicians. Qual Health Res 2007;17:149–61.

[42] Parker PA, Baile WF, de Moor C, Lenzi R, Kudelka AP, Cohen L. Breaking bad news about cancer: patients' preferences for communication. J Clin Oncol 2001;19:2049–56.

[43] Parkes CM. Accuracy of predictions of survival in later stages of cancer. BMJ 1972;2:29–31.

[44] Petticrew M, Bell R, Hunter D. Influence of psychological coping on survival and recurrence in people with cancer: systematic review. BMJ 2002;325:1066–76.

[45] Pistrang N, Barker C. Partners and fellow patients: two sources of emotional support for women with breast cancer. Am J Community Psychol 1998;26:439–56.

[46] Pistrang N, Solomons W, Barker C. Peer support for women with breast cancer: the role of empathy and self-disclosure. J Community Applied Soc Psychol 1999;9:217–29.

[47] Pollak KI, Arnold RM, Jeffreys AS, Alexander SC, Olsen MK, Abernethy AP, Skinner CS, Rodriguez KL, Tulsky JA. Oncologist communication about emotion during visits with patients with advanced cancer. J Clin Oncol 2007;25:5748–52.

[48] Ramirez AJ, Graham J, Richards MA, Cull A, Gregory WM. Mental health of hospital consultants: the effects of stress and satisfaction at work. Lancet 1996;347:724–8.

[49] Rask MT, Jensen ML, Andersen J, Zachariae R. Effects of an intervention aimed at improving nurse-patient communication in an oncology outpatient clinic. Cancer Nurs 2009;32:E1–11.

[50] Razavi D. Physicians, team work and the cancer patient: the acquisition of skills as a promoter of care quality and as a professional stress antidote. Psycho-Oncology 2009;18:S6.

[51] Saarela MV, Hlushchuk Y, Williams AC, Schürmann M, Kalso E, Hari R. The compassionate brain: humans detect intensity of pain from another's face. Cereb Cortex 2007;17:230–7.

[52] Simon K, Robb A. Cancer: breast. In Ayers S, Baum A, McManus C, Newman S, Wallston K, Weinman J, West R, editors. Cambridge handbook of psychology, health & medicine, 2nd edition. Cambridge: Cambridge University Press; 2007. p 577–80.

[53] Singer T, Frith C. The painful side of empathy. Nat Neurosci 2005;8:845–6.

[54] Sontag S. Illness as metaphor. Harmondsworth: Penguin; 1977.

[55] Stepien KA, Baernstein A. Educating for empathy: a review. J Gen Intern Med 2006;21:524–30.

[56] Strong V, Waters R, Hibberd C, Rush R, Cargill A, Storey D, Walker J, Wall L, Fallon M, Sharpe M. Emotional distress in cancer patients: the Edinburgh Cancer Centre symptom study. Br J Cancer 2007;96:868–74.

[57] Surbone A. Telling the truth to patients with cancer: what is the truth? Lancet Oncol 2006;7:944–50.

[58] Taylor C, Graham J, Potts HW, Richards MA, Ramirez AJ. Changes in the mental health of UK hospital consultants since the mid-1990s. Lancet 2005;366:742–4.

[59] Velikova G, Booth L, Smith AB, Brown PM, Lynch P, Brown JM, Selby PJ. Measuring quality of life in routine oncology practice improves communication and patient well-being: a randomized controlled trial. J Clin Oncol 2004;22:714–24.

[60] de Waal FBM. Putting the altruism back into altruism: the evolution of empathy. Annu Rev Psychol 2008;59:279–300.

[61] Williams AC. Facial expression of pain: an evolutionary account. Behav Brain Sci 2002;25:439–88.
[62] Wright EB, Holcombe C, Salmon P. Doctors' communication of trust, care, and respect in breast cancer: qualitative study. BMJ 2004;328:864–8.

***Correspondence to:*** Amanda C. de C. Williams, PhD, CPsychol, Research Department of Clinical, Health and Educational Psychology, University College London, Gower Street, London WC1E 6BT, United Kingdom. Email: amanda.williams@ucl.ac.uk.

# A Global Perspective on Patient and Family Cancer Pain Education

Jean C. Yi,[a] Samantha B. Artherholt,[a] and Karen L. Syrjala[a,b]

[a]Biobehavioral Sciences, Clinical Research Division, Fred Hutchinson Cancer Research Center; [b]Department of Psychiatry and Behavioral Sciences, University of Washington, Seattle, Washington, USA

Regardless of the type or the duration of cancer pain, patients and their family members often have uncertainty regarding the pain and the best way to treat it. In all cases they require education about what to expect, how to communicate about symptoms related to pain, and how to manage their pain. Education in itself is a method demonstrated to improve pain outcomes [6]. In this chapter, we review simple yet effective communication and educational methods that can be used in any medical practice by any professional treating cancer patients with pain in any country or location.

Even carefully implemented clinical trials or specialist consultations indicate that pharmacological or invasive treatments do not eliminate all cancer-related pain, but can make it manageable for most patients [14,34]. Explanations for less-than-adequate pain relief include numerous nonmedical reasons: patients' reluctance to take prescribed medications because of fears of side effects, their reluctance to discuss their pain, insufficient assessment leading to poor treatment, patients' inadequate knowledge about what is appropriate to discuss and treat, myths that disrupt communication between patients and health care providers, and real-world limitations such as cost or accessibility of medications [7,57,60]. As the vast majority of cancer patients are treated in ambulatory clinics, their adherence to treatment cannot be assumed. When they leave their appointments, they return home and may or may not treat themselves as instructed. Because patient factors can entirely undo an optimal treatment plan and some pain usually remains unrelieved even with the best treatment, methods to educate patients and their family members are critical not only for specialists, but for all clinicians who treat patients with cancer pain.

While extensive discussion has taken place regarding training needs of physicians, nurses, and pharmacists, far less effort has been directed toward understanding patient and family education needs. The literature on adherence makes it clear just how difficult this area is to assess, much less to intervene. When patients' beliefs do not fit what they are instructed to do, they often will not argue or even ask questions, but will nod their heads and then proceed to act on their beliefs or concerns [13,15,40,55].

While cancer treatment adherence may be fairly complete with chemotherapy, pain treatment is rarely so well defined. Lack of adherence to treatment is recognized as threatening the health and even survival of patients. Meanwhile, analgesics are less well recognized as having the potential for major health risks as a result of inadequate understanding or follow-through with prescribed pain treatment [31,44]. In spite of increased public and media attention to medical errors, adherence to cancer pain treatment by well-intentioned patients is an underaddressed problem. Most patients are given relatively loose parameters for medications, leaving them free to adjust dosing as needed. Patients act on their own beliefs or those of their families; they adjust doses, skip doses, and simply stop taking a medication because they do not like a side effect. Increasingly patients do not even fill prescriptions because costs are not covered by insurance. Health care providers usually do not hear about this unless they specifically ask about cost coverage or actual medication behaviors of patients. Conversely, patients may take too much medication simply because they do not realize what the drugs are for, or that they are supposed to stop taking one drug when they start another one. Adherence data indicate that up to 40% of cancer patients do not take their pain medications as prescribed [13,39,55]. These same data indicate that adherence is an important factor contributing to level of pain; better adherence improves pain relief. It is clear, then, that effective patient and family education is crucial to adherence and adequate control of cancer pain. Fig. 1 shows a model through which patient and family education can decrease barriers, increase adherence to pain management, decrease pain and related symptoms, and ultimately increase patients' function and overall quality of life.

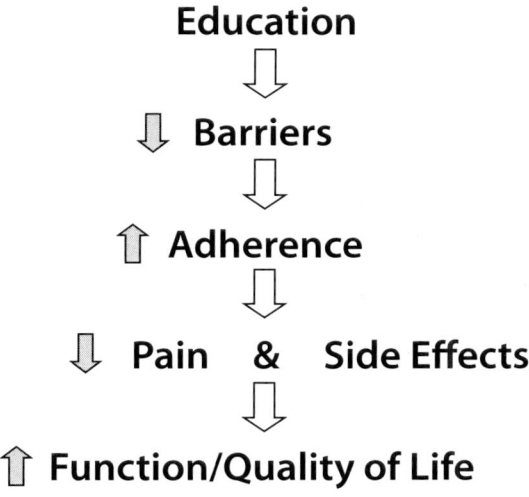

**Fig. 1.** Model of the hypothesized mechanism for the benefits of patient and family education.

## What Is Patient and Family Education?

True patient and family education requires an interactive process in which patients first learn, and then practice using their new knowledge to direct their own behavior. Education allows patients to take the information presented to them, adapt it to their changing situations, and then adjust their thoughts and behaviors accordingly. It is distinct from information provision, which essentially just tells patients what providers think they need to know, and does not require patient follow-through on the new learning. Education involves the telling of facts, but it also includes training in how to accomplish goals, along with addressing patients' questions, concerns, and problem-solving around potential obstacles [53]. For reluctant patients or those with strong beliefs about pain or medications, it is extremely helpful, after describing a pain treatment plan, to ask what they will do when they have pain and then discuss barriers to successfully implementing the prescribed plan. This rehearsal can facilitate patient adherence to treatment and can point out to the clinician where the patient may have difficulty following the prescribed plan.

A framework summarizing the education needs of patients and their family members is listed in Table I [50,53]. These targets for education ideally would be addressed when disease-related pain is mild and when opioids are first needed. At that time patients are interested, are motivated to take charge of their care, and usually have the energy to focus on and learn new information and strategies. If patients are in severe pain or have other major symptoms, education needs to be more focused and limited until symptoms are better controlled [22].

Education involves several levels, and all are important. In this section, we will discuss three elements we believe are essential for effective patient and family education: assessment, information, and communication. Goals of each aspect of patient and family education are summarized in Table II.

## Assessment Provides a Shared Language for Patients and Clinicians

Pain assessment is the cornerstone of both pharmacological and nonpharmacological intervention and provides a framework for effective communication. Adequate pain assessment is an essential step toward providing effective treatment and facilitating patient adherence. Rating pain severity via a simple method, such as on a numerical rating scale of 0–10 or using the Faces Pain Rating Scale [23], is recommended by several groups, including the National Comprehensive Cancer Network [22] and the Joint Commission on Accreditation of Healthcare Organizations [27]. Proper pain assessment begins the process of communication that determines medical treatment, while also beginning to teach patients how to think about and report their pain. When the same questions are asked at each assessment and patients learn some options for responses, patients begin to recognize different qualities in their pain, and physicians begin to

Table I
Education needs of patients and family members

*Assessment Messages*

Tell us about problems with pain or treatment. Do not just stop treatment.

Tell us about side effects. We can change the medication or treat the side effect.

Tell us about your pain in the last 24 hours and currently:

    Teach the patient how to report pain intensity, using a 0–10 numerical rating scale or the Faces Pain Rating Scale [23,27,50].

    What does the pain feel like? (suggest possible words to describe the pain)

    What is the pain pattern?

        When do you have pain?

        How long does the pain last?

        What time of day and what kind of activity makes the pain worse or better?

Use an example (practice) to assure understanding: What was your worst pain ever, how would you rate it, what did it feel like, what made it better or worse?

*Information to Convey*

Your pain is important to us.

Pain can be treated effectively, usually with pills.

    If the current treatment doesn't work, we have *many* other options.

    We will keep working with you to treat your pain until it is managed.

There is no benefit from suffering with pain.

    "Use your energy to fight the disease or to recover, not to fight the pain."

    Untreated pain has negative effects on your health.

Strong medications like morphine are often used, and they don't mean you are dying.

Addiction is almost never a problem if you have never had alcohol or drug problems. (More discussion is needed if patient has a drug or alcohol history.)

If you take the medication now, it will still work later if the pain is worse (tolerance).

Pain medications should be taken only as prescribed and by the person for whom the medication is prescribed.

What concerns do you have?

*Communication: WRITE DOWN and DATE the Treatment Plan and Review with Patient and Family*

Medications: What to take (name and color of pill)/What to take for/When to take/ How much to take

Medications to stop taking

Potential side effects

Cautions about operating machinery or motor vehicles while taking potentially sedating medications

What symptoms to be concerned about; what symptoms not to be concerned about

Who to call (name and number)/Phone number to call/When to call for:

    Problems getting medications (cost or availability)

    New pain, change in pain, no relief from pain treatment

    Side effects or new symptoms

Answer questions about treatment

Define follow-up plan

CHECK BACK on adherence (after 24 or 72 hours, depending on pain severity)

    What has the patient done, or what medications were taken, to manage pain and related symptoms?

    What has worked for pain relief?

    What has gotten in the way of pain relief?

    What are the usual and worst levels of pain?

learn about how patients communicate important elements of their pain and related symptoms. Through these regular assessments, the physician and patient also begin to develop a common language for communication, such as: "Does your pain feel like burning, shooting, pins and needles, or is it an aching, sharp, or throbbing kind of pain, or how would you describe it?" This communication process leads to improved prescribing and increased likelihood of adherence.

Table II
Goals of patient and family education

| Element of Education | Goals |
| --- | --- |
| *Assessment* | |
| Assess understanding of pain | Ensure comprehension of concepts; give the message that pain is important |
| Use 0–10 scale for usual and worst pain | Define pain and identify treatment needs; enable tracking of symptoms over time |
| Repeat words to describe pain; ask the same questions about pain at each visit | Begin use of a shared language and understanding; educate patients in the concepts needed to determine adequate treatment |
| *Information* | |
| Describe predictable quality and intensity of sensations | Make the unknown normal and predictable; decrease threat; increase tolerance; validate experience |
| Define time frame for treatment- and procedure-related pain | Remind patients that pain is time-limited |
| Explain that pain can be treated with medication | Let patients know they do not have to suffer with pain |
| Use booklets, videos | Patients can refer back to these materials as needed |
| *Communication* | |
| Write down information | Patients can refer back to this material |
| Explain how to use the treatment prescribed | Improve adherence and pain relief |
| Dispel myths that disrupt treatment | Reduce fears; improve adherence |
| Explain what side effects to expect, when to call the doctor | Enhance control while improving understanding |
| Check with the patient and family members to ensure understanding; allow time for questions or concerns | Enhance understanding; improve adherence; ensure that providers are aware of the patient's concerns about treatment; create a "team approach" with the patient and family |

## Information Provides Understanding, Familiarity, and Predictability

It always helps to make the unfamiliar more predictable by informing patients of what is going to happen, thus reassuring them that their experience is "normal." Uncertainty is known to increase distress and threaten perceptions of one's ability to cope [41]. By definition, then, uncertainty can decrease self-efficacy—the belief that one has the ability to manage the difficulties one faces. Of all psychological concepts related to pain, none are as consistently and significantly shown to influence pain level and treatment outcome as elevated distress and lowered self-efficacy [4,45,52,54].

Some of the overall uncertainty about cancer pain can be countered by providing specific information about what is known. Information also gives patients a way of "reframing" or thinking about their situation from a less threatening or more in-control perspective. It indicates that pain is important to the health care provider and not only to the patient, decreasing the patient's sense of isolation. It also conveys the message that pain is treatable. Information addresses plans, myths, and expectations for what the pain will feel like and, when possible, its duration. Sensation and duration information about pain is invaluable in relieving fears of patients whose symptoms are likely to be short-term but intense, as with procedures or treatment-related side effects.

With time demands on clinical practice, it is important to note that written materials, websites, and videos are effective strategies for reducing the face-to-face interaction time with nurses or physicians. Numerous booklets, books, and videotapes are available to use as educational tools with patients. Data consistently indicate that patient training, augmented with print, video, or audio materials, should be incorporated into routine oncology practice [6,38,50,51,64]. Written materials are useful because they reduce the burden of having to retain information solely in memory for both patient and caregiver. However, we are aware of no data to indicate that print material or videotapes alone are effective in improving pain outcomes, without some review and tailoring to the patient's needs by the provider.

## Communication Is Important for All Patients

Communication is the most basic intervention used in patient care. When illness-related concerns become the focus of a patient and family's thinking, communications with the health care team are given enormous significance. Families use the medical team's words as a primary source to define their unspoken and spoken rules, beliefs, and behaviors [46]. Research has demonstrated that effective communication between physician and patient can lead to improved health outcomes [17,20,48].

There are two sides to every communication; in the cancer clinic these two sides are represented by the patient (and family) and the health care provider. Difficulties can arise from either of these directions [17], and thus both deserve attention when educating patients and families about pain.

## Patient Barriers to Communication

Clinicians are often frustrated by patients who are given information, but seem not to hear it. Anxiety, unfamiliarity, and the numerous amnestic medications used in cancer treatment may affect patients' ability to retain material that has been discussed. Research indicates that opioids, while they have minimal effects on most areas of function, do affect long-term retention of new information [30,47]. Thus, while patients may appear to comprehend information during their office visit, they may not be able to recall this information later at home. In addition to these physiological aspects of learning interference, the distress and helplessness brought about by a cancer diagnosis, compounded by the acute experience of pain, can disrupt long-term retention. With these limitations in mind, it seems an obvious solution to write down important instructions or details so they can be recalled later. It helps to have standard prescribing sheets and pain report forms so that this information does not have to be written anew each time. Patients can also use symptom diaries to track pain level and medication use between appointments.

## Provider Barriers to Communication

Health care providers routinely convey information, listen, reassure patients and family members, and actively educate patients about both the pain and potential treatments. Each of these interactions can enhance patients' beliefs in their ability to cope with the symptoms they have, can foster adherence to the medical plan, or conversely, can escalate patient fear or helplessness—often without signaling the medical team that this is happening [17,53]. Providers, however, often lack explicit training in effective communication, and they are unsure of how much information to provide to patients and families, particularly about difficult topics such as pain management. Providers may incorrectly assume that patients will ask questions if they are unclear about physician directions [17,20]. These potential barriers, in combination with the above-mentioned difficulties on the patient side, underscore how important it is for providers to check in frequently with patients to ensure that they understand what they are being instructed to do and that they have an opportunity to ask any questions or raise concerns they may have.

# Evidence for or against Patient Education

Education has conclusively demonstrated improvement in many medical outcomes, including pain, in many types of patients. Patient education increases knowledge and improves attitudes toward cancer pain [1].

Clinical trials document the efficacy of patient education in improving cancer pain knowledge [8,12,33,63] and outcomes [11,38,43], although these efforts are not universally successful in reducing pain [12,59]. In a more recent meta-analysis of 19 randomized controlled studies, average pain intensity had moderate effect sizes that decreased from pre- to post-intervention [6]. However, five studies did not find that the intervention had any effect. There were no improvements in quality of life or mood with these interventions, and the effect of the interventions were limited to increasing knowledge and attitudes to pain and pain medication, in addition to improving pain relief. But these changes did not lead to changes in medication adherence in all studies [42]. The mechanism by which increases in knowledge can lead to reductions in pain is still unclear. Perhaps changes in beliefs also are needed to promote and sustain change [58]. However, it is clear that effective strategies are needed that have sustained impact while requiring feasible amounts of professional time.

Nearly all clinical trials have had relatively brief endpoints of 2 to 6 weeks, whereas cancer pain often continues for much longer. Our research group tested print and video materials for patient training in a study that followed patients for 6 months [51]. Patients watched a video that was followed by a 20-minute session with an oncology nurse to review the materials and answer any questions patients may have had. A follow-up phone call after 72 hours reinforced the use of communication with the patients' health care providers and the use of pain intensity ratings. Patients reported a decrease in usual pain and in barriers to pain relief, along with increased concordance of patient and physician/nurse ratings of the patient's pain intensity, suggesting improved communication. The efficacy of this study, as reflected in reduction of both barriers and pain level, has not been seen in some other studies that used similar methods. Success with this procedure may be attributable to the combination of providing standard material that all patients need through the use of videotape and print material, followed by tailoring of the face-to-face time to individual patient needs using a manualized procedure. Other studies also have used videos to standardize pain training. They have reported improved knowledge and self-efficacy, but less success in reducing pain [10,29,33].

Still other studies have used extensive tailoring to enhance patient education and improve outcomes [32,43]. Interventions have been tailored by using the baseline assessment to understand the patient's misconceptions and barriers and address them in the session. In one of these studies, patients in the tailored intervention group had reduced average pain, pain-related impairment, and pain frequency when compared with the control group that received standard care [43]. However, there were no differences in knowledge gains or adherence to pain medication. In another study using a tailored intervention, communication between patients and physicians increased as patients in the intervention group were more likely to discuss pain-related concerns [49]. However, the study did not test whether this increase in communication led to a corresponding decrease in pain.

While the environment of these educational interventions generally has been clinical settings, home visits also have been tested as a way to deliver educational material [5,29,38]. van der Peet and colleagues tested a home-based intervention using nurses [56]. Three one-and-a-half hour home visits by nurses included a brochure on pain, instruction in how to record level of pain in a diary, and encouragement for patients to seek help if needed. Caregivers could be included if they wanted to participate. The visits were spaced so that they occurred every 3 weeks. Consistent with other research in this area, patients in the intervention group increased their knowledge and had short-term decreases in pain (at 4 months), but these gains were not sustained over longer follow-up (8 months). Also, increased knowledge did not correlate with a decrease in pain.

# Challenges and Questions

### Education Dose

In published studies on cancer pain education, the education doses tend to be small, with brief interventions. Overall, results suggest that brief patient training is highly specific and does not generalize to changing pain. Some studies have reported success in reducing patients' level of "worst" pain when using longer training periods and more extended professional time in training [33,38]. Worst pain may be more difficult to treat because of its fluctuating and sometimes very brief nature and may require more intensive interventions. On the other hand, opioids are the mainstay of analgesics for moderate to severe pain and consequently are the focus for many guidelines and training efforts [9,13,51]. Opioids primarily target persistent pain and longer-lasting breakthrough pain. More specifically targeted interventions may be needed to reduce worst pain, interference of pain with sleep or other activities, and side effects of pain treatment.

To date, little is known about what constitutes a pain education dose that is appropriate, feasible, and has lasting effects [36]. Because of the complicated nature of pain, more intensive interventions may be necessary to see long-term decreases in pain. As an example, motivational interviewing can be used to address and decrease barriers to cancer pain management and could be a method to promote more durable changes in behavior on the part of patients when beliefs are primary barriers to adherence [16]. For example, if a patient is concerned about side effects, the pros and cons of taking analgesics can be discussed, along with options for steps to take in response to side effects. The challenge, of course, is that larger doses of education are difficult to administer in any medical setting where resources are limited. The issue of need for, but difficulty providing, larger doses of education is particularly notable when cancer is progressive and is complicated by multiple concurrent symptoms. In this case, the energy of patients and caregivers to learn new strategies and adapt learning to new situations can stress even the most collaborative patients and caregivers. In this situation, palliative care or hospice is needed along with education to assist families in adapting to rapidly changing situations.

Future efforts that combine patient- and provider-targeted methods may improve broader long-term outcomes [1,14]. The methods tested in cancer pain education may be more effective and the outcomes more sustained if provided by, and reinforced by, the nurses and physicians at the clinic where patients receive treatment. In this case, the dose may be more frequent, but it can remain brief and targeted to the current pain situation. This clinic integrated approach could assist patients in applying the training information when disease progresses and as treatment or side effects change.

While we believe that the opportunity for reinforcement and follow-up from patients' health care providers might help to maintain the effectiveness of training, we also note that intensity and repetition of educational content has not, in itself, ensured improved outcomes. Pain education studies of longer intervention duration or covering areas other than pain have found less consistent pain relief benefits [12,18,29]. This may be a case where fewer targets for training result in better outcomes. Although more extensive training has, in some cases, shown broadly improved pain outcomes, the follow-up periods were shorter [38]. In summary, the results on dose and focus of educational strategies have been inconsistent, although notably, these results have not been demonstrated to differ by country in which the intervention was provided.

## Other Methodological Issues

There are a few other important issues to consider with these interventions. A barrier to the adoption of routine pain training for patients is the professional time required. Providing printed materials and including caregivers can reinforce face-to-face training [10,18,19,33]. Videos or DVDs help both providers and patients by presenting information in a standardized yet engaging manner, allowing face-to-face time to be individualized. Videos have been used in clinical trials with varying, modest success [2,10,29,63]. The challenge is to determine methods and materials that optimize professional time while achieving sustained, effective cancer pain control.

There is a lack of consensus on endpoints to use in clinical trials [42]. What level of pain should be assessed? Usual? Worst? What about medication adherence, and functional impairment? While it is critical to assess and manage pain appropriately, should interventions address other related issues? Regarding responder analysis, some research has pointed to changes in quality of life and interference of pain with activities [37]. However, most studies do not find a broader impact of these interventions. Because different studies use different endpoints, it can be difficult to compare the efficacy of interventions and the mediators that contribute to change.

## Adherence

It has been difficult to track adherence to education interventions. Those studies that have tracked adherence have found varying rates after pain education [8,38,51,59]. These conflicting findings need to be reconciled through further research. Patients and physicians not only need to learn how to communicate about pain, but they also need to communicate more effectively about analgesics, analgesia-related side effects, and pain interfering with sleep or activities. Side effects are a common reason for discontinuing analgesics according to patients, yet they frequently do not tell their physicians about the side effects or tell them they have stopped analgesics [15,39]. In sum, adherence can be improved through patient training, but patients will still depend on their physicians and nurses to reinforce the use of communication strategies so that adherence is evaluated as pain and analgesic use change.

## Use of Family Caregivers

Caregivers are affected by cancer pain and often assist with administering medications, and so their attitudes about pain can influence the patient's attitudes and behaviors. Aranda and colleagues conducted a study with Australian caregivers to assess their barriers to pain management [3]. Similar to patients, caregivers were concerned about addiction and worried that pain would mean that the cancer had progressed. They also expressed concerns about side effects. Caregivers were least concerned with tolerance to opioids. Thus, caregivers have their own barriers to pain management, and it could be helpful to have targeted education programs to address these issues. Keefe and colleagues have trained caregivers in helping their patients cope with pain, along with more traditional components that include education and coping strategies [29]. Caregivers in the intervention group reported greater self-efficacy and there was a trend toward a decrease in caregiver strain. Other research that incorporated caregivers found decreases in barriers, increases in patients' adherence to medication, and lower pain scores [33].

Growing recognition of the role of caregivers has led to research that has included caregivers in educational interventions designed for patients. However, in two randomized trials of cancer pain education, patients who were accompanied by a caregiver did not do any better than patients who participated without one [51,62].

## Health Care Providers

Most existing research has focused on patients and changing their behaviors and communication, with some studies including or focusing on caregivers. However, patients and their families are not the only groups that need education about cancer pain. In a review of studies focusing on nurses, nurses' knowledge increased and their misperceptions about analgesics were corrected after an educational intervention, but these changes have not influenced patients' report of pain [21]. This finding mirrors research with patients and caregivers in that an increase in knowledge does not necessarily translate into a reduction in pain. To date, we are not aware of any randomized controlled trials on cancer pain education with physicians isolated from other outcome targets such that it is possible to evaluate the efficacy of education alone.

# Implications and Dissemination

## Cultural and Global Factors

The meta-analysis by Bennett and colleagues included studies from Taiwan, Europe, and Australia [6]. Pain education was effective in those countries. However, there is a need for research in less developed countries. In the United States, Hispanic/Latino and African American patients receive poorer pain treatment and consequently report more pain than whites

[9]. In a secondary analysis of a randomized controlled trial to educate patients about cancer pain, a brief session (20 minutes) over the phone was enough to decrease pain report by 1.73 points on a 10-point scale [28]. As expected, the minority participants reported higher pain levels prior to the intervention, but had greater pain reductions than their Caucasian counterparts in the study. This result indicates that patient education is very effective for diverse ethnically and racially identified patients and can reduce disparities in pain.

It may or may not be important to culturally tailor patient education programs, as the above study did not tailor the education program for minority patients. Important cultural differences are evident in a study of online forums for different ethnic groups to express their thoughts regarding cancer pain [24]. For example, Latino patients may underreport their levels of pain because they may think that the pain is part of their fate and nothing can be done. African Americans may feel stigmatized and thus be less likely to report pain, as cancer may be perceived as equivalent to death [25]. Asian Americans may be more likely to want to use positive thinking to cope with the pain [26]. Of course, for each of these generalizations there are likely to be exceptions, and individual tailoring is always preferred for optimal impact.

Although there may be culture-specific beliefs about pain, some research would suggest that culturally tailored interventions can have limited impact. Anderson and colleagues tested a culturally specific intervention for African American and Latino patients [2]. The African Americans in the pain education group reported significant decreases in pain intensity compared to the control group at 2 and 4 weeks, but this decrease was not maintained over time. The Latino patients in the education group and the control groups reported decreases in pain intensity and were not significantly different from one another. The authors recommend caution in interpreting these results because of the small sample sizes and advanced disease of the participating patients. More research is needed in this area because a subanalysis did not find any ethnic differences [28].

## Technology

Various applications of technology have the potential to reduce the burden of cancer pain education on health care professionals, but their efficacy needs to be demonstrated. While videos have been effectively used in cancer pain education, other modalities have yet to be tested. The telephone can be used to deliver educational interventions and may be more amenable to patients than coming early to a doctor visit, which is more typical of the interventions tested [16]. In a study that delivered education by telephone to people with cancer-related pain who called the Cancer Information Service, negative attitudes about reporting pain decreased, as did the use of analgesics [61]. Technology, such as the Internet and handheld computers, can be used to assess patients and their symptoms and has been shown to increase the rates of pain assessment by health care professionals [35]. But other modes of technology need to be tested as a way to deliver education as well as assess symptoms. The Internet can be a tool to reach people and provide access to individualized education, as well as allowing use on an as-needed basis. This tool could assist with patient adaptation to changes in pain and fluctuating education needs. Online access to health care providers, as is now being offered or tested in numerous health care systems, may also offer opportunities to clarify learning or assist with adjusting to new pain and concurrent symptom treatments.

# Conclusions

While cancer pain education can be effective for patients and even caregivers, the gains appear to be modest and difficult to maintain over time. Perhaps interventions need to include booster sessions as a way to retain or extend gains. These interventions also need to be tested with more diverse populations as the studies generally have mostly Caucasian and middle-class participants from the United States. While pain education programs have been effective in most studies, the mediators of change have yet to be elucidated. These interventions can be improved to be more effective, to reach more people, and also reduce the burden on health care professionals by using technology. Cancer pain education is a core principle of cancer pain relief. The limited number of studies completed to date offer encouragement, but do not clarify the mediators of effectiveness or the necessary elements to assure success. These are worthy targets for future research.

# Acknowledgments

Funded by National Cancer Institute grants CA 112631, CA 68139, and CA 57807.

# References

[1]   Allard P, Maunsell E, Labbé J, Dorval M. Educational interventions to improve cancer pain control: a systematic review. J Palliat Med 2001;4:191–203.

[2]   Anderson KO, Mendoza TR, Payne R, Valero V, Palos GR, Nazario A, Richman SP, Hurley J, Gning I, Lynch GR, Kalish D, Cleeland CS. Pain education for underserved minority cancer patients: a randomized controlled trial. J Clin Oncol 2004;22:4918–25.

[3]   Aranda S, Yates P, Edwards H, Nash R, Skerman H, McCarthy A. Barriers to effective cancer pain management: a survey of Australian family caregivers. Eur J Cancer Care 2004;13:336–43.

[4]   Asghari A, Nicholas MK. Pain self-efficacy beliefs and pain behaviour. A prospective study. Pain 2001;94:85–100.

[5]   Aubin M, Vezina L, Parent R, Fillion L, Allard P, Bergeron R, Dumont S, Giguere A. Impact of an educational program on pain management in patients with cancer living at home. Oncol Nurs Forum 2006;33:1183–8.

[6]   Bennett MI, Bagnall AM, Jose CS. How effective are patient-based educational interventions in the management of cancer pain? Systematic review and meta-analysis. Pain 2009;143:192–9.

[7]   Bonomi AE, Ajax M, Shikiar R, Halpern M. Cancer pain management: barriers, trends, and the role of pharmacists. J Am Pharm Assoc (Wash) 1999;39:558–66.

[8]   Chang MC, Chang YC, Chiou JF, Tsou TS, Lin CC. Overcoming patient-related barriers to cancer pain management for home care patients: a pilot study. Cancer Nurs 2002;25:470–6.

[9]   Cleeland CS, Gonin R, Hatfield AK, Edmonson JH, Blum RH, Steward JA, Pandya KJ. Pain and its treatment in outpatients with metastatic cancer. New Engl J Med 1994;330:592–6.

[10]  Clotfelter CE. The effect of an educational intervention on decreasing pain intensity in elderly people with cancer. Oncol Nurs Forum 1999;26:27–33.

[11]  Devine EC. Meta-analysis of the effect of psychoeducational interventions on pain in adults with cancer. Oncol Nurs Forum Online 2003;30:75–89.

[12]  deWit R, vanDam F, Zandbelt L, vanBuuren A, van der HK, Leenhouts G, Loonstra S. A pain education program for chronic cancer pain patients: follow-up results from a randomized controlled trial. Pain 1997;73:5569.

[13]  Du Pen AR, DuPen SL, Hansberry J, Miller-Kraybill B, Millen J, Everly R, Hansen N, Syrjala KL. An educational implementation of a cancer pain algorithm for ambulatory care. Pain Manage Nurs 2000;1:116–28.

[14]  Du Pen SL, Du Pen AR, Polissar N, Hansberry J, Kraybill BM, Stillman M, Panke J, Everly R, Syrjala K. Implementing guidelines for cancer pain management: results of a randomized controlled clinical trial. J Clin Oncol 1999;17:361–70.

[15]  Ersek M, Kraybill BM, Du Pen A. Factors hindering patients' use of medications for cancer pain. Cancer Pract 1999;7:226–32.

[16]  Fahey KF, Rao SM, Douglas MK, Thomas ML, Elliott JE, Miaskowski C. Nurse coaching to explore and modify patient attitudinal barriers interfering with effective cancer pain management. Oncol Nurs Forum 2008;35:233–40.

[17]  Fallowfield L, Jenkins V. Effective communication skills are the key to good cancer care. Eur J Cancer 1999;35:1592–7.

[18]  Ferrell BR, Grant M, Chan J, Ahn C, Ferrell BA. The impact of cancer pain education on family caregivers of elderly patients. Oncol Nurs Forum 1995;22:1211–8.

[19]  Ferrell BR, Rhiner M, Ferrell BA. Development and implementation of a pain education program. Cancer 1993;72:3426–32.

[20]  Gattellari M, Butow PN, Tattersall MH. Sharing decisions in cancer care. Soc Sci Med 2001;52:1865–78.

[21] Goldberg GR, Morrison RS. Pain management in hospitalized cancer patients: a systematic review. J Clin Oncol 2007;25:1792–1801.

[22] Grossman SA, Benedetti C, Payne R, Syrjala KL. NCCN practice guidelines for cancer pain. NCCN Proc 1999;13:33–44.

[23] Hicks CL, Von Baeyer CL, Spafford PA, van Korlaar I, Goodenough B. The Faces Pain Scale-Revised: toward a common metric in pediatric pain measurement. Pain 2001;93:173–83.

[24] Im EO, Guevara E, Chee W. The pain experience of Hispanic patients with cancer in the United States. Oncol Nurs Forum 2007;34:861–8.

[25] Im EO, Lim HJ, Clark M, Chee W. African American cancer patients' pain experience. Cancer Nurs 2008;31:38–46.

[26] Im EO, Liu Y, Kim YH, Chee W. Asian American cancer patients' pain experience. Cancer Nurs 2008;31:E17–23.

[27] Joint Commission on Accreditation of Heathcare Organizations. Improving the quality of pain management through measurement and action. Oakbrook Terrace, IL: Joint Commission Resources; 2003.

[28] Kalauokalani D, Franks P, Oliver JW, Meyers FJ, Kravitz RL. Can patient coaching reduce racial/ethnic disparities in cancer pain control? Secondary analysis of a randomized controlled trial. Pain Med 2007;8:17–24.

[29] Keefe FJ, Ahles TA, Sutton L, Dalton J, Baucom D, Pope MS, Knowles V, McKinstry E, Furstenberg C, Syrjala K, et al. Partner-guided cancer pain management at the end of life: a preliminary study. J Pain Symptom Manage 2005;29:263–72.

[30] Kerr B, Hill H, Coda B, Calogero M, Chapman CR, Hunt E, Buffington V, Mackie A. Concentration-related effects of morphine on cognition and motor control in human subjects. Neuropsychopharmacology 1991;5:157–66.

[31] Kohn LT, Corrigan JM, Donaldson MS, editors. To err is human: building a safer health system. Washington, DC: National Academy Press; 2000.

[32] Kravitz RL, Tancredi DJ, Street RL Jr, Kalauokalani D, Grennan T, Wun T, Slee C, Evans DD, Lewis L, Saito N, Franks P. Cancer Health Empowerment for Living without Pain (Ca-HELP): study design and rationale for a tailored education and coaching intervention to enhance care of cancer-related pain. BMC Cancer 2009;9:319.

[33] Lin CC, Chou PL, Wu SL, Chang YC, Lai YL. Long-term effectiveness of a patient and family pain education program on overcoming barriers to management of cancer pain. Pain 2006;122:271–81.

[34] Manfredi PL, Chandler S, Pigazzi A, Payne R. Outcome of cancer pain consultations. Cancer 2000;89:920–4.

[35] Mark TL, Fortner B, Johnson G. Evaluation of a tablet PC technology to screen and educate oncology patients. Support Care Cancer 2008;16:371–8.

[36] Miaskowski C. Patient education about cancer pain management: how much time is enough? Pain 2008;135:1–2.

[37] Miaskowski C, Dodd M, West C, Paul SM, Schumacher K, Tripathy D, Koo P. The use of a responder analysis to identify differences in patient outcomes following a self-care intervention to improve cancer pain management. Pain 2007;129:55–63.

[38] Miaskowski C, Dodd M, West C, Schumacher K, Paul SM, Tripathy D, Koo P. Randomized clinical trial of the effectiveness of a self-care intervention to improve cancer pain management. J Clin Oncol 2004;22:1713–20.

[39] Miaskowski C, Dodd MJ, West C, Paul SM, Tripathy D, Koo P, Schumacher K. Lack of adherence with the analgesic regimen: a significant barrier to effective cancer pain management. J Clin Oncol 2001;19:4275–9.

[40] Miaskowski C, Zimmer EF, Barrett KM, Dibble SL, Wallhagen M. Differences in patients' and family caregivers' perceptions of the pain experience influence patient and caregiver outcomes. Pain 1997;72:217–26.

[41] Mishel MH. Perceived uncertainty and stress in illness. Res Nurs Health 1984;7:163–71.

[42] Oldenmenger WH, Sillevis Smitt PA, van Dooren S, Stoter G, van der Rijt CC. A systematic review on barriers hindering adequate cancer pain management and interventions to reduce them: a critical appraisal. Eur J Cancer 2009;45:1370–80.

[43] Oliver JW, Kravitz RL, Kaplan SH, Meyers FJ. Individualized patient education and coaching to improve pain control among cancer outpatients. J Clin Oncol 2001;19:2206–12.

[44] Phillips DP, Christenfeld N, Glynn LM. Increase in US medication-error deaths between 1983 and 1993. Lancet 1998;351:643–4.

[45]  Porter LS, Keefe FJ, Garst J, McBride CM, Baucom D. Self-efficacy for managing pain, symptoms, and function in patients with lung cancer and their informal caregivers: associations with symptoms and distress. Pain 2008;137:306–15.

[46]  Rait D, Lederberg M. The family of the cancer patient. In: Holland JC, Rowland JH, editors. Handbook of psychooncology. New York: Oxford University Press; 1989:585-597.

[47]  Sjogren P, Thomsen AB, Olsen AK. Impaired neuropsychological performance in chronic nonmalignant pain patients receiving long-term oral opioid therapy. J Pain Symptom Manage 2000;19:100–8.

[48]  Stewart MA. Effective physician-patient communication and health outcomes: a review. CMAJ 1995;152:1423–33.

[49]  Street RL Jr, Slee C, Kalauokalani DK, Dean DE, Tancredi DJ, Kravitz RL. Improving physician-patient communication about cancer pain with a tailored education-coaching intervention. Patient Educ Couns 2009; Epub Dec 3.

[50]  Swarm R, Anghelescu DL, Benedetti C, Boston B, Cleeland C, Coyle N, Deleon-Casasola OA, Eidelman A, Eilers JG, Ferrell B, et al.; National Comprehensive Cancer Network (NCCN). Adult cancer pain. J Natl Compr Canc Netw 2007;5:726–51.

[51]  Syrjala KL, Abrams JR, Polissar NL, Hansberry J, Robison J, DuPen S, Stillman M, Fredrickson M, Rivkin S, Feldman E, et al. Patient training in cancer pain management using integrated print and video materials: a multisite randomized controlled trial. Pain 2008;135:175–86.

[52]  Syrjala KL, Chapko ME. Evidence for a biopsychosocial model of cancer treatment-related pain. Pain 1995;61:69–79.

[53]  Syrjala KL, Roth-Roemer SL. Nonpharmacologic approaches to pain. In: Berger A, editor. Principles and practices of supportive oncology. Philadelphia: Lippincott-Raven; 1998. p. 79–93.

[54]  Taylor WJ, Dean SG, Siegert RJ. Differential association of general and health self-efficacy with disability, health-related quality of life and psychological distress from musculoskeletal pain in a cross-sectional general adult population survey. Pain 2006;125:225–32.

[55]  Valeberg BT, Miaskowski C, Hanestad BR, Bjordal K, Moum T, Rustoen T. Prevalence rates for and predictors of self-reported adherence of oncology outpatients with analgesic medications. Clin J Pain 2008;24:627–36.

[56]  van der Peet E, van den Beuken-van Everdingen M, Patijn J, Schouten H, Courtens A. Randomized clinical trial of an intensive nursing-based pain education program for cancer outpatients suffering from pain. Support Care Cancer 2008; Epub Dec 23.

[57]  Von Roenn JH, Cleeland CS, Gonin R, Hatfield AK, Pandya KJ. Physician attitudes and practice in cancer pain management: a survey from the eastern cooperative oncology group. Ann Intern Med 1993;119:121–6.

[58]  Ward S, Donovan H, Gunnarsdottir S, Serlin RC, Shapiro GR, Hughes S. A randomized trial of a representational intervention to decrease cancer pain (RIDcancerPain). Health Psychol 2008;27:59–67.

[59]  Ward S, Donovan HS, Owen B, Grosen E, Serlin R. An individualized intervention to overcome patient-related barriers to pain management in women with gynecologic cancers. Res Nurs Health 2000;23:393–405.

[60]  Ward SE, Goldberg N, Miller-McCauley V, Mueller C, Nolan A, Pawlik-Plank D, Robbins ASD, Weissman DE. Patient-related barriers to management of cancer pain. Pain 1993;52:319–24.

[61]  Ward SE, Wang KK, Serlin RC, Peterson SL, Murray ME. A randomized trial of a tailored barriers intervention for Cancer Information Service (CIS) callers in pain. Pain 2009;144:49–56.

[62]  Ward SE, Serlin RC, Donovan HS, Ameringer SW, Hughes S, Pe-Romashko K, Wang KK. A randomized trial of a representational intervention for cancer pain: does targeting the dyad make a difference? Health Psychol 2009;28:588–97.

[63]  Wells N, Hepworth JT, Murphy BA, Wujcik D, Johnson R. Improving cancer pain management through patient and family education. J Pain Symptom Manage 2003;25:344–56.

[64]  West CM, Dodd MJ, Paul SM, Schumacher K, Tripathy D, Koo P, Miaskowski C. The PRO-SELF pain control program: an effective approach for cancer pain management. Oncol Nurs Forum 2003;30:65–73.

***Correspondence to:*** Karen L. Syrjala, PhD, Biobehavioral Sciences, Clinical Research Division, Fred Hutchinson Cancer Research Center, 1100 Fairview Ave. N., D5-220, Seattle, WA 98109, USA. Email: ksyrjala@fhcrc.org.

# Teaching Medical Students about Cancer Pain

## Karen Forbes and Jane Gibbins

*Department of Palliative Medicine, Bristol Haematology and Oncology Centre,*
*University of Bristol, United Kingdom*

If we are to improve quality of life for patients with pain due to cancer, their physicians need to be confident in their ability to manage cancer pain. Traditionally, physicians have received most of their training about managing cancer pain after graduation. However, it is recognized increasingly that physicians will need to know how to manage pain for many of their patients as soon as they qualify and take up practice, and therefore basic training in medical school is both desirable and necessary.

## Medical School Education about Cancer Pain

Education about pain management can occur in two main situations in medical school curricula. The management of noncancer pain, including acute, chronic, and postoperative pain, is often taught within courses on anesthesia, and the management of cancer pain within courses on oncology and palliative care. The principles of pain management in these two courses are similar, but the context of pain management in the two clinical situations differs widely, necessitating different teaching approaches.

*Cancer Pain: From Molecules to Suffering*
edited by Judith A. Paice, Rae F. Bell, Eija A. Kalso, and Olaitan A. Soyannwo
IASP Press, Seattle, © 2010

Unfortunately, the evidence suggests that few medical students receive extensive training about pain within either setting.

In an editorial published in *Pain* in 1988, Pilowsky reported the work of an International Association for the Study of Pain ad hoc subcommittee on medical school courses and curricula [27]. The group produced a model outline pain course setting out the subjects that should be covered within a medical school curriculum. Despite this recommendation, an Association of American Medical Colleges survey in 2000–2001 reported a specific pain management course in only 3% of their schools, and in April 2009 Vadivelu and colleagues were still lamenting the ongoing "urgent need for pain management training" for American medical students [36]. The literature suggests that teaching about pain elsewhere is not substantially different [22,23,28,32,35].

The management of cancer pain is, necessarily, a major component of teaching about palliative care. Three themes emerge on reviewing the literature on education in palliative care, perhaps giving some indication of the development of a new specialty over the last 30 years. Early reports focus on the inadequacy of teaching and the need for inclusion of palliative care teaching in medical school curricula [3,9,14]. Subsequent publications are surveys of the teaching available [5,6,7,8,19,26]. Further papers argue either for the inclusion of palliative care teaching in medical school curricula, or present the case for including such teaching and then describe the course developed in the authors' institution. Once the need for such teaching was established, authors discussed how such teaching should be delivered and by whom. As early as 1980, Smith and colleagues observed that while the objectives of palliative care teaching were relatively consistent in all U.S. medical schools providing such coursework, the "course content, faculty and patient roles, learning resources, and involvement in curriculum research did not evidence a systematic development" [33]. The authors also noted that the clinical implications of the teaching were unknown.

One approach to the heterogeneity of teaching was for national or governmental bodies to derive curricula to guide the teaching of palliative care. The Association for Palliative Medicine for the United Kingdom and Ireland published its curriculum for medical students and doctors in training in 1993 [2]. In the same year, the deans of the six Canadian medical schools developed a curriculum for the teaching of palliative care to medical students [18]. The American Academy of Hospice and Palliative

Medicine published *Hospice and Palliative Medicine: Core Curriculum and Review Syllabus* in 1998 [1]. The assessment and management of pain features significantly in all of these curricula.

Regulatory authorities have also recognized the need for pain education; for instance, in the United Kingdom, the General Medical Council's publication *Tomorrow's Doctors* set out the knowledge, skills, attitudes, and behavior expected of new graduates in medicine and included the recommendation that "graduates must know about and understand the principles of treatment including 'relieving pain and distress' and 'palliative care, including care of the terminally ill'" [13]. While the provision of teaching about pain and palliative care has increased over the periods surveyed, there is little evidence that these curricula have been fully implemented into the medical school curricula of their respective countries, despite such recommendations [7].

In 2000, Oneschuk and colleagues carried out a questionnaire survey of all 16 medical schools in Canada, all 30 in the United Kingdom, and 129 randomly selected medical schools in the United States and Western Europe, with a response rate of 76%. Whereas 64% of schools in the United Kingdom reported that palliative medicine experience was part of the core curriculum, this was only the case for 11% of schools in the United States, 14% in Canada, and 19% in Western Europe. Optional experience in palliative medicine was offered in 82% of U.K., 71% of Canadian, 62% of U.S., and 30% of Western European schools [25].

More recently there has been some attempt to evaluate the teaching programs described in the literature. The evaluations reported are commonly students' evaluations of satisfaction with the teaching or their perceptions of educational benefit. Where factual knowledge is assessed following palliative care teaching, often in junior doctors rather than medical students, it is often changes in students' and doctors' ability to prescribe pain relief that is explored [24,34].

# Knowledge and Attitudes in Teaching about Cancer Pain

The ability to prescribe pain relief is only one part of successfully managing a patient with pain due to cancer. In the literature, knowledge about opioids is often treated as a "proxy" for both knowledge of and attitudes toward managing patients with pain due to cancer. Much pain education concentrates on improving knowledge and teaching "appropriate" attitudes, with an assumption that this training will improve professionals' performance in assessing and managing pain, and therefore improve pain for patients. Projects have been conducted that are designed assiduously, executed carefully, and evaluated appropriately, yet they still fail to demonstrate that such teaching programs result in improved pain management for patients [11]. Indeed, when presenting a study evaluating knowledge, attitudes, and self-reported pain management behavior, Levin and colleagues suggest that "education will not effect significant behavioral changes in the care of terminally ill patients solely by the traditional approach of attempting to modify knowledge and attitudes" [16]. "Technical" knowledge alone is insufficient; once such knowledge is achieved it is argued that a broad range of skills—including communication skills—and appropriate attitudes and beliefs are needed to manage patients with cancer pain successfully in clinical practice [23,35].

In 2002 Turner and Weiner published the results of a modified Delphi process used to design a curriculum for medical students on chronic pain management in older adults. The management of cancer pain was not included in this study, but it is significant to note that the resulting curriculum consisted of 18 knowledge items (11 pain assessment and seven pain management units), 12 skills items, and 12 pain attitude items; both skills and attitudes were therefore seen as integral to managing pain successfully [35]. Attitudinal items included, for example, awareness that self-report of pain is reliable, openness to the role of the multidisciplinary team, and understanding that opioid addiction is rare and should not influence prescribing.

Medical students are likely to have preconceived ideas about their ability to manage pain successfully and whether or not interacting with patients with chronic pain will be worthwhile [37]. We know that medical students and qualified physicians have negative attitudes and beliefs about pain, and particularly about strong opioids—believing, for example, that pain is inevitable in patients with cancer, morphine has a narrow therapeutic dose range, tolerance to analgesia is common, side effects are common and cannot be managed adequately, and respiratory depression limits dose escalation [10,31]. It is argued that students take on their teachers' negative attitudes through the hidden curriculum [15]; however, it is also likely that students bring lay perceptions about morphine and the use of opioids for cancer pain with them into their medical school training. Patients see morphine as the last resort when they are dying, at a point when their pain means they have no choice but to accept it, even though they think it will hasten their death [29]. Medical students' views will be compounded by the fact that having patients with cancer pain requiring opioids also forces them to confront the issue of caring for patients who are very sick and may die. We must therefore assume our students have lay attitudes toward pain and its management and will be anxious about caring for people near the end of their lives; we must tailor our teaching accordingly.

# Can Education Change Attitudes Relevant to Managing Cancer Pain?

As long ago as 1992, Wilson and colleagues reported the effect on students' attitudes toward pain after a brief 6-hour course, a single module of which was about cancer pain. An evaluation questionnaire 5 months after the course showed that students' previously negative attitudes about patients with chronic pain had reversed and that they were more likely to think that looking after patients with pain could be worthwhile [37]. Similarly, Niemi-Murola and colleagues have shown that medical students' attitudes toward managing patients with pain can improve during their medical studies, in terms of not accepting pain as, for instance, a normal part of aging and being willing to manage pain actively, although they found more senior students to be more, rather than less, anxious about meeting a patient with pain and about their ability to manage pain. These authors suggest that this increased anxiety is due to students' increasing empathy, particularly in female students, and that this is appropriate. They recommend that students need help in dealing with their own emotions and anxieties about caring for people with pain [22].

Assessing and managing a patient in pain thus requires knowledge, skills, and appropriate attitudes and beliefs. The *Concise Oxford English Dictionary* defines "attitude" as "a settled way of thinking or feeling" and belief as "a feeling that something exists or is true, especially one without proof" or "a firmly held opinion" [30]. If attitudes are "settled" ways of thinking, and beliefs "firmly held" views that do not necessarily require "proof," then we would be naive to assume that a teacher telling a student that opioids do not hasten death will inevitably lead the student (or indeed patient) to accept this statement as fact. Our approaches to teaching and learning need to take this consideration into account.

# Gaining Relevant Clinical Experience

Miller's pyramid (Fig. 1) provides a framework for analyzing how students demonstrate competence [20]; at the lowest level, "knows," the student merely needs to reproduce information that has been taught. At the highest level, "does," the student knows the information, understands and believes it, and integrates it into practice—such as, in the medical student or physician's situation, in the care of a patient. This pyramid can also shape our approaches to teaching. To tell students something at the "knows" level may allow them to pass an assessment, but may not improve patient care. We therefore need to give students evidence to back up our assertions, so they "know how" knowledge can be put into practice and we will need to "show how" we put the knowledge we are teaching into caring for our patients. Ultimately, students will need involvement in clinical experience so that they can reach the "does" level of the pyramid. Possible strategies necessary to assess competence at each of these levels are shown in Fig. 1.

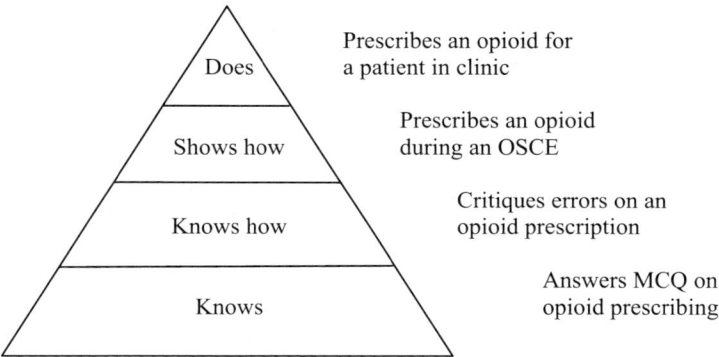

***Fig. 1.*** Miller's pyramid. Adapted from Miller [20]. OSCE, objective structured clinical examination; MCQ, multiple choice question examination.

This pyramid is helpful in understanding why knowledge-based teaching and instruction about "appropriate" attitudes might not lead to improved pain control for patients.

Clinical experience is a critical element in enabling students to develop competence at the "shows how" and "does" levels of Miller's pyramid. At the University of Bristol medical school, students have a 4-week course in oncology and palliative care, the assessment and management of cancer pain being significant learning outcomes required from the course. As part of the evaluation of this course we have interviewed final-year medical students about their experiences [K. Forbes, EdD thesis, University of Bristol, 2006].

Patients with cancer pain and palliative care needs are challenging for students. Students are often frightened of the questions patients might ask, or the things they might want to talk about; many students doubt they have the communication skills to cope with the potential conversations. They therefore need support and encouragement to interact with these patients. We must remember, however, that students meet such patients most frequently during their general clinical attachments in medicine and surgery, rather than during placements in oncology and palliative care. At the University of Bristol, students often come across these clinical situations during a 2-week course when they "shadow" the physician whose post they will take up a short time later when they qualify. These experiences are thus gained when students start to take on greater clinical responsibility [12]. However, our interviews with students suggest that they are not supported fully in meeting these patients until their oncology or palliative care attachments. Staff state that they do not wish to burden patients with seeing students when they are very ill. However, our data also suggest that general staff appear less confident with these exchanges and avoid facilitating students' interactions with palliative care patients because they might unmask the qualified professionals' weaknesses or insecurities. As one student explained:

> Palliative Care and Oncology were a bit of a shock ... the completely different approach, and it actually makes you think about it rather than just being aware of it. It is in the background the rest of the time. I think that's very much the approach for the rest of the medical school ... you go through all the treatments and that will

be that. I mean we'd had the occasional outpatient clinic where someone is breaking news on cancer, and that makes you look at it in a different way. And even things like terminal medical illnesses, you never really approach it with a palliative intent … or no one has ever explicitly mentioned it anyway. And it probably sounds a bit naive, but if no one mentions it you don't think about it, so you think "Oh, they're just doing oxygen therapy," and you don't think that that might be because it's terminal.

Broadly, students fall into three groups: students (the minority) who have sought and gained experience, students who have sought experience but were denied it, and students who have not sought experience. The first group of students either feel comfortable talking to patients who are ill and might die and therefore gain useful clinical experience, or they are in the right place at the right time and find that the interaction is less frightening than they thought it would be. For example, in talking about patients dying of cancer, a student said:

I felt I should stay. And I didn't positively want to leave. I think every medical student in their final year … unless of course they've got personal difficulties … if it's going on, you shouldn't really shy away from it. Because it's better to see it, surely, when it's not actually your responsibility than when you're in your first week and it is. And so any doctor who is shooing away a fifth year medical student because they feel they can't handle it, they need to question … really, that they should be able to handle it, and then the student should be questioning, "What am I doing if I can't handle it?"

I was around, I was staying throughout, so they do let you, which is good. And I'm really glad that I was allowed to, because it turns a hypothetical situation into a reality and you start to look at, not only the practical issues for when you are the doctor, but how are you going to react, rather than seeing it for the first time and panicking. It also gives you a chance to think about how you felt afterwards, and how the team worked as well.

Students from the second group were shielded from seeing patients with pain and palliative care needs. Some would have wanted to gain the experience; others were content to allow themselves to be prevented from seeing patients.

I've done a lot of [nursing assistant] work and I think that's actually prepared me more than medical school, because no one at medical school takes you by the hand and says: "That's what a patient looks like when they're sick." It's just recognition, but no one ever tells you and looking back, I've walked past patients on wards … and now I know. But no one ever said to me "Just go and have a look." And it's probably because they think that when you're sick and dying you don't want 15 medical students traipsing in and out of the cubicle.

The last group of students had failed to gain experience; some seemed unaware that this was experience they would need to gain.

I remember when we were doing vascular surgery there was a lady with a lot of pain who had a gangrenous leg, and she was quite old and she didn't want surgery. And so the doctor said, very quietly, "I'm afraid she's going to die." Not to the patient, you know, just telling us. I've always been surprised how few experiences I've ever had. Most people on the ward seem to be getting better.

Students often commented that experiential learning was a "lottery," particularly when the nature of the patients' problems meant that qualified professionals were inclined to "protect" patients from students and/or shield students from complex and emotive situations: "If you're on a ward and something happens, then if you were there then you'd see it, but if you were in [the operating room] then you missed it."

Our analysis was that students were concerned about burdening patients, but also anxious that they might not cope if they did interact with them, and that professionals wanted to protect patients from being burdened, although sometimes this consideration allowed them also to protect themselves. As teachers, therefore, we need to both prepare and support students through the experience of meeting and learning from patients who have cancer pain and other symptoms and are very sick or dying. It is possible to do so by being explicit about the issues, by providing tutor and peer support for students, and by encouraging students to reflect upon the experiences they have. When giving feedback on our course, students frequently reflect upon being apprehensive before the course, noting that they found the course useful, and that they were surprised at finding it enjoyable. We also have a responsibility, however, to seek ways to help our colleagues support students in interacting with patients with cancer pain who need palliative care.

## The Role of E-Learning in Teaching about Pain and Palliative Care

We have discussed the importance of experiential learning for students and the need to recognize the role of attitudes in managing cancer pain. The discussion thus far has not differentiated between explicit and implicit attitudes and beliefs. The Johari window (Fig. 2) is a framework that can be used to analyze self-awareness [17]. The window has four "panes" representing areas of which we are, or are not, aware and areas of which others are, or are not, aware in interacting with us. Our role as teachers is to help students to become aware of their blind areas through observation and feedback and for us to develop strategies to unearth issues in the "unknown area," particularly if these areas involve attitudes about prescribing opioids, for example, that might alter students' abilities to manage patients in pain once qualified. An example of a Johari window, with possible issues related to opioids, is seen in Fig. 2.

We wondered whether e-learning might help in tackling issues pertinent to cancer pain and palliative care. Our hypothesis was that e-learning might bring to the surface attitudes that could affect future

|  | Known to self | Unknown to self |
|---|---|---|
| Known to others | Is aware that opioids are often helpful for cancer pain<br><br>**AWARE** | Prescribes incorrectly<br><br><br>**BLIND SPOT** |
| Unknown to others | **FAÇADE**<br>Prescribes cautiously because of fear of making mistakes | **UNKNOWN**<br>Prescribes unaware of patients' fears about opioids |

**Fig. 2.** The Johari window. Adapted from Luft [17] to show possible levels of awareness in opioid prescribing.

patient care and might even change, i.e., teach, attitudes. We developed a series of "maze" tutorials designed to engage with attitudes such as opioiphobia, therapeutic nihilism in cancer, unwillingness to diagnose patients as dying, and reluctance to withdraw treatment at the end of life. A "maze" tutorial presents students with a number of decision-making points within a clinical case. At each decision point students can take a variety of paths. A simplified version of a small portion of the information behind a maze tutorial exploring opioiphobia is shown in Fig. 3. We have introduced these tutorials within a research project. Preliminary results from the focus group aspect of the evaluation suggest that attitudes can come to the surface in these tutorials, i.e., students see the "blind spots" from their Johari window, and that for some students, understanding their previously "unknown" attitude has changed their perspective on clinical care. Students' comments included:

> I always thought I would know when to stop treating a patient when it was not working, but this tutorial made me realise that I wanted to keep going, just in case there was a chance. What if I stopped and it was the wrong thing to do? It would be my responsibility.

> I know it is important to manage pain properly, but I realised I was frightened of giving too much morphine.

A positive outcome we had not anticipated was students finding that they could try options and even take risks because they were managing a "virtual" patient via a computer screen, unobserved, often in the privacy of their own home. As a student explained:

> You protect us too much by telling us we are going wrong and giving us the option to try again. You need to build more dead ends in. Let us make mistakes … let us get it wrong … let us kill the patient if that's what we are going to do.

Students felt they would prefer to learn through mistakes in a safe (virtual) environment, rather than bear the responsibility of making these difficult decisions with patients and have to bear the emotional consequences of getting it wrong in the real world.

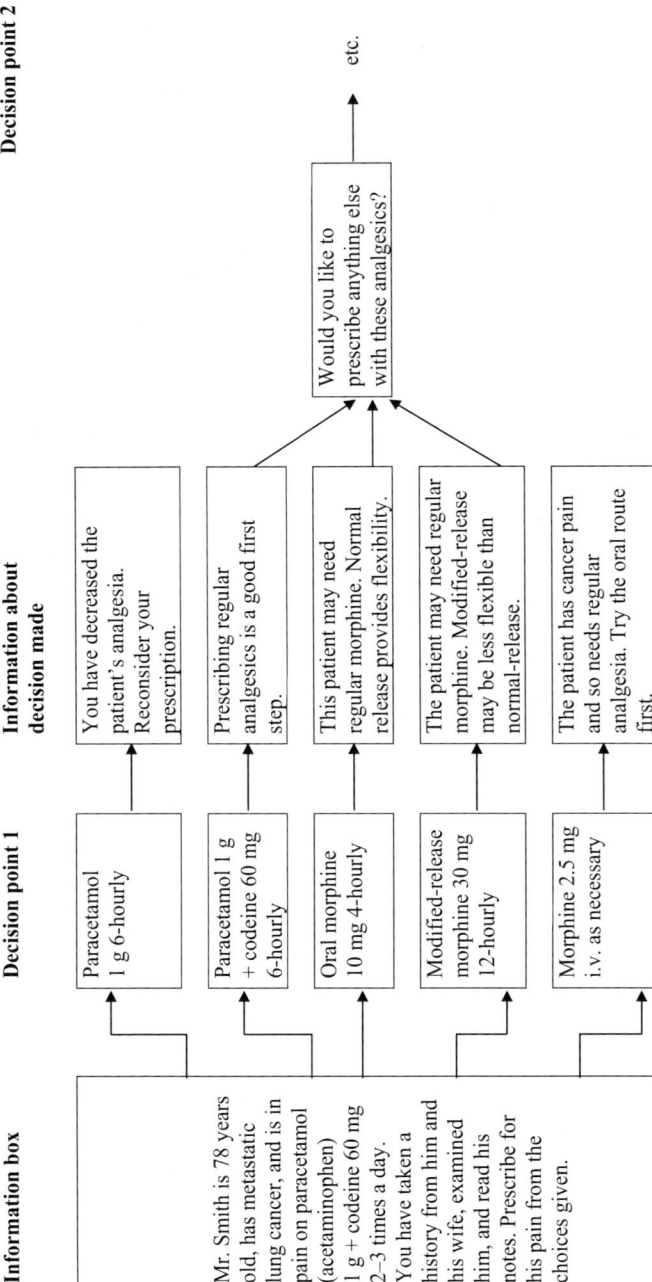

**Fig. 3.** Information embedded within a small portion of a "maze" tutorial on opioiphobia. Students view only one decision point at a time and see only information relevant to the path they choose to follow through the "maze."

It may seem counterintuitive to introduce e-learning when students lack clinical experience. Indeed one of our students objected to completing the e-learning tutorials, stating:

> Sitting in front of a computer is not the way to learn about these issues. You learn this from being on the wards. We have already done this.

This student was a mature student with very varied previous experience who had spent a lot of extra time on the wards and clearly was confident about seeking clinical experience. His colleagues' responses included:

> You may have done it, but we haven't. We haven't seen these patients. We haven't seen these situations. For us these tutorials were really useful.

Other authors have suggested that a combination of approaches, computer-based and clinical, will be most effective in educating students [32]. Our preliminary results suggest that the e-learning tutorials need to be more sophisticated to mirror clinical practice more realistically, but they also indicate that e-learning can be used to reveal attitudes and to facilitate discussion about them, which will allow some students to adopt new attitudes. We hope that this change in attitude, in turn, will encourage and enable medical students to spend more time with, and learn from, patients with pain due to cancer and those who have palliative care needs.

# Summary

Newly qualified physicians will meet patients with pain due to cancer as soon as they begin to practice. In order to give their patients optimal care, they require good education that must include attention to attitudes, skills, and behavior as well as knowledge. For this to occur, schools need to implement the curricula already available, to explore different ways of providing students with relevant teaching materials, and to ensure that students are supported in obtaining the sometimes difficult clinical experience they need. The majority of faculty members currently teaching students will not have received training in managing patients with cancer pain and palliative care needs. Supporting these teachers will enhance the education of our teachers of the future, and we can have confidence in these future professionals when, as final year medical students, they have the reflective and compassionate way of thinking indicated by this closing quote:

> I have wondered "Could there have been an introduction earlier in the course?" Because we've been doing medicine for five years, and we've been seeing patients who were sick and in pain and dying all the past five years, and no one's really dealt with that. But with some sort of introduction I think you'd be more open to the experience, you'd be more open to seeing patients that perhaps you would have overlooked on your ward in other specialties or other attachments because you simply didn't know how to deal with it, or how to approach it. I'm sure there have been patients where I've been told that they're dying, and I've shied away. Or someone's said, "Oh they're dying, you can't go in there." Which, if I'd had an introduction I might feel slightly more confident to say: "Well, actually, I'd quite like to go in and see this patient and just see how they're getting on, and how they're feeling." It's only a patient sitting around waiting for something to happen, be it a test or an operation, or death, and you can give them something … you can always give something.

## Acknowledgments

The authors would like to thank the students who agreed to be interviewed and took part in focus groups evaluating our teaching, and also Dr. Jane Williams, Jules Cook, and Dominic Alder for their input into the research project evaluating the e-learning tutorials.

## References

[1] American Academy of Hospice and Palliative Medicine. Hospice and palliative medicine: core curriculum and review syllabus. Illinois: American Academy of Hospice and Palliative Medicine; 1998.
[2] Association for Palliative Medicine of Great Britain and Ireland. Palliative medicine curriculum. Southampton: Association for Palliative Medicine of Great Britain and Ireland; 1993.

[3] Barton D. The need for including instruction on death and dying in the medical curriculum. J Med Ed 1972;47:169–75.

[4] Bloch S. Teaching medical students how to care for the dying. Med J Aust 1975;2:902–3.

[5] Bloch S. Instruction on death and dying for the medical student. Med Ed 1976;10:269–73.

[6] Dickinson GE. Death education in US medical schools. J Med Ed 1976;51:134–6.

[7] Dickinson GE, Field D. Teaching end-of-life issues: current status in United Kingdom and United States medical schools. Am J Hosp Palliat Care 2002;19:181–6.

[8] Dickinson GE, Mermann AC. Death education in US medical schools 1975–1995. Acad Med 1996;71:1348–9.

[9] Doyle D, Parry KM, MacFarlane RG. Education in terminal care. J R Coll Gen Pract 1982;32:335–8.

[10] Elliott T, Elliott BA. Physician attitudes and beliefs about the use of morphine for cancer pain. J Pain Symptom Manage 1992;7:141–8.

[11] Elliott TE, Murray DM, Oken MM, Johnson KM, Braun BL, Elliott BA, Post-White J. Improving cancer pain management in communities: main results from a randomized controlled trial. J Pain Symptom Manage 1997;13:191–203.

[12] Feest K, Forbes K. Today's students, tomorrow's doctors: reflections from the wards. Oxford: Radcliffe; 2007.

[13] General Medical Council. Tomorrow's doctors. London: General Medical Council; 2003.

[14] Hull FM. Death, dying and the medical student. Med Ed 1991;25:491–6.

[15] Klein S, Tracy D, Kitchener HC, Walker LG. The effects of the participation of patients with cancer in teaching communication skills to medical undergraduates: a randomised study with follow-up after 2 years. Eur J Cancer 2000;36:273–81.

[16] Levin ML, Berry JI, Leiter J. Management of pain in terminally ill patients: physician reports of knowledge, attitudes and behavior. J Pain Symptom Manage 1998;15:27–40.

[17] Luft J. Of human interaction. Palo Alto, CA: National Press; 1969. p 177.

[18] MacDonald N, Mount B, Boston W, Scott JF. The Canadian palliative care undergraduate curriculum. J Cancer Ed 1993;8:197–201.

[19] Mermann AC, Gunn DB, Dickinson GE. Learning to care for the dying: a survey of medical schools and a model course. Acad Med 1991;66:35–8.

[20] Miller GE. The assessment of clinical skills/competence/performance. Acad Med 1990;65(Suppl 9):63–7.

[21] Mitka M. 'Virtual textbook' on pain developed. JAMA 2003;290:2395.

[22] Niemi-Murola L, Nieminen J, Kalso E, Pöyhiä R. Medical undergraduate students' beliefs and attitudes towards pain: How do they mature? Eur J Pain 2007;11:700–6.

[23] Niemi-Murola L, Pirkko H, Pyörälä E, Kalso E, Pöyhiä R. Training medical students to manage a chronic pain patient: both knowledge and communication skills are needed. Eur J Pain 2006;10:167–70.

[24] Oneschuk D. Undergraduate medical palliative care education: a new Canadian perspective. J Palliat Med 2002;5:43–7.

[25] Oneschuk D, Hanson J, Bruera E. An international survey of undergraduate medical education in palliative medicine. J Pain Symptom Manage 2000;20:174–9.

[26] Perez EL, Gosselin JY, Gagnon A. Education on death and dying: a survey of Canadian medical schools. J Med Ed 1980;55:788–9.

[27] Pilowsky I. An outline curriculum on pain for medical schools. Pain 1988;33:1–2.

[28] Pöyhiä R, Kalso E. Pain related undergraduate teaching in medical faculties in Finland. Pain 1999;79:1121–5.

[29] Reid CM, Gooberman-Hill R, Hanks GW. Opioid analgesics for cancer pain: symptom control for the living or comfort for the dying? A qualitative study to investigate the factors influencing the decision to accept morphine for pain caused by cancer. Ann Oncol 2008;19:44–8.

[30] Soanes C, Stephenson A, editors. Concise Oxford English dictionary. Oxford: Oxford University Press; 2004.

[31] Sloan P, Montgomery C, Musick D. Medical student knowledge of morphine for the management of cancer pain. J Pain Symptom Manage 1998;15:359–64.

[32] Sloan PA, Plymale M, Johnson M, LaFountain P, Johnson M, Snapp J, Sloan D. Equipping medical students to manage cancer pain: a comparison of three educational methods. J Pain Symptom Manage 2004;27:333–42.

[33] Smith MD, McSweeney M, Katz BM. Characteristics of death education curricula in American medical schools. J Med Ed 1980;55:844–50.
[34] Tiernan E, Kearney M, Lynch A, Holland N, Pyne P. Effectiveness of a teaching programme in pain and symptom management for junior house officers. Support Care Cancer 2001;9:606–10.
[35] Turner GH, Weiner DK. Essential components of a medical student curriculum on chronic pain management in older adults: Result of a modified Delphi process. Pain Med 2002;3:240–52.
[36] Vadivelu N, Kombo N, Hines RL. The urgent need for pain management training. Acad Med 2009;84:408.
[37] Wilson JF, Brockopp GW, Kryst S, Steger H, Witt WO. Medical students' attitudes towards pain before and after a brief course on pain. Pain 1992;50:251–6.

***Correspondence to:*** Prof. Karen Forbes, Department of Palliative Medicine, Bristol Haematology and Oncology Centre, Horfield Road, Bristol BS2 8ED, United Kingdom. Email: k.forbes@bristol.ac.uk.

# Are Research and Clinical Practice Improving Management of Pain in Cancer Patients? Why Do Patients Still Suffer?

## Augusto Caraceni

*Department of Palliative Care, Pain Therapy and Rehabilitation,
IRCCS Foundation, National Cancer Institute, Milan, Italy*

## Clinical Practice and Science: The First Steps

Cancer pain is a significant clinical problem due to the high prevalence of advanced cancer both in the developed and developing world. For patients facing a poor prognosis, such pain causes physical, psychological, and existential suffering. The need to control pain satisfactorily is of paramount importance, but pain control must be part of an overall palliative care strategy built on multidisciplinary care, a holistic approach to the patient's needs, and continuity of care. The ability to provide specialized pain therapy is one of the pillars of care for the "total pain" described by Cicely Saunders [14]. Without skilled pain relief, with attention to every clinical detail, it would be impossible to address the psychological, personal, and spiritual aspects of palliative care for the patient with pain due to advanced and terminal cancer.

In the past, potentially relievable pain was often managed inappropriately, due to lack of knowledge of available pain control techniques or unavailability of fundamental drugs. The hospice movement was the first organized clinical attempt to put into practice a protocol for the relief of cancer pain. This protocol emphasized the rational use of oral morphine, which was traditionally an idiosyncratic treatment with formulations that varied from one local hospital dispensary to another, at least in England [40,52]. In fact, the contribution of the hospice movement, together with increased interest in pain research and management thanks to the work of pioneers such as John Bonica and Vittorio Ventafridda, gave a significant impetus to the World Health Organization (WHO) program for cancer pain relief in the 1980s. Given that morphine or alternative opioids were not available or were not appropriately used in most areas of the world, including both developed and developing nations, this program promoted the availability and use of opioids [3,40] by publishing and disseminating worldwide the WHO guidelines for cancer pain relief [58].

Even without formally developed evidence-based guidelines, and with its known limitations [30], it is very likely that the WHO effort and the subsequent dissemination of the cancer pain relief guidelines made an enormous impact, resulting in better pain management for many patients with advanced cancer in most parts of the world.

In reviewing why we still have patients with cancer pain who have poor pain control, we will follow a relatively simplistic scheme to try to provide the answers and perhaps raise new questions: How many patients are suffering with cancer pain because of inadequate use of the available treatments and knowledge? How many are suffering with cancer pain because their pain is difficult to control despite the adequate implementation of available treatments and knowledge?

# How to Improve Clinical Practice

The process of implementing present knowledge into clinical practice to culminate in a benefit for the patient is not a straightforward path, because in general, it involves changing attitudes and practices [38]. The implementation of guidelines and educational approaches has been empirically tested in the field of cancer pain. As mentioned above, the first attempt to implement cancer pain management guidelines was the cancer pain control program endorsed by the WHO in

1982 [57]. As part of this program, a field test of the WHO guidelines, at that time described as the WHO method for cancer pain relief, was launched in those years thanks to a strong collaboration between Jan Stjernswärd, chief of the WHO cancer unit, Vittorio Ventafridda, and the Floriani Foundation in Milan. The study was designed as a international nonrandom comparison of centers exposed to the WHO method and others that were not exposed to it. The study was coordinated by the WHO collaborating center in Milan directed by Vittorio Ventafridda. Of the 69 centers that were invited to participate, 63 accepted, representing 29 countries, and 25 centers in 15 countries contributed patients to the study. Even if attrition was very significant—particularly for centers not exposed to the WHO method, which were mostly in less developed countries—it could be demonstrated that the percentage of patients with good pain control was significantly higher in centers that were exposed to the WHO method (76%) than in those that were not (48%) [54].

A more recent study evaluated the effect of implementing a pain management algorithm for cancer pain based on the Agency for Healthcare Policy and Research (AHCPR) Clinical Practice Guidelines [1]. This study showed that in the group of patients treated according to the algorithm, the intensity of worst and usual pain measured on 0–10 numerical scales was lower than in patients treated according to standard clinical practice in oncology clinics [17].

Several educational programs were tested to identify the potential to improve clinical attitudes, clinical practice, and finally patient outcomes. A recent systematic review showed that while educational interventions can be successful in changing specific aspects of how pain is managed and how care is delivered, it could not be proven that they could change patients' reported pain experiences [23]. The same review showed instead that the provision of care by specialized palliative care services could reduce patients' subjective symptom burden. The authors pointed out that the methodology of most studies should be improved and that more homogeneous and standardized systems for pain assessment and classification should be applied to this patient population.

# How to Assess the Appropriateness of Clinical Practices

Despite the availability of numerous clinical guidelines for the treatment of cancer pain [25,47,48], it is not clear how widespread their use is in clinical practice and how clinical practice may differ from the guidelines. The popularity of the WHO guidelines and of the WHO analgesic ladder (which matches pharmacological treatment to pain severity in a stepwise approach) over the last few decades led to the development of the Pain Management Index (PMI) to score pain management as either appropriate (PMI scores from 0 to +3) or inappropriate (PMI scores from −1 to −3) [15]. A number of survey studies have used the PMI, which can be considered a very rough and conservative estimate of appropriate pain management. The PMI is indeed strongly influenced by prompt recourse to "strong" opioids (morphine and morphine-like opioids). With these limitations in mind, use of the PMI can show that pain management practices still vary according to aspects such as the setting of care (a pain clinic, oncology department, or palliative care).

In a review by De Andrea et al. [16], a weighted mean of 43% of negative PMI scores was calculated across 26 different studies. Factors associated with undertreatment (negative PMIs) were year of publication, showing an improving trend for undertreatment in more recent times, sociodemographic status, residence in Asian countries, less advanced disease, and the discrepancy between the patient's and physician's assessment of pain intensity. Other factors highlighted in the past in U.S. data include belonging to a minority group and age. In a recent Italian survey of 1,461 patients, the percentage of negative PMI was 25%, and PMI score was influenced by the type of center and the level of pain management expertise. The frequency of a negative PMI score was associated with being referred to oncology clinics and pain clinics, whereas more aggressive treatment was shown in hospices [2].

Overall, these findings support the concept that better and homogeneous standard approaches to the treatment of cancer pain can still ameliorate individual patients' suffering caused by undertreatment, although the causes and the patterns of undertreatment have significant regional variations. In some countries, lack of knowledge about opioid use and even more significant problems in the availability of opioids for medical use [13a] should still be viewed as basic unresolved barriers against adequate pain control for patients with advanced cancer and other uncurable diseases. One of the most effective interventions to improve the management of pain is likely to be the specific allocation of professional resources to palliative care and pain management [23].

# International Research in Cancer Pain

International efforts to identify a global research agenda for improving the assessment, classification, and treatment of cancer pain have been limited and have met with only partial success. The Task Force on Cancer Pain of the International Association for the Study of Pain was able to finalize a survey study that tested a clinical classification of cancer pain in an international group of experts, but it did not achieve its goal of implementing observational studies or clinical trials with a common methodology [9,10].

The Research Network of the European Association for Palliative Care produced a number of working groups and one European survey on the characteristics of pain and its management in a palliative care population. However, it did not establish any durable internationally based research activity that could sponsor the task of performing longitudinal trials in large numbers of patients or identify updated priorities in this field [7,13,32,34,36].

A group of researchers from Canada have consistently applied a clinically based classification system for cancer pain, known as the Edmonton Classification System for Cancer Pain, which has identified some patient-related factors such as neuropathic pain, incident pain, psychological distress, and addictive behavior as potential risk factors for poor pain relief [20,21].

Recently the European Union funded a research consortium, the European Palliative Care Research Collaborative (www.epcrc.org), which endorsed systematic revisions of a number of unresolved issues in cancer pain research related to the lack of international consensus about assessment and classification. Another related effort, the European Pharmacogenetic Opioid Study, was launched to identify the contribution of genetic variance to the variability of opioid analgesia in cancer pain [27,28,31]. The

EPCRC effort is presently trying to integrate the activities of the European Association for Palliative Care Research Network into a new initiative, the European Palliative Care Research Center (www.ntnu.no.prc), which will tackle the current shortcomings in cancer pain research.

Significant efforts have been made or are underway to introduce the use of patient-reported outcomes, especially pain intensity, within the objectives of clinical oncological trials [19,22].

# Specific Areas for Future Research

It is impossible to give a comprehensive description of the knowledge gaps that must be addressed to improve pain control in this population of patients, but I can try to address the areas that to my knowledge and in my experience can be considered relevant and are already the object of international research efforts.

## Identify a Minimum Data Set for Classification and Assessment Measures

Systematic literature reviews have shown that we lack common criteria by which to classify patients with cancer pain and to assess pain with standardized methods that allow comparison across studies and meta-analyses [27,28,33].

Another systematic literature review of oncological trials that included pain control as a primary or secondary study endpoint demonstrated that many aspects of pain assessment and measurement were of insufficient quality in a surprising number of published papers [6].

Several international groups are attempting to create consensus on how to classify and assess cancer pain to make it possible to obtain homogeneous data from clinical practice and research that are clinically relevant and comparable across populations and cultures [18,22,31]. One international consensus panel recently tried to link these initiatives and is working on a protocol for a minimum data set [31].

## Neuropathic Pain in Cancer

Clinical experience has shown that neuropathic pain due to cancer is more difficult to control than other types of cancer-related pain. This type of pain, which is included in the Edmonton Classification System, is often managed with adjuvant drugs in addition to opioids. Although this widely accepted strategy has guided clinical practice for at least 30 years [24], very little scientific evidence has been produced to describe how patients with neuropathic pain due to cancer differ from other patients with nonmalignant pain, how this type of pain should be diagnosed [53], and how different treatments can benefit patients. One cross-sectional assessment of a large patient population recently showed that neuropathic pain is independently associated with a less favorable response to treatment [5]. The few controlled clinical trials specifically addressing this problem have significant methodological problems due to the lack of a homogeneous clinical classification [4,11,42].

## Incident Bone Pain

Bone pain is an important source of suffering in cancer patients. Pain that is exacerbated by movement—incident pain—is often difficult to treat with acceptable side effects, even with careful use of appropriate pharmacological interventions. Incident pain due to bone lesions has consistently been found to be difficult to alleviate with the available treatment strategies [41,44], thus justifying emerging interest in new, more effective drugs for breakthrough cancer pain. Standard diagnostic methods and clinical approaches should also be improved [26].

Increased understanding of the pathophysiology of bone cancer pain has led to the development and widespread use of drugs that interfere with the process of osteolysis [29]. The use of bisphosphates has been shown to improve the complications of metastatic bone cancer lesions, but many trials of these drugs did not focus on pain. The available clinical trials are not helpful in identifying the analgesic effects of these interventions, mainly due to methodological limitations in evaluating pain [56,59]. Therefore, our knowledge about the role of bisphosphonates and their appropriate use for improving pain, particularly in the most advanced cases, is limited to uncontrolled observational data from a few patients [37].

Clinical trials to identify the role of other nonopioid drugs to improve the analgesia obtained with opioids in incident bone pain are being conducted to confirm uncontrolled clinical observations [12]. Nonsteroidal anti-inflammatory drugs were once thought to have important analgesic properties in bone pain due to cancer, but this impression was never proven to be true. The relative importance of these drugs in the overall treatment strategy is largely unknown from a research point of view. The meager evidence base consists of older data [43,45,50] and uncontrolled clinical observations [8].

## Opioid Response Variability

The undeniable main role of opioids in the treatment of cancer pain should drive more research on the sources of individual opioid response variability. One promising area of research is opioid pharmacogenomics. However, preliminary results from ongoing research were criticized recently [55], showing that this type of research requires special attention and collaboration between basic scientists and clinicians to fulfil its potential to address relevant clinical questions [39]. Not only experts in genetics but researchers from the full range of neuroscience and neuropharmacological sciences have been looking at the mechanisms of opioid analgesia and at pathophysiological conditions and other factors that can modify opioid analgesia.

Complicating the obstacles described above is a lack of new drugs in development to treat cancer pain. We are beginning to see the clinical application of anti-nerve growth factor antibodies in cancer pain [49], and cannabinoids are being studied in clinical trials. However, the lack of new drugs is another disadvantage for the field of cancer pain and for patients with the most difficult pain conditions.

## A Comprehensive Patient-Centered Approach

To provide good pain relief to patients with pain due to advanced cancer, it is not sufficient to provide adequate analgesia. Pain associated with progressive uncurable disease is a more complex condition, first because it must be considered in the context of cancer treatment and comorbidities, and second, because it involves a full range of psychological, social, and existential problems, as highlighted in the powerful model of total pain mentioned at the beginning of this chapter. The impact of psychological distress in complicating cancer pain and in worsening pain therapy outcomes is another complex area of research. Indeed, psychological distress is one of the domains that are considered relevant in classifying the complexity of cancer pain [46]. At the same time, we lack systems for the recognition and evaluation of psychological distress as an indicator of pain complexity in this patient population, which could be used for clinical classification both in clinical practice and in research [51].

These important issues show that the full range of symptoms and comorbidities must be considered together with pain because they will define specific populations from the point of view of their ability to participate in clinical trials, for instance, thus affecting the generalizability of data from such trials, and because they call for appropriate assessment tools [31]. It is also mandatory that specialized acute pain services collaborate with dedicated palliative care programs and services and that palliative care and oncology services collaborate in formally organized networks to establish and integrated pathways of care, as suggested by some models [35]. The suffering and avoidable pain due to lack of collaboration and integration of services can equal the suffering caused by insufficient availability of services.

# Conclusion

To answer the question, why do patients still suffer, I have summarized how the failure to implement existing knowledge, as well as insufficient research and knowledge about the pathophysiology, classification, assessment, and therapy of cancer pain, may explain why we still fail to control all pain due to cancer (Table I).

Table I
Obstacles to cancer pain relief

Lack of implementation of existing knowledge
    Available guidelines are not followed
    Available guidelines are old and need to be updated
Lack of knowledge to improve existing therapeutic strategies
    Standard assessment and classification systems need improvement
    Difficult pain pathophysiology is poorly understood
    Individual variability of opioid analgesic response is not explained
    Clinical trials to answer the relevant clinical questions are lacking
Lack of service integration and research policy
    Insufficient integration between pain, palliative care, and oncology specialists
    Insufficient integration between cancer control research and pain/palliative care research
    Insufficient resources on clinical research in cancer pain and palliative care
    Lack of new drug development

One aspect of pain relief that cannot be solved by science and research is the interest of health care professionals in the patient's pain and suffering. Suffering is more than pain, and relief of suffering is the mainstay of palliative care. No health care professional can pretend to be interested in relieving suffering without being interested in relieving pain. All clinicians involved in palliative care know that they cannot completely resolve suffering, even after taking away the pain, and yet they shall be interested in being there to ease their patients' suffering to the best of their ability.

# References

[1] American Pain Society Quality of Care Committee. Quality improvement guidelines for the treatment of acute pain and cancer pain. JAMA 1995;274:1874–80.

[2] Apolone G, Corli O, Caraceni A, Negri E, Deandrea S, Montanari M, Greco M; Cancer Pain Outcome Study Group (CPO SG) Investigators. Pattern and quality of care of cancer pain management. Results from the Cancer Pain Outcome Study Group. Br J Cancer 2009;100:1566–74.

[3] Bonica JJ, Ventafridda V, editors. International symposium on pain of advanced cancer. Advances in pain research and therapy, Vol. 2. New York: Raven Press; 1979.

[4] Bruera E, Ripamonti C, Brenneis C, McMillan K, Hanson J. A randomized double-blind crossover trial of intravenous lidocaine in the treatment of neuropathic cancer pain. J Pain Symptom Manage 1992;7:138–40.

[5] Caraceni A, Brunelli C, Greco M, Montanari M, Apolone G, Knudsen A, Kaasa S. Predictive validity of an abbreviated version of the Edmonton Classification System for cancer pain. Proceedings of the 11th Congress of the European Association for Palliative Care. European Association for Palliative Care; 2009. p. 186.

[6] Caraceni A, Brunelli C, Martini C, Zecca E, De Conno F. Cancer pain assessment in clinical trials. A review of the literature. J Pain Symptom Manage 2005;29:507–19.

[7] Caraceni A, Cherny N, Fainsinger R, Kaasa S, Poulain P, Radbruck L, De Conno F; Steering Committee of the EAPC Research Network. Pain measurement tools and methods in clinical research in palliative care: recommendations of an expert working group of the European Association of Palliative Care. J Pain Symptom Manage 2002;23:239–55.

[8] Caraceni A, Gorni G, Zecca E, De Conno F. More on the use of nonsteroidal anti-inflammatories in the management of cancer pain. J Pain Symptom Manage 2001;21:89–92.

[9] Caraceni A, Martini C, Zecca E, Portenoy RK; Working Group of the IASP Task Force on Cancer Pain. Breakthrough pain characteristics and syndromes in patients with cancer pain. An international survey. Pall Med 2004;18:177–83.

[10] Caraceni A, Portenoy RK; Working Group of the IASP Task Force on Cancer Pain. An international survey of cancer pain characteristics and syndromes. Pain 1999;82:263–74.

[11] Caraceni A, Zecca E, Bonezzi C, et al. Gabapentin as adjuvant to opioid analgesia in neuropathic cancer pain. A multicenter randomized controlled clinical trial. Proceedings of the 8th Congress of the European Association for Palliative Care. The Hague: European Association for Palliative Care; 2003.

[12] Caraceni A, Zecca E, Martini C, Pigni A, Bracchi P. Gabapentin for breakthrough pain due to bone metastases. Pall Med 2008;22:392–3.

[13] Cherny N, Ripamonti C, Pereira J, Davis C, Fallon M, McQuay HJ, Mercadante S, Pasternak G, Ventafridda V. Strategies to manage the adverse effects of oral morphine: an evidence-based report. J Clin Oncol 2001;19:2542–54.

[13a] Cherny NI, Baselga J, de Conno F, Radbruch L. Formulary availability and regulatory barriers to accessibility of opioids for cancer pain in Europe: a report from the ESMO/EAPC Opioid Policy Initiative. Ann Oncol 2010;21:615–26.

[14] Clark D. "Total pain," disciplinary power and the body in the work of Cicely Saunders, 1958–1967. Soc Sci Med 1999;49:727–36.

[15] Cleeland CS, Gonin R, Hatfield AK, Edmonson JH, Blum RH, Stewart JA, Pandya KJ. Pain and its treatment in outpatients with metastatic cancer. N Engl J Med 1994;330:592–6.

[16] De Andrea S, Montanari M, Moja L, Apolone G. Prevalence of undertreatment in cancer pain. A review of published literature. Ann Oncol 2008;19:1985–91.

[17] Du Pen SL, Du Pen AR, Polissar N, Hansberry J, Kraybill BM, Stillman M, Panke J, Everly R, Syrjala K. Implementing guidelines for cancer pain management: results of a randomized controlled clinical trial. J Clin Oncol 1999;17:361–70.

[18] Dworkin DS, Turk DC, Farrar JT, Haythornthwaite JA, Jensen MP, Katz NP, Kerns RD, Stucki G, Allen RR, Bellamy N, et al. Core outcome measures for chronic pain in clinical trials: IMMPACT recommendations. Pain 2005;113:9–19.

[19] European Organization for Research and Treatment of Cancer. Home page. Available at: http://www.eortc.be/.

[20] Fainsinger R, Fairchild A, Nekolaichuk C, Lawlor P, Lowe S, Hanson J. Is pain management a predictor of the complexity of cancer pain management. J Clin Oncol 2009;27:585–90.

[21] Fainsinger R, Nekolaichuk CL, Lawlor PG, Neumann CM, Hanson J, Vigano A. A multicenter study of the revised Edmonton Staging System for classifying cancer pain in advanced cancer patients. J Pain Symptom Manage 2005;29:224–37.

[22] Garcia S, Cella D, Clauser S, Flynn K, Lad T, Lai J, Reeve B, Wilder Smith A, Stone A, Weinfurt K. Standardizing patient-reported outcomes assessment in cancer clinical trials: a patient-reported outcomes measurement information system initiative. J Clin Oncol 2007;25:5106–12.

[23] Goldberg GR, Morrison RS. Pain management in hospitalized cancer patients: a systematic review. J Clin Oncol 2007;25:1792–1801.

[24] Grond S, Radbruch L, Meuser T, Sabatowski R, Loick G, Lehman KA. Assessment and treatment of neuropathic cancer pain following WHO guidelines. Pain 1999;79:15–20.

[25] Hanks G, De Conno F, Cherny N, Hanna M, Kalso E, McQuay H, Mercadante S, Meynadier J, Poulain P, Ripamonti C, et al. Morphine and alternative opioids in cancer pain: the EAPC recommendations. Br J Cancer 2001;84:587–93.

[26] Haugen D, Hjermstad M, Hagen N, Caraceni A, Kaasa S. Assessment and classification of cancer breakthrough pain. A systematic literature review on behalf of the European Palliative Care Research Collaborative (EPCRC). Pain; in press.

[27] Hjermstad M, Gibbins J, Haugen D, Caraceni A, Loge J, Kaasa S; European Palliative Care Research Collaborative. Pain assessment tools in palliative care: an urgent need for consensus. Palliat Med 2008;22:895–903.

[28] Hølen JC, Polit C, Hjermstad MJ, Loge JH, Fayers PM, Caraceni A, De Conno F, Forbes K, Fürst CJ, Radbruch L, Kaasa S. Pain assessment tools: is the content appropriate for use in palliative care? J Pain Symptom Manage 2006;32:567–80.

[29] Honore P, Mantyh PW. Bone cancer pain: from mechanism to model to therapy. Pain Med 2000;1:303–9.

[30] Jadad AR, Browman GP. The WHO analgesic ladder for cancer pain management. Stepping up the quality of its evaluation. JAMA 1995;274:1870–3.

[31] Kaasa S, Loge JH, Fayers P, Caraceni A, Strasser F, Hjermstad M, Higginson I, Radbruch L, Haugen DF. Symptom assessment in palliative care: a need for international collaboration. J Clin Oncol 2008;26:3867–73.

[32] Kaasa S, Torvik K, Cherny N, Hanks G, De Conno F. Patient demographic and centre description in European palliative care units. Palliat Med 2007;21:15–22.

[33] Knudsen A, Aass N, Fainsinger R, Caraceni A, Klepstad P, Jordhøy M, Hjermstad M, Kaasa S. Classification of pain in cancer patients: a systematic literature review. Palliat Med 2009;23:295–308.

[34] Lugsand EA, Kaasa S, De Conno F, Hanks G, Klepstad P; Research Steering Committee of the EAPC. Intensity and treatment of symptoms in 3,030 palliative care patients: a cross-sectional survey of the EAPC Research Network. J Opioid Manage 2009;5:11–20.

[35] Maltoni M, Amadori D. Palliative medicine and medical oncology. Ann Oncol 2001;12:443–50.

[36] Maltoni M, Caraceni A, Brunelli C, Boeckaert B, Christakis N, Eychmuller S, Glare P, Nabal M, Viganò A, Larkin P, De Conno F, Hanks G, Kaasa S. Prognostic factors in advanced cancer patients: evidence-based clinical recommendations: a study by the Steering Committee of the European Association for Palliative Care. J Clin Oncol 2005;23:6240–8.

[37] Mancini I, Dumon J, Body J. Efficacy and safety of ibandronate in the treatment of opioid-resistant bone pain associated with metastatic bone disease a pilot study. J Clin Oncol 2004;22:3587–92.

[38] Max MB. Improving the outcome of analgesic treatment: Is education enough? Ann Intern Med 1990;11:885–9.

[39] Max MB. Moving pain genetics into the genome-wide association era. In: Castro-Lopes J, editor. Current topics in pain: 12th World Congress on Pain. Seattle: IASP Press; 2009. p. 185–97.

[40] Meldrum M. The ladder and the clock: cancer pain and public policy at the end of the twentieth century. J Pain Symptom Manage 2005;29:41–54.

[41] Mercadante S. Malignant bone pain: pathophysiology and treatment. Pain 1997;69:1–8.

[42] Mercadante S, Arcuri E, Tirelli W, Villari P, Casuccio A. Amitriptyline in neuropathic cancer pain in patients on morphine therapy: a randomized placebo-controlled, double-blind crossover study. Tumori 2002;88:239–42.

[43] Mercadante S, Casuccio A, Agnello A, Pumo S, Kargar J, Garofalo S. Analgesic effect of nonsteroidal anti-inflammatory drugs in cancer pain due to somatic and visceral mechanisms. J Pain Symptom Manage 1999;17:351–6.

[44] Mercadante S, Maddaloni S, Roccella S, Salvaggio L. Predictive factors in advanced cancer pain treated only by analgesics. Pain 1992;50:151–5.

[45] Mercadante S, Sapio M, Caligara M, Serretta R, Dardanoni G, Barresi L. Opioid-sparing effect of diclofenac in cancer pain. J Pain Symptom Manage 1997;14:15–20.

[46] Nekolaichuk C, Fainsinger R, Lawlor P. A validation study of a pain classification system for advanced cancer patients using content experts: the Edmonton Classification System for Cancer Pain. Palliat Med 2006;19(6):466–76.

[47] Pigni A, Brunelli C, Gubbins J, Hanks G, De Conno F, Kaasa S, Klepstad P, Radbruch L, Caraceni A. Content development from European guidelines on the use of opioids for cancer pain: a systematic review and expert consensus study. Minerva Anestesiol 2010; in press.

[48] Scottish Intercollegiate Guidelines Network. Control of pain in adult patients with cancer. 2008. Available at: http://www.sign.ac.uk/guidelines/fulltext/106/index.html.

[49] Sevcik M, Ghilardi J, Peters C, Lindsay T, Halvorson K, Jonas B, Kubota K, Kuskowski M, Boustany L, Shelton D. Anti-NGF therapy profoundly reduces bone cancer pain and the accompanying increase in markers of peripheral and central sensitization. Pain 2005;115:128–41.

[50] Stambaugh JE, Drew J. The combination of ibuprofen and oxycodone/acetaminophen in the management of chronic cancer pain. Clin Pharmacol Ther 1988;44:665–9.

[51] Turk DC, Sist T, Okifuji A, Miner M, Florio G, Harrison P, Masse J, Lema M, Zevon M. Adaptation to metastatic cancer pain, regional/local cancer pain and non-cancer pain: role of psychological and behavioral factors. Pain 1998;74:247–56.

[52] Twycross RG. The equipotent dose ratio of diamorphine and morphine administered by mouth. Br J Pharmacol 1972;46:554–5.

[53] Ventafridda V, Caraceni A. Cancer pain classification: a controversial issue. Pain 1991;46:1–2.

[54] Ventafridda V, Caraceni A, Gamba A. Field-testing of the WHO guidelines for cancer pain relief. In: Foley KM, Ventafridda V, Bonica JJ, editors. 2nd International Congress on Cancer Pain. Advances in pain research and therapy, Vol. 16. New York: Raven Press; 1990. p. 451–64.

[55] Walter C, Lotsch J. Meta-analysis of the relevance of the OPRM1 118A>G genetic variant for pain treatment. Pain 2009;146:270–5.

[56] Wong R, Wiffen P. Bisphosphonates for the relief of pain secondary to bone metastases. Cochrane Database Syst Rev 2002;2:CD002068.

[57] World Health Organization. Report of a WHO consultation, Milan, 14–16 October 1982. WHO draft interim guidelines handbook on relief of cancer pain (for research purposes only). Geneva: World Health Organization; 1982.

[58] World Health Organization. Cancer pain relief. Geneva: World Health Organization, 1986.

[59] Yuen KK, Sze WM, Wilt T, Mason MD. Bisphosphonates for advanced prostate cancer. Cochrane Database Syst Rev 2006;18(4):CD006250.

**Correspondence to:** Augusto Caraceni, MD, Division of Palliative Care, Pain Therapy and Rehabilitation, Fondazione IRCCS, Istituto Nazionale dei Tumori, Via Venezia 1 20133, Milan, Italy. Email: augusto.caraceni@istitutotumori.mi.it.

# How to Make a Difference in the Developing World: Organizing Resources

Olaitan A. Soyannwo

*Department of Anaesthesia, College of Medicine, University of Ibadan, Ibadan, Nigeria*

Cancer has become a more common occurrence worldwide, largely due to the growth of the world's population, along with significant increases in life expectancy, especially in the developed world. The recorded number of cases has also increased due to improvements in cancer detection and diagnosis. The International Agency for Research on Cancer (IARC) estimated that in 2008 there were 12.4 million incident cases of cancer, 7.6 million deaths from cancer, and 28 million people living within the median 5-year survival prognosis. The IARC also estimated that just over half the incident cases and two-thirds of cancer deaths occurred in low- and middle-income countries [1]. These countries are identified as "developing countries" for convenience, as defined by the World Bank's classification of economies of countries according to gross national income per capita [25]. By 2020 the World Health Organization (WHO) estimates that 70% of new cancer cases will be in developing countries, with most patients presenting with late stages of cancer [16]. Even when patients seek early care, diagnosis and treatment may be delayed, unaffordable, or unavailable. Approximately half of the patients diagnosed with cancer in

*Cancer Pain: From Molecules to Suffering*
edited by Judith A. Paice, Rae F. Bell, Eija A. Kalso, and Olaitan A. Soyannwo
IASP Press, Seattle, © 2010

developed countries die of advanced disease; in developing countries this figure reaches 70% [25].

Another issue of concern is the prevalence of pain associated with the disease. Cancer pain is often problematic for patients and their families. Reports from the developed world indicate that the frequency of pain at the time of diagnosis and at early stages is approximately 50%, increasing to 75% at advanced stages. A recent meta-analysis found the prevalence of pain in cancer survivors to be 33% [22]. Most patients referred for cancer-related symptom management have at least two anatomically distinct pain sites. The pain may be caused by several mechanisms, including direct tumor involvement, cancer therapy (chemotherapy, surgery, or radiation therapy), and non-cancer-related problems such as preexisting disease. Despite the paucity of published data from developing countries, the situation there is unlikely to be any better than in the developed world [17].

More than 5 billion people (85% of the world's population) reside in developing countries. Low-income countries have an annual gross national income per capita of less than US$765, and the corresponding amount for middle-income countries is less than US$9300 [10]. Such countries often have a limited health budget and a high incidence of communicable disease. As a result, the available resources remain grossly inadequate to deal with various health issues such as cancer and its associated pain. In order to improve cancer pain management in the developing world, it is essential to create strategies for equality in access to care through careful organization of the scarce available resources. This chapter will discuss the reasons for unresolved issues in pain and suffering in the developing world, along with the strategies and resources required to meet these needs.

# Resources and Priorities for Health Care in Developing Countries

The developing countries are heterogeneous, with social, economic, and health system differences. There is often a sharp disparity between the poor majority and the wealthy minority, who have access to a level of health care comparable to that in developed and affluent countries. Given that most nations lack the resources to meet all the health needs of the community, an assessment of the available resources and their proper allocation and utilization are of particular concern in developing countries.

The basic resources necessary for providing health care are manpower, money and materials, and time. In developing countries, manpower (professional and auxiliary staff) is often in short supply and is disproportionate between rural and urban areas. Although the majority of the population resides in rural areas, the absence of amenities discourages health professionals from working in these areas. As a result, when rural dwellers have serious illnesses such as cancer, they are referred to urban specialist centers for diagnosis and treatment.

Lack of money and materials limits the availability of health care for populations at need. Existing priorities on health often coincide with the 2000 United Nations Millennium Development Goals, which emphasize "areas that cause widespread illness and death amongst the population." These priorities are eradication of poverty and hunger; universal primary education; gender equality; reduction of child mortality; improvement in maternal health; combating HIV/AIDS, malaria, and other life-threatening diseases; environmental sustainability; and developing global partnerships [21]. Due to the low gross national income in developing countries, funds are often allocated to other issues, limiting resources for issues such as cancer. Cancer and disease management must be made visible in order to receive the resources necessary to expand treatment for cancer and the associated pain.

# Resources for Cancer Control and Management

The concept of cancer control has been developed to attack the cancer problem at various points. This concept includes primary prevention strategies aimed to determine risk factors associated with the development of cancer [27]. Other goals include detecting cancers at an early, asymptomatic stage (secondary prevention), which would lead to decreased mortality rates for certain cancers.

Effective control of cancer and the related pain requires a major commitment to public education programs, training of health care professionals, and provision of adequate facilities for treatment. National policies

must be established based on the pattern of cancer within a specific country. For example, during the 1990s, the cancers with the highest incidence
in Ugandan men were Kaposi's sarcoma, prostate cancer, and esophageal
cancer. The most common cancers affecting women in Uganda were Kaposi's sarcoma and breast and cervical cancers [23]. However, along with
the AIDS epidemic has come a significant increase in the incidence of
Kaposi's sarcoma, squamous cell carcinoma of the conjunctiva, and non-
Hodgkin's lymphoma [15].

The publication of the 1993 world cancer report demonstrated
how a low-income country can provide a minimum package of cost-effective public health care and clinical interventions for its population
with a budget of US$12 per capita [1]. The WHO also stated that "an
initial priority, especially in developing countries, should be the development of national diagnostic and treatment guidelines to establish a
minimum standard of care, and promote the rational use of existing resources and greater equity in access to treatment services" [27]. Such
guidelines for breast cancer treatment and allocation of resources have
been developed for limited-resource countries [5]. The guidelines were
based on the stage of breast cancer. A "minimum standard of care" was
established as a foundation on which to build an incremental model for
improving care, designated as basic, limited, enhanced, and maximal.
Appropriate pain control for each stage of the disease—from basic to enhanced pain management techniques—was built into this model. Thus
for each cancer type, pain management and research should be an integral part of policy considerations.

## Educational Resources for Cancer Pain Management

A survey of 189 respondents from 46 developing countries conducted by
the International Association for the Study of Pain (IASP) identified the
barriers to good pain management as lack of education in pain management, low priority given to pain management by government agencies,
limited drug availability as a result of cost implications, and poor patient
compliance [9]. Although adequate pain treatment is now considered a
human right, health care systems in many developing countries have yet to
view pain management in this context. Pain management awareness, education, and training are essential if health care providers are to help their

patients. Pain education, especially for medical students, is an important step in addressing current issues in clinical practice. Patients must also be properly educated.

Over an 18-month period, the University of Toronto Center for the Study of Pain's Interfaculty Pain Education Committee developed a 20-hour undergraduate pain curriculum to be delivered during a 1-week period. This integrated undergraduate pain curriculum was based on the existing IASP curricula for health care professionals. Six health science faculties (dentistry, medicine, nursing, pharmacy, physical therapy, and occupational therapy) implemented this curriculum during their second- or third-year program. Students who participated in this program demonstrated improvement in pain knowledge and beliefs [24].

Adequate resources on cancer pain and skills management are currently available in the developed world that might be translated into evidence-based, cost-effective, and culturally appropriate interventions for developing countries. Relevant materials on cancer pain within the IASP's core curriculum for professional education in pain can be included under existing courses of study (e.g., physiology, pharmacology, nursing assessment, oncology, psychiatry, and anesthesia) [3]. IASP's members and chapters in developing countries could play leadership roles in curriculum review and in ensuring that pain education is included in both undergraduate and postgraduate courses, with grant support from IASP's Developing Countries Project.

It is important to educate and motivate health professionals to assess and treat pain according to local protocols. Available educational resources such as Web-based materials on cancer pain can be disseminated through local courses and clinical training. Training programs should encourage discussion of clinical scenarios of pain management and include detailed information on pain assessment, therapeutic options, and how to address psychosocial, spiritual, cultural, ethical, and legal issues as part of the holistic care of the patient.

The results of the IASP survey support the decision to develop "bottom-up" education programs in developing countries, addressing local needs and using local trainers and local facilities. Such an approach could also be used to develop clinical training support. Education is also needed for patients. Compared with standard educational materials and counseling, a brief individualized education and coaching intervention for outpatients with cancer-related pain was associated with greater improvement in average pain levels [14].

In order to build up a sufficient number of trainers, out-of-country training must be encouraged. Those who have received training must be empowered to return to their own countries to continue to work. In this era of global interdependence, collaboration should be explored between wealthier countries and those with fewer resources to establish trained workers for effective cancer pain management and research in developing countries. Establishment of regional centers designed specifically for this purpose can be facilitated by major international organizations such as WHO, IASP, the World Federation of Societies of Anesthetists (WFSA), the International Union Against Cancer (UICC), and the International Association for Hospice and Palliative Care (IAHPC), with support from donor agencies, the industrial sector, and governments. Such regional programs will encourage future collaborative endeavors for pain treatment and research between centers with poor resources and those with better resources.

## Costs

Pain is a multidimensional problem that requires several approaches to its management. Recommended approaches to cancer pain management, involving the use of drugs and alternative resources, are as follows [28]. (1) Psychological support (understanding, companionship, and cognitive-behavioral therapies). (2) Modification of the pathological process (radiotherapy, hormone therapy, chemotherapy, and surgery). (3) Drugs (analgesics, antidepressants, anticonvulsants, anxiolytics, and neuroleptics). (4) Interruption of pain pathways (local anesthetics, neurolytic agents, and neurosurgery). (4) Modification of daily activities (physical therapy, occupational therapy).

The cost of treatment and care will vary based on the severity and complexity of the pain and the use of basic or advanced therapies to manage symptoms (Table I). In addition, indirect costs are associated with cancer morbidity, such as days lost from work for the patient or caregiver. Nonmonetary costs associated with pain, suffering, or loss of companionship are difficult to measure, but they are very real to patients and their families.

Table I
Pain treatment methods and required resources
for implementation in developing countries

| Pain Treatment Methods | Resources Required | | |
|---|---|---|---|
| | Trained Personnel | Infrastructure and Equipment | Cost Implications |
| Nonopioid drugs | Trained personnel | Minimal | Cheap |
| Opioid analgesic drugs | Trained nurses, doctors, pharmacists | Minimal for oral route | Relatively cheap in many countries (when available) |
| Adjuvant drugs (antidepressants, anticonvulsants, steroids) | Trained nurses, doctors, pharmacists | Minimal | Relatively cheap (many are used for other medical conditions) |
| Surgery | Surgeons, anesthesiologists, nurses, others | Operating room facilities (including water and electricity), patient beds, anesthetics, and sterile surgical equipment | Expensive |
| Chemotherapy | Oncologists | Chemotherapy drugs, delivery pumps, disposable catheters | Expensive |
| Radiotherapy | Radio-oncologist | Radiotherapy machines, special suites | Expensive |
| Nondrug therapies (physical and rehabilitative therapy, psychotherapy, spiritual support, social support) | Physiotherapists, psycho-oncologists, psychologists, spiritual caregivers, social workers | Specialized training, equipment for physical therapy | Less expensive and more affordable |
| Palliative care (drug and nondrug modalities) | Trained professionals | Family, volunteers | Home-based care cheaper than hospice care |
| Advanced therapies (intrathecal drugs, nerve blocks, radiofrequency lesions, neurosurgery) | Specialist doctors, pain teams | Specialized infusion pumps, disposable items, radiodiagnostic equipment, treatment rooms | Expensive |

Another monetary issue that patients face is the cost of drugs to manage their pain. De Lima and colleagues [4] compared retail prices and availability of potent opioids in the developing countries of Argentina, Colombia, India, Mexico, and Saudi Arabia to similar data from the developed countries of Australia, Canada, Denmark, Italy, Japan, Spain, and the United States. In U.S. dollars, the median cost of opioids differed between developed and developing countries ($53 and $112, respectively). The median costs of all opioid preparations as a percentage of gross national product per capita per month were 36% for developing and 3% for developed nations; the difference was statistically significant ($P < 0.001$). In developing countries, 23 of 45 opioid dosage forms (51%) cost more than 30% of the monthly gross national product per capita, versus only 3 of 76 (4%) in developed countries. These data suggest that for most patients in developing countries, access to opioids is likely to be limited by cost. Another recommendation from this study is that the development of palliative care programs will require heavy or total subsidization of opioid costs, as is the case for antiretroviral drugs. In Uganda, an oral morphine solution, the major opioid analgesic available for cancer pain treatment, is prepared from powder. This opioid is affordable and provides pain relief to those in urban and rural areas [11,20]. Expensive medications and treatments may overburden patients who have very limited resources, which results in compromises between compliance with the prescribed regimen and other financial responsibilities.

Although research has produced new cytotoxic and biological agents that can increase survival rates for cancer patients, most of them carry a substantial cost. In the past decade, the cost of a standard treatment regimen for a patient with advanced colon cancer has risen from US$500 to $250,000, and survival has increased by about 12 months [12]. Such costs are unaffordable for most patients in developing countries. National health insurance schemes and social security arrangements are hard to come by, and out-of-pocket expenses accumulate, leading to poor survival rates along with pain and suffering in the terminal stages of cancer.

## Resources for Research: From the Laboratory to the Bedside

Evidence from research laboratories involving diverse animal models and clinical trials provides great opportunities for understanding pain mechanisms, appropriate interventions for cancer pain management, and new drug targets. Researchers have uncovered genes that affect the processes of pain, while several polymorphisms of genes have been shown to significantly affect opioid efficacy. Multicenter research including developing countries will be necessary to further elucidate opioid dosages and determine responders and nonresponders within different groups. Unfortunately, research centers are very scarce in developing countries, and a research career is often unattractive because of relatively poor funding, lack of interest in the findings, and low remuneration and limited appreciation for investigators. Research grants from external sources are highly competitive and are not readily available. Research also allows for implementation of findings in clinical practice, but due to the lack of research in pain management and other fields, standard practices are unable to improve existing procedures [8]. Given the constraints of funding in developing countries, research in palliative care and pain management is not seen as a priority. Research must be translated into clinical practice so that all levels of health care providers, from doctors and nurses to patients and care providers, can experience its benefits [6,8].

With few exceptions, low- and middle-income countries invest relatively little in health research and development, despite encouragement by the Global Forum for Health Research to increase research efforts [2,18]. The Millennium Development Goals urged governments of developing countries to provide resources necessary for essential research, to spend at least 2% of their national health budgets on health research, and to strengthen their research capacity. Donors were also urged to allocate 5% of their funding for similar purposes. More proactive efforts are required by organizations that sponsor effective pain relief strategies to promote international collaborations for research and development in developing countries [18].

# Public Health Approach for Optimization of Resources

Palliative care, including pain control, is increasingly being recognized and promoted as a public health issue, especially through units of WHO that focus on cancer, AIDS, aging, and mental health. The World Health

Assembly Cancer Prevention and Control Resolution of 2005 emphasized the need for reinforcing comprehensive cancer control programs
worldwide. This resolution also recognized the provision of palliative care
as an urgent humanitarian responsibility and stressed the need for improving opioid availability [26]. In the early 1980s, the WHO Cancer Unit
began to develop a global initiative to advocate for cancer pain relief and
opioid availability worldwide. WHO later pioneered a public health strategy that includes palliative care for all (Fig. 1). The strategy starts with four
essential components: appropriate government policies; adequate drug
availability; education of the public, policy makers, and health professionals; and implementation of palliative care services at all levels of society.
Although cancer pain was a target symptom and cancer was the disease
identified when the strategy was developed, the same policies and strategies could benefit those with other life-threatening illnesses, including
HIV/AIDS [19].

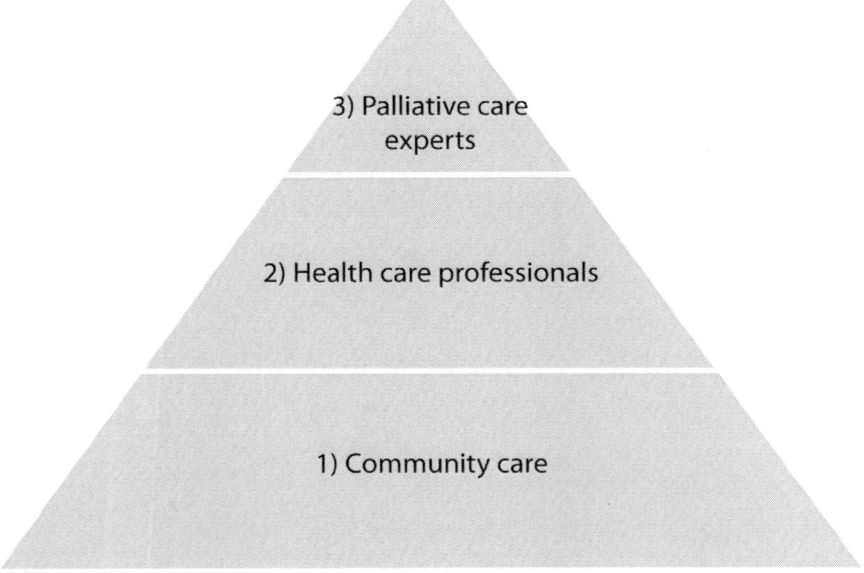

**Fig. 1.** Palliative care for all. Adapted from Stjernswärd et al. [20].

Public health systems should provide an effective link between the three levels of health care in developing countries (primary, secondary, and tertiary). Pain management, education, and research should be emphasized. Community strategies should involve collective and social action to promote palliative care for all [20]. The plan is to integrate palliative care into all levels of health care—from the community level upward and from the palliative care expert downward (Fig. 1). India, with more than one-sixth of the world's population and fewer than 100 palliative care specialists, followed the WHO's public health and primary health recommendations to initiate a people's movement to enhance palliative care [13]. The same principle can be applied to the goal of "cancer pain relief for all" by training health care professionals to provide appropriate pain service at various levels, from pain diagnosis and basic interventions to treatment of complex pain problems, teaching, and research at the tertiary level (Fig. 2).

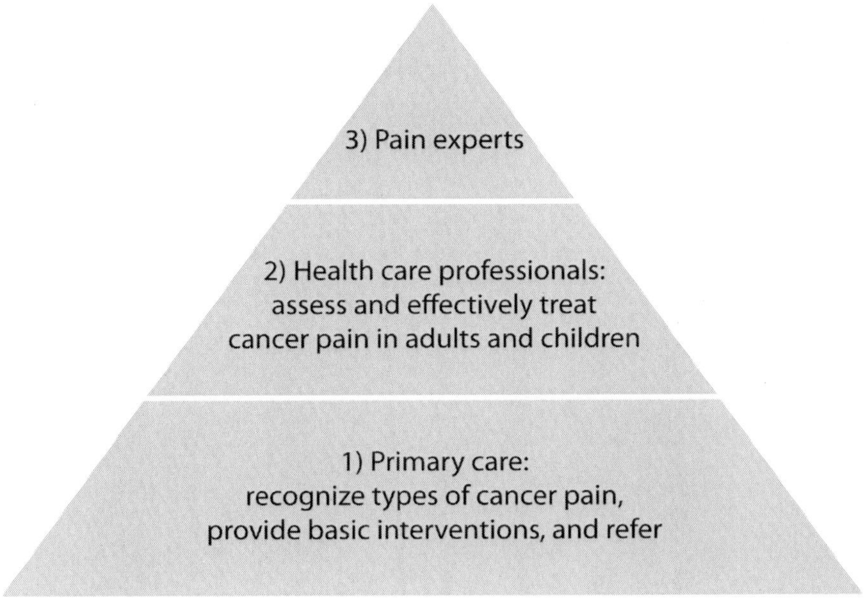

3) Pain experts

2) Health care professionals:
assess and effectively treat
cancer pain in adults and children

1) Primary care:
recognize types of cancer pain,
provide basic interventions, and refer

*Fig 2.* Cancer pain relief for all. On the tertiary level, pain experts can assess pain, treat pain (including complex pain problems), teach, and conduct research. Adapted from Stjernswärd et al. [20].

In response to increasing awareness of palliative care, research findings can help identify potential outcomes of palliative care measures to ensure the proper utilization of scarce resources [7]. Research to determine cost-effective treatments could help provide financial relief for patients and their families, who have already incurred the burden of heavy costs related to treatment. Without high-quality, persuasive research findings, it is difficult to develop an adequate palliative care program or to secure future funding for palliative care and pain management [8].

Cancer pain is devastating for patients, and the suffering is extended to their caregivers and families, especially in developing countries, where most patients present with advance disease. Every effort must be made to improve resources for education, research, and treatment of cancer and the associated pain.

# References

[1]   Boyle P, Levin B, editors. World cancer report 2008. Lyon: International Agency for Research on Cancer; 2008.
[2]   Commission on Health Research for Development. Health research essential link to equity and development. New York: Oxford University Press; 1990. p. xvii–xix.
[3]   Charlton JE, editor. Core curriculum for professional education in pain, 3rd ed. Seattle: IASP Press; 2004.
[4]   De Lima L, Sweeney C, Palmer JL, Bruera E. Potent analgesics are more expensive for patients in developing countries: a comparative study. J Pain Palliat Care Pharmacother 2004:S18;59–70.
[5]   Eniu A, Carlson RW, Aziz Z, Bines J, Hortobagyi GN, Bese NS, Vikram B, Kurkure A, Anderson BO. Breast cancer in limited-resource countries: treatment and allocation of resources. Breast J 2006;12:S38–S53.
[6]   Gomes B, Harding R, Foley K, Higginson I. Optimal approaches to the health economics of palliative care: report of an international think tank. J Pain Symptom Manage 2009;38:4–10.
[7]   Harding R, Gomez B, Foley KM, Higginson L. Research priorities in health economics and funding for palliative care: views of an international think tank. J Pain Symptom Manage 2009;38:11–14.
[8]   Harding R, Powell RA, Downing J, Conner SC, Mwangi-Powell F, Defilippi K, Cameron S, Garanganga E, Kikule E, Alexander C. Generating an African palliative care evidence base: the context, need, challenges, and strategies. J Pain Symptom Manage 2008;36:304–9.
[9]   IASP Developing Countries Taskforce. Education and training for pain management in developing countries: a report by the IASP Developing Countries Taskforce. Available at: www.iasp-pain.org. Accessed July 20, 2009.
[10]  International Network for Cancer Treatment and Research. Cancer: an increasingly important cause of death in developing countries. Available at: www.inctr.org. Accessed December 24, 2008.
[11]  Jagwe J, Merriman A. Uganda: delivering analgesia in rural Africa: opioid availability and nurse prescribing. J Pain Symptom Manage 2007;33:547–51.
[12]  Marcus AD. Price becomes factor in cancer treatment. Wall Street J 2004;September 7:D1–D7.
[13]  McDermott E, Selman L, Wright M, Clark D. Hospice and palliative care development in India: a multi-method review of services and experiences. J Pain Symptom Manage 2008;35:583–93.
[14]  Oliver JW, Kravitz RL, Kaplan SH, Meyers FJ. Individualized patient education and coaching to improve pain control among cancer outpatients. J Clin Oncol 2001;19:2206–12.

[15] Parkin DM, Wabinga H, Namboozes S, Wabwire-Mangen F. AIDS-related cancers in Africa: maturation of the epidemic in Uganda. AIDS 1999;13:2563–70.

[16] Ramsey S. Raising the profile of palliative care for Africa. Lancet 2001;358:734.

[17] Soyannwo OA. Cancer pain management in developing countries. Pain: Clin Updates 2009;XVII.

[18] Stjernswärd S. Uganda: initiating a government public health approach to pain relief and palliative care. J Pain Symptom Manage 2002:24;257–64.

[19] Stjernswärd J, Colleau S, Ventafridda V. The World Health Organization Cancer Pain and Palliative Care Program. Past, present and future. J Pain Symptom Manage 1996:12;65–72.

[20] Stjernswärd J, Foley KM, Ferris FD. The public health strategy for palliative care. J Pain Symptom Manage 2007;33:486–93.

[21] United Nations. The millennium development goals report 2008. Available at: www.un.org/millenniumgoals/. Accessed March 23, 2009.

[22] Van den Beuken-van Everdingen MH, de Rijke JM, Kessels AG, Schoulten HC, van Kleef M, Patijn J. Prevalence of pain in patients with cancer: a systematic review of the past 40 years. Ann Oncol 2007;18:1437–49.

[23] Wabinga HR, Parkin DM, Wabwire-Mangen F, Nambooze S. Trends in cancer incidence in Kyadondo County, Uganda, 1960–1997. Br J Cancer 2000;82:1585–92.

[24] Watt-Watson J, Hunter J, Pennefather P, Librach L, Raman-Wilms L, Schreiber M, Lax L, Stinson J, Dao T, Gordon A, Mock D, Salter M. An integrated undergraduate pain curriculum, based on IASP curricula, for six health science faculties. Pain 2004;110:140–8.

[25] World Bank. World Bank classification of economies of countries. Available at: www.nationsonline.org/oneworld/countriesclassification.htm. Accessed January 6, 2008.

[26] World Health Assembly. Cancer prevention and control resolution of 2005. Available at: http://apps.who.int/gb/ebwha/pdf-files/WHA 58.22-en.pdf. Accessed June 15, 2009.

[27] World Health Organization. Executive summary. In: National cancer control programmes: policies and managerial guidelines. Geneva: World Health Organization; 2002. p. I–XXIV.

[28] World Health Organization. Cancer pain relief, 2nd edition: with a guide to opioid availability. Geneva: World Health Organization; 1996.

*Correspondence to:* Olaitan Soyannwo, MMed, FWACS, FAS, Department of Anaesthesia, College of Medicine, University College Hospital, University of Ibadan, PMB 5116, Ibadan, Nigeria. Email: folait2001@yahoo.com.

# Index

Page numbers followed by f refer to figures; page numbers followed by t refer to tables.